Hegde'
PocketGuide to
Assessment in
Speech-Language Pathology

Second Edition

NOTICE TO THE READER

Hegde's PocketGuide to Assessment in Speech-Language Pathology

Second Edition

M. N. Hegde, Ph.D.
Department of Communicative
Sciences and Disorders
California State University-Fresno

SINGULAR

★

THOMSON LEARNING

Australia   Canada   Mexico   Singapore   Spain   United Kingdom   United States

MT

SINGULAR
THOMSON LEARNING

Hegde's PocketGuide to Assessment in Speech-Language Pathology, Second Edition
by M. N. Hegde, Ph.D.

Business Unit Director:
William Brottmiller

Acquisitions Editor:
Marie Linvill

Development Editor:
Kristin Banach

Executive Marketing Manager:
Dawn Gerrain

Channel Manager:
Tara Carter

Production Manager:
Barbara Bullock

Production Editor:
Sandy Doyle

Library of Congress Cataloging-in-Publication Data

Hegde, M. N. (Mahabalagiri N.), 1941-
Hegde's pocketGuide to assessment in speech-language pathology/by M.N. Hegde—2nd ed.
  p. ; cm.
Rev. ed. of: PocketGuide to assessment in speech-language pathology. c1996.
Includes bibliographical references.
ISBN 0-7693-0158-4 (soft cover: alk. paper)
1. Speech Disorders—Diagnosis—Handbooks, manuals, etc. I. Title: Pocket-Guide to assessment in speech-language pathology.
II. Hegde, M. N. (Mahabalagiri N.) 1941- PocketGuide to assessment in speech-language pathology. III. Title.
[DNLM: 1. Speech Disorders—Diagnosis—Handbooks. 2. Language Disorders—Diagnosis—Handbooks. WL 39 H462h 2001]
RC423 .H38286 2001
616.85'5075—dc21
                                00-049225

rel. 7/16/12

ABBREVIATED CONTENTS: MAJOR ENTRIES

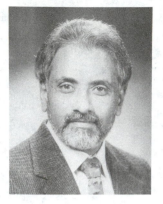

M. N. (Giri) Hegde is Professor of Communicative Sciences and Disorders at California State University-Fresno. He holds a master's degree in Experimental Psychology from the University of Mysore, India, a post-master's diploma in Medical (Clinical) Psychology from Bangalore University, India, and a doctoral degree in Speech-Language Pathology from Southern Illinois University at Carbondale.

A specialist in fluency disorders, language disorders, research designs, and treatment procedures in communicative disorders, Dr. Hegde has made numerous scientific and professional presentations to national and international audiences. He has extensive clinical and research experience and has published research articles on a wide range of subjects, including fluency and language, their disorders, and treatment. Dr. Hegde has authored or co-authored several highly regarded and widely used scientific and professional books, including *Clinical Research in Communicative Disorders, Introduction to Communicative Disorders, Treatment Procedures in Communicative Disorders, Treatment Protocols in Communicative Disorders, A Coursebook on Scientific and Professional Writing in Speech-Language Pathology, Clinical Methods and Practicum in Speech-Language Pathology, A PocketGuide to Treatment in Speech-Language-Pathology, A Singular Manual of Textbook Preparation, A Coursebook on Language Disorders in Children, An Advanced Review of Speech-Language Pathology,* and *Assessment and Treatment of Articulation and Phonological Disorders in Children.* He is the Editor of the Singular Textbook Series and has served on the editorial boards of several scientific and professional journals. Dr. Hegde has received many honors and awards, including the Distinguished Alumnus Award from Southern Illinois University Department of Communication Sciences and Disorders, Outstanding Professor Award from California State University-Fresno, Outstanding Professional Achievement Award from District Five of California Speech-Language-Hearing Association, and Fellowship in the American Speech-Language-Hearing Association.

Preface

The second edition of this PocketGuide to assessment procedures in speech-language pathology has been updated and expanded by more than 60 pages. Information on ethnocultural variables that affect assessment have been added. Simultaneous revision of the companion volume, *Hegde's PocketGuide to Treatment in Speech-Language Pathology* has also helped to streamline the information in the two books.

This PocketGuide to assessment procedures in speech-language pathology has been designed as a companion volume to the *PocketGuide to Treatment in Speech-Language Pathology.* The two PocketGuides combine the most desirable features of a specialized dictionary of terms, clinical resource book, textbook, and manual. PocketGuides are meant to be quick reference books like a dictionary because the entries are alphabetized; but they offer more than a dictionary because they specify assessment or treatment procedures in a "do this" format. The two PocketGuides are like resource books in that they avoid theoretical and conceptual aspects of procedures presented; but they offer more than a resource book by clearly specifying the steps involved in assessing or treating clients. The PocketGuides are like standard textbooks that describe assessment or treatment procedures; but the guides organize information in a manner conducive to more ready use. By avoiding theoretical background and controversies, PocketGuides give the essence of assessment or treatment in a step-by-step form that promotes easy understanding and ready reference just before beginning clinical work. The PocketGuides do not suggest that theoretical and research issues are not important in clinical work; rather they assume that the user is familiar with them.

How the PocketGuide Is Organized

This PocketGuide summarizes basic information on disorders of communication and specifies steps involved in assessing them. Each main entry is printed in bold and blue color. Each main disorder of communication is entered in its alphabetical order; in most cases, the immediately following entry describes types or varieties of that disorder. For example, after the main entry Aphasia the reader will find Aphasia: Specific Types; after the main entry Dysarthria, Dysarthria: Specific Types follows.

To avoid repetition under each main entry, common assessment techniques (e.g., case history, interview, hearing screening, orofacial examination) are described as one main entry (Common/Standard Assessment Procedures). However, certain aspects of these common/standard procedures that are unique to a given disorder are described under the entry for that disorder.

How to Use This PocketGuide

The guide may be used very much like a dictionary. A clinician who wants to read about assessment of a particular disorder will find it by its main alphabetical entry. An abbreviated table of contents will quickly direct the clinician to the major entries in the book; most of these are names of various disorders. Under each main entry, the clinician may be referred to certain concepts, assessment techniques, or assessment tools that are cross-referenced. All cross-referenced entries are underlined in blue. Thus, throughout the guide, an underlined term means that the reader can find more about it in its own main alphabetical entry.

The clinician also may look up certain assessment methods by name. Two such entries, Speech and Language Sample and Standard/Common Assessment Procedures have been noted. Other such entries that are not disorders but assessment targets, concepts, or techniques include Augmentative and Alternative Communication (AAC), Phonological Processes, Grammatic Morphemes of Language, Computerized Axial Tomography, Maximum Phonation Duration, and so forth.

Serious attempts have been made to include most assessment techniques described in the literature. However, the author is aware that not all techniques have been included. The guideline used in selecting techniques has been the most common usage in the context of frequently encountered disorders.

I would like to thank Celeste Roseberry-McKibbin, Ph.D. and Donald Freed, Ph.D.—two of my expert colleagues and good friends—who have reviewed various parts of the manuscript. While deficiencies are my own responsibility, their scholarly review and constructive comments have been very helpful in improving and clarifying the presentations. I also would like to thank Deanna Garvin for her excellent help in researching standardized assessment instruments included in this guide. Her competent assistance has helped me complete the project in a timely manner. Finally, and most importantly, my wife Prema's help in editing, cross-referencing the entire manuscript, and her unconditional support throughout the writing period have been invaluable.

Abbreviation Used Throughout the Book

PGTSLP: Hegde's PocketGuide to Treatment in Speech-Language Pathology, 2nd ed., by M. N. Hegde (2001). San Diego, CA: Singular Thomson Learning.

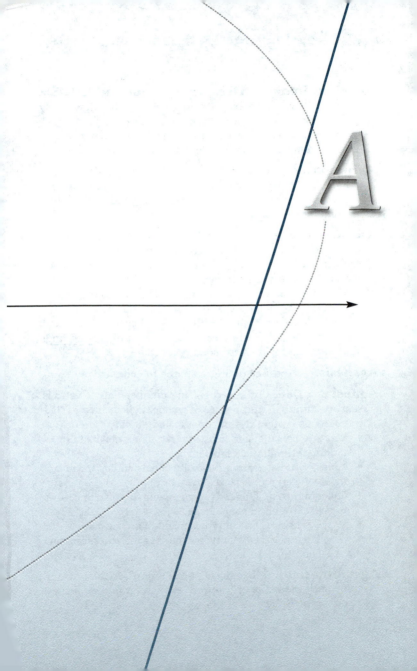

Acquired Immune Deficiency Syndrome

Acquired Immune Deficiency Syndrome (AIDS). A syndrome caused by human immunodeficiency virus; destruction of white blood cells that reduce cell-mediated immunity; currently no cure; several experimental drugs under evaluation; some recent drugs appear promising.

Acrocephaly. A cranial abnormality resulting in high-domed skull; part of certain genetic syndromes including Waardenburg syndrome (see Syndromes Associated With Communicative Disorders).

Adaptation Effect. Progressive decrease in the frequency of stuttering when a printed passage is orally read repeatedly; maximum decrease often on the second reading; decrease is progressively less on subsequent readings; little or no decrease after the fifth reading; reduced or eliminated by rest pause between readings; shows no transfer across passages; contrasts with Consistency Effect; marked effect suggests relatively weak stimulus control of stuttering; see Stuttering for the assessment procedure.

Agenesis. Absence of an organ due to genetic defect.

Agnosia. Difficulty in recognizing the meaning of various sensory stimuli in the absence of sensory deficits; due to central nervous system dysfunction; includes many varieties:
- Auditory agnosia: Difficulty in recognizing the meaning of auditory stimuli including language
- Auditory verbal agnosia: Difficulty understanding the meaning of spoken words (also known as pure word deafness)
- Finger agnosia: Difficulty recognizing or discriminating objects through finger contact
- Prosopagnosia: Difficulty recognizing familiar faces
- Visual agnosia: Difficulty recognizing or discriminating visual stimuli

Agrammatism. Language production with omitted grammatic elements or features; deficient grammar; a characteristic of Aphasia.

Agraphia. A general term to describe writing problems of clinical significance; in children, developmental writing problems typically are associated with learning disorders; in adults, problems of writing often are associated with aphasia, dementia, and other neurological disorders; speech-language pathologists assess and treat writing problems in the context of aphasia and other language disorders; see Aphasia.

AIDS Dementia Complex. *Dementia* associated with acquired immune deficiency syndrome; resembles subcortical dementia in the beginning and cortical dementia in the advanced stages.

Etiology
- Human immunodeficiency virus
- Depletion of white blood cells
- Impaired immune system

Early Symptoms
- Memory problems
- Attention deficits relative to conversation and writing
- Slow reaction time
- Disorientation to time and space
- Progressive deterioration in balance
- Weakness in legs
- Deterioration in handwriting
- Apathy and social withdrawal
- Reduced verbal output

Advanced Symptoms
- Serious and general cognitive deterioration
- Severe deterioration in motor skills and performance
- Ataxia
- Hypertonia
- Incontinence
- Confusion and indifference

Assessment Objectives/General Guidelines
- The same as those of Dementia and Alzheimer's Disease

AIDS Dementia Complex

Case History/Interview Focus
- See **Case History** and **Interview** under Standard/Common Assessment Procedures
- Concentrate on history of AIDS and conditions that support its diagnosis

Ethnocultural Considerations
- See Ethnocultural Considerations in Assessment

Assessment
- Assess the major symptoms listed
- Use procedures described under Dementia and Alzheimer's Disease
- Be aware that in some patients, dementia may be the only presenting symptom of undiagnosed AIDS

Standardized Tests
- Use the Clinical Dementia Rating and the Global Deterioration Scale to rate the severity of dementia into mild, moderate, and severe (see Dementia)

Related/Medical Assessment Data
- Medical diagnosis of AIDS essential

Standard/Common Assessment Procedures
- Complete the Standard/Common Assessment Procedures

Diagnostic Criteria
- The same as those for Dementia or Alzheimer's Disease

Differential Diagnosis
- Relatively early onset for symptoms of dementia (as early as late 20s, unlike dementia associated with degenerative neurological diseases)
- History of AIDS

Prognosis
- Guarded; the same as that for Dementia of other types

Recommendations
- Treatment for the patient in the early stages of dementia; clinical management of problems the main goal
- Working with the family in all stages, and especially in the final stages

Alexia

- See the cited sources and *PGTSLP* for details

Larson, C. R. (1998). *HIV-1 and communication disorders*. San Diego: Singular Publishing Group.

Lubinski, R. (Ed.). (1991). *Dementia and communication*. Philadelphia: B. C. Decker.

Ripich, D. N. (1991). *Handbook of geriatric communication disorders*. Austin, TX: Pro-Ed.

Alexia. A general term to describe reading problems; in children, such problems are often associated with learning disabilities; in adults, deteriorated writing problems typically are due to aphasia, dementia, and other neurological disorders; also called Dyslexia; speech-language pathologists assess and treat reading problems because of their frequent association with Aphasia; need to rule out peripheral visual problems in making a diagnosis of alexia associated with central pathology; includes *Alexia With Agraphia; Alexia Without Agraphia; Deep Dyslexia,* and *Frontal Dyslexia;* take note of their symptoms under this entry and see Aphasia for their assessment procedures.

Alexia With Agraphia. Coexistence of reading and writing problems often found in patients with aphasia; also called parietal-temporal alexia; see Agraphia for associated writing problems; due to lesions in the dominant parietal and temporal lobes.

Symptoms
- Reading and writing problems associated with Wernicke's aphasia and Broca's aphasia (see Aphasia: Specific Types)
- Reading difficulties reflect problems of oral expression
- Reading comprehension deficits more serious in Wernicke's patients; generally related to the degree of auditory comprehension of spoken language
- Better reading of concrete nouns than abstract words by patients with Broca's aphasia
- Better comprehension of read material by Broca's patients than by Wernicke's patients

Differential Diagnosis
- Distinguish alexia associated with aphasia from poor premorbid reading skills
- Distinguish alexia from pure motor difficulties in oral reading
- Distinguish reading comprehension problems from motor speech difficulties in expressing what may have been comprehended
- Consider attention deficits and fatigue in making a differential diagnosis
- Rule out visual neglect and peripheral visual problems

Alexia Without Agraphia. Reading difficulties with relatively intact writing skills; associated with various neuropathologies; also known as <u>Occipital Alexia</u> and <u>Pure Alexia</u>; causes include various neuropathologies associated with <u>Aphasia</u> and, more specifically, a disassociation between occipital association cortex and the dominant angular gyrus.

Symptoms
- Variety of reading problems as in alexia with agraphia
- Patients cannot read what they write well
- Right visual field deficits in many clients
- Difficulty naming visually presented colors (color agnosia)

Differential Diagnosis
- Distinguish pure alexia from alexia with agraphia; document writing skills comparable to those at the premorbid levels in patients with pure alexia to make this differential diagnosis; see <u>Agraphia</u>
- Distinguish alexia without agraphia from frontal alexia by documenting symptoms of Broca's aphasia associated with the latter
- Distinguish pure alexia from deep dyslexia by documenting semantic errors in oral reading associated with the latter; see *Deep Dyslexia* in this section

Deep Dyslexia. A reading disorder characterized by a variety of semantic reading errors; semantic reading errors are those that are in some way related to meaning of the printed word being misread; etiology not well understood, although involvement of right hemisphere has been suggested.

Symptoms

- General semantic errors (e.g., misreading the printed word *close* as *"shut"*; and printed *tall* as *"long"*)
- Derivational errors (e.g., misreading printed word *wise* as *"wisdom"*; and *entertain* as *"entertainment"*; deletion of suffixes as in misreading the printed word *hardest* as *"hard'* or *walking* as *"walk"*)
- Errors based on visual similarity of printed words and misreading (e.g., printed word *crocus* as *"crocodile"*; *crowd* as *"crown"*)
- Misreading of grammatic function words (e.g., misreading the printed word *the* as *"yes"*)
- Inability to read nonsense syllables or misreading them as meaningful words (e.g., responding with *"I don't know"* for the printed syllable *wux*; or misreading *dup* as *"dump"*)

Differential Diagnosis

- The highest number of errors on grammatic function words, followed by adjectives, verbs, and abstract nouns; and the lowest number of errors on concrete nouns help identify deep dyslexia
- Distinguish aphasia without deep dyslexia by documenting the dominant symptom complex of semantic errors in the latter
- Distinguish deep dyslexia from frontal alexia by documenting the association of Broca's aphasia with the latter

Frontal Alexia. A reading disorder associated with Broca's aphasia; also called the third alexia or anterior alexia; cause is anterior cerebral neuropathology as in Broca's aphasia.

Symptoms

- Greater difficulty with abstract nouns and function words than with concrete nouns
- Relatively better reading comprehension of content words

- Difficulty in comprehending words spelled aloud
- Absence of letter-by-letter reading (the patient uses the whole word approach to reading)
- Difficulty in deriving meaning of sentences from their syntactic structures

Differential Diagnosis
- Differential reading difficulties as listed
- Distinguish frontal alexia from deep dyslexia by documenting semantic errors in the latter

Alternating Motion Rates (AMRs). The same as diadochokinetic rates; a measure of the speed and regularity with which repetitive movements of the articulatory structures are made; help assess the functional and structural integrity of the lips, jaw, and the tongue; of diagnostic value in assessing motor speech disorders; in assessment, usually followed by Sequential Motion Rates (SMRs) which require rapid movement from one articulatory posture to another by having the client produce different syllables as rapidly and as steadily as possible.

Procedure
- Ask the client to "take a deep breath and say puh-puh puh-puh for as long and as steadily as possible"
- Model the response for 2 to 3 seconds
- Ask the patient to stop when a 3- to 5-second sample has been recorded
- Ask the client to take a deep breath and "say tuh-tuh tuh-tuh for as long and as steadily as possible"; model if necessary- record a 3- to 5-second sample
- Ask the client to take a deep breath and "say kuh-kuh kuh-kuh for as long and as steadily as possible"; model if necessary; record a 3- to 5-second sample
- Move on to measure the SMRs by asking the client to say "puh-tuh-kuh-puh-tuh-kuh-puh-tuh-kuh-puh-tuh-kuh for as long and as steadily as possible"; model if necessary; record the sample

Analysis
- Analyze the response rates in relation to normative data

- The normative data for AMRs range from 5 to 7 repetitions per second in normal adults
- The normative data for SMRs range from 3.6 to 7.5 repetitions per second in normal adults
- Slowness or accelerated speech may both suggest neuromotor problems

Alzheimer's Disease (AD).   A degenerative neurological disorder characterized by deterioration in behavior, cognition, memory, language, communication, and personality; AD is responsible for 65% of dementias; more common in women than in men; associated with a family history of Down syndrome (see <u>Syndromes Associated With Communicative Disorders</u>); patients with Down syndrome are more likely than those without to develop AD later in life; first described in 1906 by the German neurologist Alois Alzheimer.

Etiology
- Pathology and laboratory findings
  - <u>Neurofibrillary Tangles</u>, especially in pyramidal cells of the hippocampus and the amygdaloid nucleus
  - <u>Neuritic (Senile) Plaques</u>, especially in the outer half of the cortex
  - <u>Granulovacuolar Degeneration</u>, especially in the hippocampus
  - neuronal loss especially of large neurons in the frontal and temporal regions and in deeper structures; brain weight about 10% less than that in age-matched healthy individuals
  - amyloid angiopathy
  - decreased dendritic branches
  - neurochemical deficits, primarily cholinergic deficit, resulting in reduced neurotransmission
  - diffused slowing of the electroencephalogram (EEG)
  - reduced cerebral blood flow, the degree consistent with the level of dementia; especially noted in parietotemporooccipital area of the brain
  - reduced cortical glucose metabolism as measured by <u>Positron Emission Tomography</u>

Alzheimer's Disease (AD)

Theories
- Infection, such as the one found in scrapie, a disease that affects sheep; need more evidence
- Toxicity; note that aluminum toxicity, which was frequently mentioned in the past, has recently been questioned
- Genetic transmission because of greater Familial Incidence, higher Concordance Rate for monozygotic twins than for ordinary siblings, and AD's association with Down syndrome; still, need more evidence

Onset/Early Symptoms
- Typically gradual onset
- Memory problems are the earliest and the most frequently noted; both recent and remote memory impaired
- Difficulty in learning and retaining new material
- Work-related problems
- Behavioral (personality) changes including irritability, hostility, apathy, suspiciousness, frustration
- Vague and empty speech with naming problems
- Impaired inferential ability
- Impaired construction and other visual-spatial orientation

Progression/Advanced Symptoms
- More serious and obvious memory problems
- More serious behavioral changes including indifference, poor social judgment, and lack of emotional responses
- More serious communication problems including further deterioration in the content of speech and some structural problems
- Further deterioration in problem solving; needs help with simple problems
- Further deterioration in visual-spatial skills; spatial disorientation, poor construction, and misperception
- Restlessness and agitation
- Global deterioration in intellectual functioning
- Disorganized behavior
- Wandering

Alzheimer's Disease (AD)

- Globally deteriorated language skills, mutism, echolalia, palilalia, and perseveration
- Rigidity and spasticity
- Periodic incontinence
- Diurnal rhythm disturbances in some patients
- Delusions and hallucinations in some patients
- Violence and emotional lability in some patients

Assessment Objectives/General Guidelines

- To document communication deficits including memory problems
- To help plan a communication intervention program

Case History/Interview Focus

- See **Case History** and **Interview** under Standard/Common Assessment Procedures
- Concentrate on changes in cognition, general behavior, and communication skills; consider using the Alzheimer Dementia Risk Questionnaire during case history taking and interview

Ethnocultural Considerations

- See Ethnocultural Considerations in Assessment

Assessment

- Assess speech
  - record a Speech and Language Sample (see Standard/Common Assessment Procedures) to analyze articulation or phonological disorders
  - be aware that no significant errors are noted in the early stages or middle stages
  - errors of sound production may be noted in the late stages, but no sound combinations that are alien to the language
- Assess language
  - use the recorded speech and language sample to analyze language problems
  - assess language comprehension in conversational speech; take note of the number of utterances the patient correctly and incorrectly comprehends

11

- assess sentence comprehension by orally presenting a series of simple and progressively more complex sentences; use *Auditory Comprehension Test for Sentences* or the *Revised Token Test* (See Aphasia)
- assess such pragmatic skills as turn taking, topic initiation, topic maintenance, and narrative skills (see Language Disorders in Children)
- assess comprehension of word meaning (semantic feature) by presenting a series of client-specific words the client is asked to define or give meanings for; use the *Peabody Picture Vocabulary Test* (PPVT) (See Language Disorders in Children)
- assess confrontation naming by presenting a series of common objects or pictures and by asking the patient to name them; use the *Boston Naming Test* (See Aphasia)
- assess short- and long-term memory
- use such standardized tests of aphasia as the *Boston Diagnostic Aphasia Examination* (BDAE), the *Porch Index of Communicative Ability* and *Western Aphasia Battery* for an overall analysis of linguistic breakdown (See Aphasia)
- Assess fluency
  - use the conversational speech sample to calculate the percentage of dysfluencies (divide the number of dysfluencies with the number of words spoken and multiply it by 100)
  - assess word fluency by asking the client to say as many words as possible that begin with a certain letter; use the Word Fluency Measure
- Assess voice
  - make a routine analysis
  - take note of any voice disorders

Standardized Tests
- Consider using standardized tests listed under Dementia

Related/Medical Assessment Data
- Integrate available medical, neurological, psychological, behavioral, and diagnostic medical laboratory findings with the results of communication assessment

Alzheimer's Disease (AD)

Standard/Common Assessment Procedures
- Complete the Standard/Common Assessment Procedures

Diagnostic Criteria/Guidelines
- A gradual onset of a progressive and generalized memory and intellectual deterioration is a necessary condition for diagnosis of AD
- In the absence of direct pathological evidence, diagnosis is made by exclusion (ruling out dementia due to other causes)

Differential Diagnosis
- Note that the diagnosis of Alzheimer's disease is finally established only through an autopsy to document its neuropathology
- Rule out dementia due to other etiological factors including:
  - cerebrovascular diseases
  - Parkinson's disease
  - Huntington's disease
  - hypothyroidism
  - vitamin B_{12} deficiency
  - HIV infection
  - substance abuse
- Do *not* diagnose AD if
  - the symptoms are exclusively associated with delirium
  - cognitive deterioration may be explained on the basis of such other psychiatric disorders as schizophrenia
- Distinguish AD from aphasia:
  - AD is likely to be confused with Wernicke's aphasia, anomic aphasia, and transcortical sensory aphasia because of relative fluency in all of them, but not with Broca's aphasia because of nonfluent, agrammatic speech of the latter; (see Aphasia: Specific Types)
  - the greater the severity of dementia of the Alzheimer type, the more it contrasts with aphasia
- Distinguish subtypes of AD:
  - AD with early onset (65 years or under)

Alzheimer's Disease (AD)

Dementia of the Alzheimer's Type	Aphasia
Slow onset	Sudden onset
Bilateral brain damage	Damage to the left hemisphere
Diffuse brain damage	Focal brain lesions; however, some may have more diffuse damage.
May be moody, withdrawn, agitated	Mood is usually appropriate though depressed or frustrated at times
Impaired cognition, but relatively better preserved language; however, some patients may show greater impairment in language than in cognition	Impaired language, but relatively intact cognition; however, some cognitive impairment may be present in some patients
Memory is impaired to various degrees, often severely	Memory typically is intact
Behavior often irrelevant, socially inappropriate, and disorganized	Behavior generally is relevant, socially appropriate, and organized
Progression of deterioration from semantic to syntactic to phonologic performance	Semantic, syntactic, and phonologic performance simultaneously impaired
Fluent until dementia becomes worse	Fluent or nonfluent
Relatively poor performance on spatial and verbal recognition tasks	Relatively better performance on spatial and verbal recognition tasks
Relatively poor story retelling skills	Relatively better story retelling skills
Relatively poor description of common objects	Relatively better description of common objects
	(continued)

14

(continued)

Dementia of the Alzheimer's Type	Aphasia
Relatively poor silent reading comprehension	Relatively better silent reading comprehension
Relatively poor pantomimic expression	Relatively better pantomimic expression
Relatively poor drawing skills	Relatively better drawing skills

- AD with late onset (after age 65 years)
- AD with Down syndrome (see Syndromes Associated With Communicative Disorders)
- AD with Aphasia
- AD with such other diseases as Parkinson's Disease
- uncomplicated AD (with no associated clinical conditions)

Prognosis
- Poor because dementia is irreversible and there is no effective medical treatment

Recommendations
- Family counseling
- Behavioral management of patient's symptoms in the earlier stages
- Family counseling and management during the latter stages
- See the cited sources and *PGTSLP* for details

American Psychiatric Association. (1994). *Diagnostic and statistical manual of mental disorders* (4th ed.). Washington, DC: Author.

Bayles, K. A., & Kaszniak, A. W. (1987). *Communication and cognition in normal aging and dementia.* Austin, TX: Pro-Ed.

Brookshire, R. H. (1994). *An introduction to neurogenic communication disorders* (5th ed.). St. Louis, MO: Mosby Year Book.

Cummings, J. L., & Benson, D. F. (1983). *Dementia: A clinical approach.* Boston, MA: Butterworth.

Fuld, P. A. (1980). Guaranteed stimulus processing in the evaluation of memory and learning. *Cortex, 16,* 255–271.

Ripich, D. (Ed.). (1991). *Handbook of geriatric communication disorders.* Austin, TX: Pro-Ed.

Alzheimer Dementia Risk Questionnaire. A guide to conducting family interview and obtaining a comprehensive case history; helps obtain information on the patient's family, education, work, onset and course of dementia, and communication.

Breitner, J. C., & Folstein, M. (1984). A prevalent disorder with specific clinical features. *Psychological Medicine, 14,* 63–80.

Amyloid Angiopathy (Cerebral). Vascular disease in which amyloid (fatty) substance accumulates in the small and medium vessels of the brain causing microinfarcts; a pathology associated with <u>Alzheimer's Disease</u>.

Anomia. Difficulty in naming people, places, or things; the client may suggest the word in other ways, including gestures, descriptions, and writing, but cannot say it; probably due to lesions in varied cortical and subcortical structures including the angular gyrus in the parietal lobe of the left (dominant) hemisphere, left posterior superior temporoparietal region, and subcortical structures such as insula-putamen; a major characteristic of <u>Aphasia</u>; also found in <u>Dementia</u>, <u>Right Hemisphere Syndrome</u>, <u>Traumatic Brain Injury</u>; the major characteristic of anomic aphasia; for assessment procedures, see <u>Aphasia</u> and concentrate on the following symptoms:

Anomic Symptoms/Types of Anomia

- *Delayed response.* Presumably due to the slow activation of the naming process
- *Limited anomia.* Disconnection anomias; such category-specific problems as difficulty naming animals or vegetables
- *Paraphasias* or *Paraphasic Anomia.* Word-retrieval problems resulting in unintended word or sound substitutions
- *Perseveration.* Word-retrieval problems resulting in persisting errors

- *Self-corrected errors*. Word-retrieval problems resulting in relatively fast or slow self-correction of errors; self-correction partially or fully successful
- *Semantic anomia*. Failure to recognize the words not produced
- *Unrelated words*. Word-retrieval problems resulting in irrelevant responses.
- *Word production anomia:* Anomia due mainly to motor problems
- *Word selection anomia:* Clients can describe, gesture, write, and draw to suggest a word they cannot say; can correctly recognize the name when given

Chapey, R. (Ed.). (1994). *Language intervention strategies in adult aphasia*. Baltimore, MD: Williams & Wilkins.

Davis, G. A. (1993). *A survey of adult aphasia* (2nd ed.). Englewood Cliffs, NJ: Prentice-Hall.

Hegde, M. N. (1998). *A coursebook on aphasia and other neurogenic language disorders* (2nd ed.). San Diego, CA: Singular Publishing Group.

Rosenbek, J. C., LaPointe, L. L., & Wertz, R. T. (1989). *Aphasia: A clinical approach*. Austin, TX: Pro-Ed.

Anterior Isolation Syndrome.   The same as transcortical motor aphasia; see Aphasia: Specific Types.

Aphasia.   A language disorder caused by brain injury in which (a) all aspects of language comprehension and production are impaired to varying degrees (a nontypological definition); (b) one or more aspects of language comprehension and language production may be affected (a typological definition); language impairment in aphasia is more striking than other impairments; the most common cause is a stroke or cerebrovascular accident that deprives oxygen and causes lesions in the brain; a common cause of strokes is thrombosis or embolism in the middle cerebral artery; most immediate causes of strokes and aphasia have many chained events behind them, each a cause for the next effect.

Aphasia

Etiology

- Cerebrovascular Accidents (Strokes) that are either:
  - ischemic: reduced or interrupted blood supply because of a Thrombosis, often associated with Arteriosclerosis or Embolism
  - hemorrhagic: ruptured cerebral blood vessel causing Cerebral Hemorrhage
- Traumatic Brain Injury that may be either:
  - penetrating (open): the skull is fractured or lacerated and the meninges are torn
  - nonpenetrating (closed): the meninges are intact although the skull may be fractured or intact
- Brain tumors which may be:
  - primary: tumors originally grown in the brain
  - metastatic: tumors grown elsewhere in the body but migrated into the brain
  - meningiomas: tumors within the meninges
- Toxicity which includes:
  - drug overdose
  - drug interactions
  - heavy metal toxicity from lead and mercury
- Infections that attack brain tissue, which include:
  - bacterial meningitis
  - brain abscess (bacteria, fungus, or parasites migrating into the brain from sinuses, middle ear, or mastoid cells)
- Viral infections that cause brain injury, which include:
  - mumps and measles
  - equine encephalitis and rabies
- Metabolic disorders that affect brain functions, which include:
  - hypoglycemia and thyroid disorders
- Nutritional disorders that affect brain function, which include:
  - thiamin deficiency (much less common than the others)

Aphasia

Onset/Early Symptoms of Stroke
- Typically sudden, rarely slow progressive onset
- Headaches in most cases, and stupor or coma in some cases
- Vomiting in some cases
- Convulsions in some cases
- Paralysis in certain cases or flaccidity on one side of the body
- Sensory loss and memory impairment
- Confusion
- Respiratory problems
- Falling to the ground
- Communication impairments, sometimes severe
- Transient ischemic attacks (TIA) that last less than 24 hours

Stabilization/Subsequent Symptoms
- Recovery from many physical symptoms
- Improved and stabilized physical condition in the absence of multiple strokes or other illnesses
- Improved mental condition
- Some improvement in communication skills, but a constellation of communication problems emerges or becomes more apparent
- Auditory comprehension deficits in most if not all clients; varied severity ranging from very mild to very severe deficits; more severe in certain types of aphasia than in other types; problems may include:
  - auditory Agnosia (impaired recognition of sounds) in some cases
  - auditory verbal Agnosia, also known as word deafness (impaired recognition of words) in some cases
  - word comprehension deficits in some cases
  - isolated sentence comprehension deficits in many cases
  - complex discourse comprehension deficits in most cases and to varying degrees
- Fluency problems to varying degrees; more severe in certain types of aphasia than in other types; production of

five or more words without dysfluencies indicate acceptable fluency; problems may include:

- impaired word fluency (production of many words in succession as a response to a single word given as stimulus)
- impaired fluency in phrase or sentence production (speech filled with pauses, repetitions, and other forms of dysfluencies)
- reduced speaking rate (e.g., *very slow rate*: 0 to 50 words per minute [wpm]; *slow rate*: 51 to 90 wpm; *normal rate*: 90 or more wpm)
- impaired rhythm, intonation, or melodic line of speech
- impaired facility in producing phonemes and syllables
- reduced variety of grammatical forms and types
- Impaired repetition of modeled speech to varying degrees; along with other symptoms, may help support diagnosis of certain types of aphasia; problems include:
  - impaired repetition of single words
  - impaired repetition of phrases and sentences
- Word finding or naming problems; a core problem of aphasia; may be a residual problem in clients with good recovery of language skills; problems include:
  - impaired confrontation naming of objects and pictures (naming in response to "What is this?")
  - impaired naming in response to descriptions or definitions of objects (e.g., "it is a tool for writing" to evoke "pen")
  - impaired sentence completion (e.g., "you write with a . . ." to evoke "pen")
  - impaired word fluency (see under *Fluency problems* described earlier)
  - word-finding problems in discourse; measured through picture description tasks and discourse analysis; indicated often by (a) substitution of such general terms as *this, that, thing,* and *stuff* for specific terms; (b) other kinds of word substitutions; (c) still other kinds of <u>Paraphasias</u> including verbal, random, phonemic, semantic, and neologistic

(Jargon) paraphasia; (d) dysfluencies; and (e) markedly reduced speech rate

- Agrammatism; errors of grammar, found mostly in patients with nonfluent aphasia; speech consists mostly of content words (nouns, verbs, adjectives); errors include:
  - omission of such function words as articles, prepositions, and pronouns
  - omission of such grammatical morphemes as the regular plural, auxiliary verbs, and past tense inflections
- Possibly impaired use or understanding of gestures in some patients (a controversial deficit)
- Reading problems (Alexia); various kinds of reading difficulties found in most clients; problems include:
  - lack of recognition of printed words
  - dysfluent, effortful, slow reading
  - word-by-word reading of sentences
  - substitution and omission of words
  - poor comprehension of read material; more serious in Wernicke's aphasia
- Writing problems (Agraphia); various kinds of writing deficits found in most cases; some due to the necessity of using the nonpreferred left hand because of paresis or paralysis of the preferred right hand; problems include:
  - poor letter formation due to paresis of the dominant hand
  - poor word formation
  - poor script writing
  - reversed, confused, or substituted letters
  - writing nonsensical syllables
  - repeated but unsuccessful attempts at self-correction
  - perseverative writing errors
  - omission of grammatical forms (unusual in Wernicke's aphasia, common in Broca's)
  - syntactic deficiencies (short phrases, inadequate sentence structures, confused syntax, especially in Wernicke's aphasia)
  - omission or substitution of words

- wrong word order
- misspelling
- omission or misuse of punctuation marks
- disorganized writing (poor spacing between letters)
- sparse writing
- totally illegible writing (especially in global aphasia)
- Differential bilingual deficits; aphasia may differentially affect language skills of a bilingual person:
  - better performance in the native language in some clients
  - faster recovery of expressive skills in the native language in some clients
  - better performance in the most frequently used language in other clients
  - sudden recovery of few or more expressions of infrequently used or forgotten native language in some clients
- Potential pragmatic communication problems; need research substantiation of pragmatic problems; possibly, the problems include the following:
  - poor communication in spite of apparently better language skills, especially in patients with Wernicke's aphasia
  - potential topic initiation, topic maintenance, and turn-taking problems in discourse
- Potential impairments in automatic speech and singing; not found in most patients with aphasia; musical impairment suggestive of right-hemisphere pathology; possibly, the problems include the following:
  - impaired automatic speech (e.g., recitation of days of the week, number sequence)
  - impaired ordinary musical skills (e.g., failure to hum a song, sing overlearned poems or nursery rhymes)

Assessment Objectives/General Guidelines
- To make a brief assessment of language skills in the early stages
- To make a more thorough assessment of communication skills including expressive, receptive, and gestural com-

munication as the patient's physical condition improves and stabilizes
- To identify initial treatment targets

Case History/Interview Focus
- See **Case History** and **Interview** under Standard/Common Assessment Procedures
- Concentrate on the onset and recovery from stroke or other clinical condition; detailed biographic information including education, occupation, literacy, and premorbid intellectual and communication skills; current family communication patterns

Ethnocultural Considerations
- See Ethnocultural Considerations in Assessment

Assessment: Specific Communication Skills
- Obtain a language (discourse) sample
  - tape record the entire conversation and assessment session
  - ascertain information on the hearing status of the client; speak clearly or slightly loudly as the client's condition demands
  - engage the client in conversation
  - ask the client about his or her recent health problems, family, occupation and work experience, interests, hobbies, and so forth
  - ask the client to narrate experiences
  - ask the client to describe pictures
  - do not ask questions that evoke yes/no answers unless the client's communicative skills are severely impaired
  - make every attempt to evoke longer, grammatically more complete utterances by asking the client to "say more" or "say it in a sentence" and so forth
  - use personally relevant questions that evoke better responses than neutral questions
  - challenge the client whose auditory comprehension is mildly impaired with more complex sentences, stories, proverbs, logical-illogical statement, and narratives to detect subtle problems

- Assess auditory comprehension deficits
  - assess comprehension of commands
    → use common commands first; use uncommon commands to challenge a mildly impaired client
    → do not use gestures as you give your commands
    → give direct commands (e.g., "point to the pen," not "can you point to the pen?")
    → give natural commands:
    "Move your chair a bit closer"
    "Close your eyes"
    "Show me the door"
    "Please turn off the lights"
    "Please remove your glasses"
    → give multistep commands and note the number of steps completed:
    "Pick up the pencil and the comb and place them in the box"
    "Fold this paper, put it in the envelope, and place the envelope on this book"
  - assess comprehension of single words; note that single words are not necessarily easy for aphasic patients; write down the exact responses for analysis:
    → assess first comprehension of category words; include objects, actions, numbers, colors, and letters:
    "Point to books"
    "Point to colors"
    "Point to walking"
    "Point to letters"
    "Point to numbers"
    → assess comprehension of specific items within categories:
    "Point to big book"
    "Point to blue"
    "Point to the man walking"
    "Point to the letter B"
    "Point to the number seven"
    → assess comprehension of single spoken sentences and connected speech

- → take note of breakdowns in comprehension of sentences when you interview the client
- → take note of breakdowns in comprehension of global discourse meaning
- → make your sentences progressively longer or more complex
- → use a variety of sentences (e.g., active, passive, question, and so forth)
- → "Point to the man who is walking"
- → "Point to the woman who is wearing a red dress"
- → "Point to the brown dog that is chasing a black cat"
- assess comprehension of abstract and logical sentences
  - → "Will ice cubes melt in snow?"
  - → "Will a baby who can't swim drown in a pool?"
  - → "Can you drive a car with no gas?"
  - → "Why do you need a car?"
  - → "How would you find someone's phone number?"
  - → "Can a thief arrest a policeman?"
- assess comprehension of paragraph-length material
  - → tell a brief, unique, interesting story with some humor and emotionality in it; do not select a story that gives the client a special advantage
  - → ask yes/no questions about the story
  - → ask about the main ideas and specific details of the story
  - → ask about inferences one might make about the story
- Assess fluency
  - use the conversational speech sample to evaluate fluency:
    - → observe and record the type and frequency of <u>Dysfluencies</u>
    - → observe and record the length of phrases measured in words
    - → observe and record the speech rate
    - → make notes about the rhythm and intonation of speech
    - → take note of the variety of grammatical structures used

→ make notes about the ease with which the client produces sounds and words

- Assess repetition skills
  - assess repetition of single words; model the words and ask the client to imitate (repeat)
    → present a variety of single-syllable words with visible consonants that are commonly used (nouns, verbs, numbers, and letters; start with common words):
    "Say *bed*"
    "Say *pen*"
    "Say *men*"
    "Say *baking*"
    "Say *five*"
    "Say *B*"
    → present blends and multi-syllable words; present progressively longer and less familiar words until breakdowns occur
    "Say *basket*"
    "Say *bubble*"
    "Say *truck*"
    "Say *gingerbread*"
    "Say *fraternity*"
    "Say *refrigerator*"
    "Say *pediatrician*"
    → write down the responses, including errors for later analysis
  - assess repetition of sentences
    → present common, simple, short sentences and ask the client to imitate; present progressively longer and more complex sentences:
    "Say *I like it*"
    "Say *he is here*"
    "Say *I am hungry*"
    "Say *it is getting dark*"
    "Say *who did this?*"
    "Say *I can do it if you tell me*"

"Say *let us go out and have dinner tonight*"
"Say *how do you do it, if you don't know anything about it*"
"Say *the man who was watching the game was hit by the ball*"

- Assess word finding and naming skills
  - assess responsive naming
    - → ask direct questions that give linguistic contexts for specific responses
    - → evoke nouns and verbs
    - → evaluate whether errors are due to auditory comprehension deficit or naming problems
      "What do you use to write?"
      "What do you use to unlock a door?"
      "What do you sleep on?"
      "What color is snow?"
      "What do you use to tell time?"
      "What do you use when you can't see well?"
      "What do you use to clean your body during a shower?"
      "What do you use to brush your teeth?"
      "What do you do with a knife?"
      "What do you do with a pen?"
      "What do you do when you are tired?"
      "What do you do when you are hungry?"
  - assess confrontation naming
    - → show an item to be named and ask "What is this?"
    - → present both common and uncommon pictures or objects
    - → present objects, picture of objects, letters, numbers, colors, and body parts and pictured actions
    - → record the stimulus presented and the actual responses for later analysis
    - → record your observations (e.g., "hesitant," "self-correction")
    - → show selected objects one at a time and ask "What is this?"

→ show selected pictures one at a time and ask "What is this?"
→ show pictures of various actions and ask the relevant question: "What is the woman doing?" or "What is the man doing?" or "What is the dog doing"
→ show selected colors and ask "What color is this?"
→ show selected letters and ask "What letter is this?"
→ show selected numbers and ask "What number is this?"
→ show selected body parts on a picture and ask "What is this?"

- assess categorical naming
  → ask the client to name words belonging to different categories; allow 1 minute for each category
  → use such common categories as animals, vegetables, fruits, furniture, and cities
    "Tell me the names of all animals you can think of"
    "Tell me the names of all vegetables you can think of"
    "Tell me the names of all furniture items you can think of"
    "Tell me the names of all cities in your state (specify)"

- assess closure naming
  → use the sentence completion procedure to assess naming
  → ask the client to complete the sentence with one word
  → first present a trial sentence and you supply the answer
    "The sky is _____"
    "You drive this _____"
    "You can fly this _____"
    "When it is night, you turn on the _____"
    "When you are hungry, you want to _____"
    "When you are tired, you want to _____"

- assess automatic serial naming
  → ask the client to produce automatic, serial words and numbers
    "Name the days of the week"

"Name the months of the year"
"Please count to 20"

- Assess the client's use of grammatic structures
  - assess the client's use of sentence structures and types; use the taped interview as well to make an analysis of language structures the client uses, misuses, and omits
    → take an extended language sample; use pictures if necessary to stimulate connected speech
    → tape-record the sample
    → analyze the average length of utterances and sentences measured in words; analyze the types and variety of sentences the client correctly uses and those that the client misuses
  - assess the client's use of morphologic features
    → use the language sample to analyze the correct and incorrect use of <u>Grammatic Morphemes of Language</u>; take note of omissions and substitutions
    → use the protocol provided in Shipley and McAfee (1992) for assessment of morphologic skills
- Assess understanding or usage of gestures
  - assess understanding of gestures
    → present a few common gestures (e.g., drinking from a glass, writing, looking at a distant object)
    → ask the client to say what the gestures mean
  - assess the use of gestures
    → take note of whether the client uses appropriate hand and facial gestures along with verbal expressions
    → take note of whether the client can gesture the words he or she cannot say
    → take note of whether the client has acquired any formal signs (such as those from the American Sign Language)
- Assess reading problems
  - assess comprehension of silently read material
    → select a prose passage that is appropriate to the client's age, education, and cultural background
    → ask the client to read the passage silently

  → ask the client specific questions about the material to assess comprehension
- assess errors in oral reading
  → to rule out peripheral visual problems, ask the client to match a few pictures with printed words and to match a few spoken words with printed words
  → select a prose passage that is appropriate to the client's age, education, and cultural background
  → ask the client to read the passage
  → on a copy of the passage mark the errors the client makes in reading (e.g., omission and substitution of sounds and words, misreading of words, self-corrections, and errors based on phonemic or semantic similarity)
  → take note of the rate of reading and dysfluencies exhibited
  → to rule out visual neglect, note whether the client ignores the printed material on the left half of the page
- Assess writing problems
  - assess graphomotor skills (letter formation)
    → find out the dominant hand the client used to write with before the onset of aphasia
    → note the hand the client uses to write (preferred but now weak right hand or nonpreferred left hand)
    → ask the client to copy printed words, sentences, and a paragraph
    → ask the client to spontaneously write about his or her family or work
    → ask the client to write a description of a picture
    → analyze the letter formation, upper- and lowercase letter usage, use of script or printed letters, overall quality of letter formation, legibility of letters, and letter formation errors
  - assess confrontation writing skills
    → ask the client to write the names of pictures shown
    → analyze the error patterns

- assess writing to dictation
  - → ask the client to write words and sentences you dictate
  - → analyze the error patterns
- assess narrative writing with obtained writing samples; ask the client to bring a premorbid writing sample for later comparison
  - → analyze the error patterns
- assess automatic or spontaneous writing
  - → ask the client to write his or her name and address
  - → ask the client to write the names of his family members
  - → ask the client to write the letters of the alphabet
  - → ask the client to fill out a check, a form, and to make a shopping list
  - → ask the client to write a brief message to a family member
  - → analyze the error pattern; be aware that automatic writing may be better preserved and may not be indicative of spontaneous and narrative writing problems
- Assess bilingual deficits
  - find out the primary language the client used before the onset of aphasia
    - → assess the client in his or her primary language or the language of strong and frequent use before the onset
    - → refer the client to a clinician who can assess the client in primary language if you cannot do it
    - → obtain an interpreter who is trained in providing assistance in assessment of aphasia if you need to provide services
    - → assess the client in his or her second language if warranted
    - → compare the communication deficits in the primary and the secondary languages

   → use culturally and linguistically appropriate assessment tools and materials
* Assess pragmatic communication problems
  * make a discourse analysis
    → use the conversational speech sample (discourse) to make an analysis of pragmatic problems
    → tell a short story to the client and ask the client to narrate it back to you
    → ask the client to narrate an experience or an event (e.g., the recent visit to hospital, the last vacation, a sports event of interest, or a hobby)
    → take note of the event/temporal sequence and the details given or missed
    → record the frequency with which the client correctly took turns during the interview and speech and language samples
    → record the frequency with which the client initiated a new topic during conversation
    → record the frequency with which the client abruptly switched from one topic to another

Aphasia Standardized Tests

* Administer a standardized test of aphasia; select the one that is appropriate for the client, practical, or preferred because of your experience with it; among others, consider one or more of the following tests:

Test	Purpose
Amsterdam-Nijemegen Everyday Language Test (L. Blomert, C. Koster, H. van Mier, & M. L. Kean)	To assess pragmatic language skills; a functional assessment tool
ASHA Functional Assessment of Communication Skills for Adults (C. M. Frattali, C. K. Thompson, A. L. Holland, C. B. Whol, & M. M. Ferketic)	To assess functional communication skills in a variety of settings and environments *(continued)*

(continued)

Test	Purpose
Assessment of Nonverbal Communication (New England Pantomime Test) (J. R. Duffy & J. R. Duffy)	To assess comprehension and expression of gestures through picture selection
Auditory Comprehension Test for Sentences (C. M. Shewan)	To assess comprehension of spoken sentences
Boston Assessment of Severe Aphasia (N. Helm-Estabrooks and associates)	To assess communication skills in severely aphasic patients
Boston Diagnostic Aphasia Examination (H. Goodglass & E. Kaplan)	To assess articulation, fluency, naming, repetition, serial speech, grammar, paraphasia, auditory comprehension, syntax, oral reading, and writing
Boston Naming Test (H. Goodglass, E. Kaplan, & S. Weintraub)	To assess naming skills through line drawings
Communicative Abilities in Daily Living (A. L. Holland)	To assess communication skills in daily living conditions; a functional assessment tool
Communicative Effectiveness Index (J. Lomas, L. Pickard, S. Bester, H. Elbard, H. A. Finlayson, & C. Zoghaib)	To assess pragmatic communication skills through a questionnaire filled out by a family member or a friend; a functional assessment tool
Examining for Aphasia (J. Eisenson)	To assess receptive and expressive language skills
Functional Auditory Comprehension Task (L. L. LaPointe & J. Horner)	To assess functional auditory comprehension of spoken language *(continued)*

(continued)

Test	Purpose
Functional Communication Profile (M. T. Sarno)	To assess various categories of communication; a functional assessment tool
Minnesota Test for Differential Diagnosis of Aphasia—Revised (H. Schuell & H. Sefer)	To assess speech, language, auditory comprehension, reading, and writing skills
Neurosensory Center Comprehensive Examination for Aphasia (O. Spreen & A. L. Benton)	To assess language comprehension and production, memory, reading, and writing skills
Porch Index of Communicative Ability (B. E. Porch)	To assess auditory comprehension, reading, oral expressive language, pantomime, visual matching, writing, and copying
Reading Comprehension Battery for Aphasia (L. L. LaPointe & J. Horner)	To assess reading comprehension of words, sentences, and paragraphs; functional reading, synonyms, and morphosyntax
Revised Token Test (M. M. McNeil & T. E. Prescott)	To assess auditory processing through token manipulation
Western Aphasia Battery (WAB) (A. Kertesz)	To assess speech content, fluency, auditory comprehension, repetition, naming, reading, writing, calculation, drawing, nonverbal thinking, and block design
Multilingual Aphasia Examination—Third Edition (A. L. Benton, K. De S. Hamsher, & A. B. Sivan)	To assess oral expression, spelling, verbal understanding, reading, articulation, and writing in English, Spanish, French, or German

Aphasia

Related/Medical Assessment Data

- Consider the results of medical neurodiagnostic techniques
- Consider the results of available psychological, cognitive, physical therapy, and related assessment information
- Consider the client's current medical condition and prognosis

Standard/Common Assessment Procedures

- Complete the Standard/Common Assessment Procedures

Analysis of Assessment Results

- Analyze results of assessment to obtain both the strengths and limitations of the client
- Summarize the communication deficits:
  - auditory comprehension deficits; levels of breakdown (e.g., intact comprehension for isolated sentences, but breakdown at paragraph level or in conversation)
  - describe the client's fluency skills and the types and number of dysfluencies
  - summarize the client's repetition skills; describe the level of breakdown (e.g., can repeat words but not phrases)
  - naming problems; describe the types of naming problems
  - syntactic and morphologic problems; describe the sentence types produced and not produced, morphologic features used, not used, or misused
  - describe the client's limitations in understanding and using gestures
  - reading and writing problems; describe the types of errors
  - describe the bilingual client's deficits in the primary and the secondary language
  - pragmatic communication deficits; summarize problems in discourse
  - summarize the results of standardized tests administered and integrate the results with client-specific procedures, observations, and the results of specific assessment procedures
  - rate the severity of aphasia if appropriate
  - specify the type of aphasia if desirable and appropriate

35

Aphasia

Diagnostic Criteria
- To diagnose aphasia, language disturbance should be due to recently acquired cerebral injury, except in some rare cases of gradual onset
- Language disturbances should outweigh any intellectual deficits observed
- Case history and available medical data (including neurological, radiological, and related data) should support the diagnosis of aphasia
- Pattern of deficits observed should help rule out related and similar disorders as specified under differential diagnosis

Differential Diagnosis
- Distinguish aphasia from normal language with some aphasic-like characteristics, apraxia, dementia, dysarthria, language of confusion, schizophrenia, right hemisphere syndrome, and traumatic brain injury; use the following grids to make a differential diagnosis (adapted from Hegde, 1998):

APHASIA OR NORMAL LANGUAGE?

Aphasia	Aphasic-like But Normal Language
Positive history of stroke, tumor, and other central neuropathology	Negative history of central neuropathology
Prior history of normal language; deterioration in language skills	Prior history of limited language; no evidence of deterioration in language skills
Lack of education does not explain the problems	Lack of education could explain the problems
Level of literacy does not explain the problem	Level of literacy could explain the problem
Current environment could not explain the problem	Current environment could explain the problem
Sudden onset	Lifelong problem

APHASIA OR DEMENTIA?

Aphasia	Dementia
Onset mostly is sudden	Onset mostly is slow
Damage in the left hemisphere	Bilateral brain damage
Focal brain lesions in most cases	Diffuse brain damage in most cases
Mood usually is appropriate, though depressed or frustrated at times	May be moody, withdrawn, and agitated
Impaired language, but cognition mostly is intact	Cognition is mildly or severely impaired, but better language skills until later stages
Memory typically is intact	Memory is impaired to various degrees, often severely
Behavior generally is relevant, appropriate, and organized	Behavior often is irrelevant, socially inappropriate, and disorganized
Alert and oriented to time and space	Confused and disoriented to time and space
No disorientation to self	Disorientation to self in later stages
Semantic, syntactic, and phonologic performance simultaneously impaired	Progression of deterioration from semantic to syntactic to phonologic performance
Fluent or nonfluent	Fluent until dementia becomes worse
Relatively better performance on spatial and verbal tasks	Relatively poor performance on spatial and verbal recognition tasks
Relatively better story retelling skills	Relatively poor story retelling skills
Relatively better description of common objects	Relatively poor description of common objects

(continued)

(continued)

Aphasia	Dementia
Relatively better silent reading comprehension	Relatively poor silent reading comprehension
Relatively better pantomimic expression	Relatively poor pantomimic expression
Relatively better drawing skills	Relatively poor drawing skills

Caution: (a) Patients with fluent aphasia are more likely to be confused with dementia than are those with nonfluent aphasia. (b) Aphasia and dementia may coexist. (c) An aphasic patient may develop a neurological disease resulting in dementia (Alzheimer's disease). (d) A patient with dementia may suffer a stroke, resulting in aphasia.

APHASIA OR THE LANGUAGE OF CONFUSION?

Aphasia	Confusion
Left hemisphere damage, focal	Bilateral damage, diffuse
Strokes are the most common cause	Traumatic brain injury and toxic and metabolic disturbances are the most common causes
Often relevant	Typically irrelevant
Attentional deficits are not the most striking	Attentional deficits are the most striking
Writing problems parallel speaking problems	Writing problems often greater than speaking problems
No confabulation	Confabulation
Syntactic difficulties	Little or no syntactic difficulties
Repetition skills often impaired	Repetition skills often intact
Significant word-finding problems	No significant word-finding problems
Varying degrees of auditory comprehension problems	Generally intact auditory comprehension

(continued)

(continued)

Aphasia	Confusion
No disorientation except for the first few hours of stroke	Disoriented to time, place, and persons
History suggests stroke	History suggests brain trauma
No significant behavioral change	Significant behavioral change
More stable or slower change in symptoms	More rapid, positive changes in symptoms

Caution: Confusion may coexist with aphasia when a patient with traumatic brain injury suffers a focal left hemisphere damage.

APHASIA OR SCHIZOPHRENIA?

Aphasia	Schizophrenia
Sudden onset	Gradual onset
Late onset (adult or old age)	Early onset (adolescence or early adulthood)
Not a psychotic disorder; no history of psychiatric disturbances	A psychotic disorder; a history of psychiatric disturbances
Due to a general medical condition (cerebral infarct)	Not due to a general medical condition
No thought disorders	Thought disorders including delusions
No such perceptual disorders as hallucinations	Perceptual disorders, especially auditory hallucinations
No confabulation, generally relevant	Confabulation, typically irrelevant
No evidence of disorganized speech	Disorganized speech
Deficits in auditory comprehension	No deficits in auditory comprehension (may be inattentive)

(continued)

(continued)

Aphasia	Schizophrenia
Reading and writing affected	Reading and writing may not be affected
Appropriate emotional responses	Lack of emotional expression and inappropriate or incongruent emotional responses
Social behavior, personal hygiene, and general behavior not affected or disorganized; any limitation due to motor problems	Social behavior, personal hygiene, and general behavior grossly disorganized; none due to physical limitations
Appropriate sexual behavior	Inappropriate sexual behavior
Absence of <u>Catatonic Motor Behavior</u>	Presence of <u>Catatonic Motor Behavior</u>

Caution: Aphasia and schizophrenia may coexist, especially when a patient with schizophrenia suffers a stroke.

APHASIA OR RIGHT HEMISPHERE SYNDROME?

Aphasia	Right Hemisphere Syndrome
Significant or dominant problems in naming, fluency, auditory comprehension, reading, and writing	Only mild problems in naming, fluency, auditory comprehension, reading, and writing
No left-sided neglect	Left-sided neglect
No denial of illness	Denial of illness
Speech is generally relevant	Speech is often irrelevant, excesive, rambling
Generally normal affect	Often lack of affect
Intact recognition of familiar faces	Possible impaired recognition of familiar faces
Simplification of drawings	Rotation and left-sided neglect

(continued)

(continued)

Aphasia	Right Hemisphere Syndrome
No significant prosodic defect	Significant prosodic defect
Appropriate humor	Inappropriate humor
May retell the essence of a story	May retell only nonessential, isolated details (no integration)
May understand implied meanings	Understands only literal meanings
Pragmatic impairments less striking	Pragmatic impairments more striking (eye contact, topic maintenance, etc.)
Though limited in language skills, communication is often good	Though possessing good language skills, communication is very poor
Pure linguistic deficits are dominant	Pure linguistic deficits are not dominant

Note: Right hemisphere damage in those few individuals whose right hemisphere is dominant for language results in aphasia, and for the same etiologic factors.

APHASIA OR APRAXIA OF SPEECH?

Aphasia Without Apraxia of Speech	Apraxia of Speech Without Aphasia
Neurogenic language problem	Neurogenic speech problem
Trial and error, groping articulatory movements are not significant	Trial and error, groping articulatory movements are significant
Misarticulations less variable, more consistent	Misarticulations more variable, more inconsistent
Some impairment in auditory comprehension	Generally, no impairment in auditory comprehension
Prosodic problems not dominant	Prosodic problems dominant

(continued)

A

(continued)

Aphasia Without Apraxia of Speech	Apraxia of Speech Without Aphasia
Difficulty in initiating utterances is less obvious	Difficulty in initiating utterances is more obvious
Omission of function words	No significant tendency to omit function words
Word-finding problems	No word-finding problems
Limb or oral apraxia not dominant	Limb or oral apraxia or both may be dominant

Note: Apraxia of speech and Broca's aphasia often coexist. Pure apraxia is rare. It often is associated with Broca's aphasia.

APHASIA OR DYSARTHRIA?

Aphasia Without Dysarthria	Dysarthria Without Aphasia
Neurogenic language problem	Neurogenic speech problem
The language problems are not due to muscle weakness	The speech problems are due to muscle weakness, spasticity, rigidity (except for ataxic dysarthria)
No consistent misarticulations	Consistent misarticulations
Intelligibility of speech not clearly related to the rate of speech	Intelligibility clearly related to the rate of speech
No respiratory problems associated with speech production	Respiratory problems associated with speech production
Phonatory problems not significant	Phonatory problems may be significant
Resonance disorders not significant	Resonance disorders significant
Prosodic disorders not as dominant	Prosodic disorders may be dominant

(continued)

Aphasia

(continued)

Aphasia Without Dysarthria	Dysarthria Without Aphasia
Abnormal voice quality not significant	Abnormal voice quality may be significant
Abnormal stress not significant	Abnormal stress may be significant

Note: Occasionally, aphasia and dysarthria may coexist. Subcortical lesions that produce aphasia are more likely to be associated with dysarthria.

APHASIA OR TRAUMATIC BRAIN INJURY?

Aphasia	Traumatic Brain Injury
Pure linguistic problems are dominant	Pure linguistic problems are not dominant
Significant grammatic errors	Grammatic errors not significant
Dysarthria not a part of the syndrome (although the two may co-exist)	Dysarthria part of the syndrome
Language not confused	Initially, confused language
Slower improvement in language	Faster improvement in language
Less serious pragmatic problems	More serious pragmatic problems
Social interaction not as seriously impaired	Social interaction seriously impaired
Not disorganized or confused	Initially disorganized and confused
Not disoriented to time and space	Initially disoriented to time and space
Not inconsistent or irrelevant	May be inconsistent or irrelevant

(continued)

(continued)

Aphasia	Traumatic Brain Injury
Attentional problems not as serious	Serious attentional problems including distractibility, impulsivity, poor social judgment, and lack of insight

Note: Traumatic brain injury may cause aphasia as well.

- Note that agrammatic writing skills help distinguish Wernicke's aphasia; suggest Broca's aphasia
- Note that severe writing skills suggest global aphasia

Prognosis

- Evidence on such biographical variables as the age (at onset), gender, education, and occupational status is contradictory or ambiguous
- Aphasia resulting from traumatic brain injury may have better prognosis than that resulting from vascular pathology which in turn may have better prognosis than that resulting from subcortical hemorrhage
- Larger lesions and bilateral lesions indicate less favorable prognosis than smaller and unilateral lesions
- More posterior lesions, especially in the temporoparietal regions, and deeper lesions suggest less favorable prognosis than more anterior and upper cortical lesions
- Better health and intact sensory modalities are associated with more favorable prognosis than poor health and sensory deficits
- More favorable prognosis for improved language without treatment during the first 3 to 6 months
- Less severe aphasia is associated with more favorable prognosis for higher level of language recovery than more severe aphasia which may show greatest improvement yet stabilizing at a lower level of language

Recommendations

- Recommend communication treatment for all patients with aphasia, at least on a trial basis

- Let the initial treatment outcome help make judgments about continued treatment
- See the cited sources and *PGTSLP* for details

Bayles, K. A., & Kaszniak, A. W. (1987). *Communication and cognition in normal aging and dementia.* Austin, TX: Pro-Ed.

Brookshire, R. (1997). *An introduction to neurogenic communication disorders* (5th ed.). St. Louis: Mosby Year Book.

Chapey, R. (1994) (Ed.). *Language intervention strategies in adult aphasia.* Baltimore, MD: Williams & Wilkins.

Darley, F. (1982). *Aphasia.* Philadelphia: W. B. Saunders.

Davis, G. A. (1993). *A survey of adult aphasia* (2nd ed.). Englewood Cliffs, NJ: Prentice-Hall.

Hegde, M. N. (1998). *A coursebook on aphasia and other neurogenic language disorders* (2nd ed.). San Diego, CA: Singular Publishing Group.

Helm-Estabrooks, N., & Albert, M. L. (1991). *Manual of aphasia therapy.* Austin, TX: Pro-Ed.

LaPointe, L. L. (Ed.) (1997). *Aphasia and related neurogenic language disorders* (2nd ed.). New York: Thieme Medical Publishers.

Lubinski, R. (1991). *Dementia and communication.* Philadelphia: B. C. Decker.

Rosenbek, J. C., LaPointe, L. L., & Wertz, R. T. (1989). *Aphasia: A clinical approach.* Austin, TX: Pro-Ed.

Ripich, D. (Ed.). (1991). *Handbook of geriatric communication disorders.* Austin, TX: Pro-Ed.

Aphasia: Specific Types. Variations in aphasia symptom complex that allow for typological classification; most commonly described types include the following:

Anomic Aphasia. A type of fluent Aphasia with persistent and severe naming problems as its dominant characteristic; varied etiologic factors including closed head injury, focal lesions in the angular gyrus or the second temporal gyrus, and Alzheimer's disease; pure anomic aphasia may be rare; chronic patients with a history of other kinds of aphasia may remain as anomic aphasic individuals; use the assessment procedures described under Aphasia and pay special attention to the following:

Major Symptoms
- Marked naming problems

- Good repetition skills
- Relatively better auditory comprehension
- Fluent speech
- Good articulation of speech sounds
- Acceptable prosody
- Near-normal syntactic and morphologic features

Diagnostic Criteria/Guidelines
- Persistent and significant naming problems that dominate the clinical picture
- Other language skills better preserved
- History and etiology consistent with aphasia

Differential Diagnosis
- Relatively better auditory comprehension skills associated with anomic aphasia distinguish it from Wernicke's aphasia and global aphasia (poor auditory comprehension)
- Fluent speech and good grammatic structures associated with anomic aphasia distinguish it from Broca's aphasia (agrammatism)
- Better repetition skills associated with anomic aphasia distinguish it from conduction aphasia (poor repetition skills)

Recommendations
- Aphasia treatment, with an emphasis on teaching naming skills

Broca's Aphasia. A type of nonfluent aphasia with lesions in the third frontal convolution of the left or dominant hemisphere (Brodman's area 44); less commonly referred to as expressive aphasia, motor aphasia, and verbal aphasia; a somewhat controversial diagnostic category because some experts believe that injury limited to Broca's area produces apraxia of speech along with transient mutism, not aphasia; in some patients, injury to Broca's area may produce transcortical motor aphasia; injury to Broca's area, though the basis for the diagnostic category, is neither necessary nor sufficient to produce aphasia; injury to other areas, and generally more extensive damage than originally thought may be involved in patients diagnosed with Broca's aphasia; use the assessment procedures described under Aphasia and pay special attention to the following:

Major Symptoms

- Obvious neurological symptoms including right-sided hemiparesis, paralysis, and initial confinement to a wheelchair
- Depression and emotional reactivity in some patients
- Nonfluent, effortful speech; limited word output
- Missing grammatical elements; speech often limited to content words (nouns and verbs)
- Impaired repetition of words and sentences
- Marked naming problems, especially with naming something or someone when asked to (confrontation naming: response to "what is this?")
- Slow rate of speech, uneven flow; long and frequent pauses in speech; lack of intonation
- Limited syntax, short sentences
- Better auditory comprehension (may have mild to moderate deficits)
- Associated Dysarthria and Apraxia of Speech
- Poor oral reading skills and writing problems including poor formation of letters, spelling errors, and letter omissions

Diagnostic Criteria/Guidelines

- Dysfluent, effortful, agrammatic speech with better receptive skills suggest Broca's aphasia
- History and etiology consistent with aphasia

Differential Diagnosis

- Relatively better auditory comprehension skills associated with Broca's aphasia distinguish it from Wernicke's aphasia and global aphasia (poor auditory comprehension)
- Nonfluent speech and limited grammatic structures associated with Broca's aphasia distinguish it from Wernicke's aphasia, transcortical sensory aphasia, anomic aphasia, and conduction aphasia (fluent speech with good grammar)

- Poor repetition skills associated with Broca's aphasia distinguish it from transcortical motor aphasia and transcortical sensory aphasia (better repetition skills)

Recommendations
- Aphasia treatment, with an emphasis on improving phrase length, fluency, and naming skills

Conduction Aphasia. A type of fluent aphasia; somewhat rare; first postulated by Wernicke; site of lesions include the supramarginal gyrus, the superior temporal lobe, and regions between Broca's and Wernicke's area; also known as central aphasia; use the assessment procedures described under <u>Aphasia</u> and pay special attention to the following:

Major Symptoms
- Paresis of the right side of the face and right upper extremity
- Oral and limb apraxia in some patients
- Marked impairment in repetition skills, the most important distinguishing feature; phonemic paraphasia
- Moderate to mild auditory comprehension deficits
- Fluent speech, good articulation, acceptable prosody
- Near-normal syntactic and morphologic features
- Severe to mild naming problems
- Recognition of errors
- Often unsuccessful efforts at self-correction
- Variable but not too severe reading problems

Diagnostic Criteria/Guidelines
- Markedly impaired repetition skills
- Other language skills better preserved
- History and etiology consistent with aphasia

Differential Diagnosis
- Severely impaired repetition skills associated with conduction aphasia distinguish it from anomic aphasia, transcortical motor aphasia, and transcortical sensory aphasia (good repetition skills)
- Relatively better auditory comprehension skills associated with conduction aphasia distinguish it from Wer-

nicke's aphasia, transcortical sensory aphasia, and global aphasia (poor auditory comprehension)
- Fluent speech, good articulation, and better grammatic structures associated with conduction aphasia distinguish it from Broca's aphasia, global aphasia, and transcortical motor aphasia (agrammatism)

Recommendation
- Aphasia treatment, with an emphasis on teaching naming skills

Crossed Aphasia. Aphasia in right-handed persons with right hemisphere injury; a somewhat rare occurrence; frequent causes include brain tumor or trauma (as against vascular pathology in the left-hemisphere injury); use the assessment procedures described under Aphasia and pay special attention to the following:

Major Symptoms
- Missing grammatical elements (Agrammatism)
- Minimal naming problems and minimal auditory comprehension problems
- Symptoms of Broca's aphasia in some cases
- May include left-sided neglect and difficulties in drawing

Diagnostic Criteria/Guidelines
- Right-hemisphere damage in right-handed individuals
- History and etiology consistent with aphasia; presence of brain tumor or trauma in most cases

Differential Diagnosis
- Right-hemisphere damage in right-handed individuals distinguish crossed aphasia from other syndromes of aphasia caused by left-hemisphere pathology
- High incidence of tumor and trauma causing right-hemisphere injury and aphasia distinguish it from left-hemisphere injury and aphasia that typically result from vascular pathology
- Minimal problems in naming and auditory comprehension, combined with drawing problems and left-sided

neglect, help distinguish crossed aphasia from aphasia resulting from left-hemisphere pathology

Recommendation
- Aphasia treatment, with an emphasis on improving grammatic skills, fluency, left-sided neglect, and drawing skills

Global Aphasia. A type of nonfluent aphasia characterized by severe deficits in comprehension and production of language; all sensory modalities may be affected; due to extensive brain damage; lesions in the frontal, temporal, and parietal lobes; lesions may extend to the white matter of the brain; Broca's and Wernicke's areas may both be involved; use the assessment procedures described under Aphasia and pay special attention to the following:

Major Symptoms
- Nonfluent, extremely limited speech and language skills
- Severely impaired naming and repetition skills
- Extreme difficulty in auditory comprehension
- Impaired gestural skills
- Impaired reading and writing skills

Diagnostic Criteria/Guidelines
- Severe deficits in all modalities of communication are essential for a diagnosis of global aphasia

Differential Diagnosis
- Extremely limited verbal expression distinguishes global aphasia from other nonfluent aphasias
- Extremely limited fluency, phrase length, grammatic skills, and prosodic features distinguish global aphasia from fluent aphasias

Recommendations
- Aphasia treatment, with an emphasis on basic and functional communication skills including the use of gestures, communication boards, simple writing, expression of basic words and phrases, and basic auditory comprehension

Isolation Aphasia. A rare type of nonfluent aphasia caused by lesions surrounding the perisylvian speech area, thus isolating language areas from other areas of the brain; resembles global aphasia; use the assessment procedures described under Aphasia and pay special attention to the following:

Major Symptoms
- Severely impaired fluency
- Severely impaired auditory comprehension
- Marked naming difficulties
- Moderate to mild problems in repetition

Diagnostic Criteria/Guidelines
- Symptoms similar to global aphasia except for the better preserved repetition skills
- Unique neuropathology

Differential Diagnosis
- All severely depressed language modalities except for repetition skills distinguish isolation aphasia from other types

Recommendations
- Aphasia treatment, with an emphasis on improved basic and functional communication skills

Subcortical Aphasias. Several newer syndromes of aphasia that are due to damage to left subcortical regions, contrasted with better known syndromes that are caused by damage to left cortical regions of the brain; damage to such subcortical structures as internal capsule, putamen, and thalamus due to vascular occlusion or hemorrhage may be involved; more research and clinical observation needed to fully understand their communication deficits and neuropathology; may still be due to impaired cortical function; the damaged subcortical structures may or may not be involved in language; decreased cortical metabolism noted in patients with subcortical damage; use the assessment procedures described under Aphasia and pay special attention to the following:

Aphasia: Specific Types

Major Symptoms
- Lesions of the anterior limb of the internal capsule and putamen cause:
- severe dysarthria
- severe writing problems
- mild to moderate problems in word repetition, naming, reading, and auditory comprehension
- normal or near-normal syntax and phrase length
- right hemiplegia
- Lesions of the left posterior limb of the internal capsule and putamen cause:
- severe problems in auditory comprehension and naming
- near-normal fluency and syntax with mild articulation problems, if any
- right hemiplegia
- Subcortical anterior and posterior lesions affecting internal capsule, putamen, and thalamus cause:
- symptoms of global aphasia (all speech-language functions severely affected)
- Left thalamic lesions cause:
- problems in initiating spontaneous speech
- sparse, fluctuating, perseverative, neologistic, and echolalic speech
- relatively intact reading and comprehension skills
- symptoms generally similar to transcortical motor aphasia

Diagnostic Criteria/Guidelines
- Diagnosis depends on the site of lesion
- Presence of specific symptoms associated with different subcortical pathology

Differential Diagnosis
- Like patients with Broca's aphasia, patients with lesions in the anterior limb of the internal capsule and putamen exhibit severe articulation problems and minimal auditory comprehension problems; unlike Broca's patients, they have good syntactic skills and fluency

- Patients with lesions in the posterior limb of the internal capsule and putamen resemble patients with Wernicke's aphasia except that they exhibit right hemiplegia (absent in Wernicke's patients)

Recommendations
- Aphasia treatment

Transcortical Motor Aphasia. A type of nonfluent aphasia; also known as *dynamic aphasia* and *anterior isolation syndrome*; resembles Broca's aphasia with intact repetition skills; compared and contrasted with transcortical sensory aphasia, which resembles Wernicke's aphasia with good repetition skills; lesions located above or below Broca's area and in the deep white matter below the supplementary motor area; neural pathology affects spontaneous speech but not repetition; lesions are supposed to disconnect the supplementary motor area from otherwise unaffected Broca's area; use the assessment procedures described under Aphasia and pay special attention to the following:

Major Symptoms
- Intact repetition; can repeat long and complex sentences
- Lack of spontaneous speech; limited speech output only when strongly urged; limited syntax, short sentences; naming problems
- Agrammatic, paraphasic, telegraphic speech as in Broca's aphasia
- Generally fluent speech, good articulation
- Better auditory comprehension (may have mild to moderate deficits)

Diagnostic Criteria/Guidelines
- Good repetition skills, lack of spontaneous speech, fluent and good articulation
- History and etiology consistent with aphasia

Differential Diagnosis
- Lack of spontaneous speech combined with limited word output in the absence of articulation problems

contrasted with excellent repetition skills distinguish transcortical motor aphasia from other types

Recommendations

- Aphasia treatment, with an emphasis on improving spontaneous speech and phrase length

Transcortical Sensory Aphasia. A type of fluent aphasia; also known as posterior isolation syndrome and Wernicke's aphasia type II; compared and contrasted with transcortical motor aphasia; similar to Wernicke's aphasia; intact repetition skills a major characteristic; lesion often located in the temporoparietal region (border zone between the middle and posterior cerebral arteries) with spared Wernicke's area; possible involvement of the angular gyrus and visual and auditory cortex; may be associated with bilateral lesions; a form of aphasia commonly associated with Alzheimer's disease; use the assessment procedures described under <u>Aphasia</u> and pay special attention to the following:

Major Symptoms

- Intact repetition; can repeat long and complex sentences; echolalia
- Auditory comprehension deficits as in Wernicke's aphasia
- Moderate to severe naming difficulties
- Generally fluent speech that is full of paraphasias; adequate phrase length, syntax, and prosody

Diagnostic Criteria/Guidelines

- Symptoms of Wernicke's aphasia with intact repetition skills
- History and etiology consistent with aphasia

Differential Diagnosis

- Intact repetition skills distinguish transcortical sensory aphasia from Wernicke's aphasia
- Generally fluent speech with severe to moderate auditory comprehension deficits distinguish transcortical sensory aphasia from transcortical motor aphasia with its

nonfluent and limited spontaneous speech; intact repetition is a common feature of both types

Recommendations

- Aphasia treatment, with an emphasis on improving naming skills

Wernicke's Aphasia. A type of fluent aphasia; a less controversial syndrome than the nonfluent Broca's aphasia, with which it contrasts; also called *receptive aphasia*; less commonly referred to as *word deafness*, *syntactic aphasia*, and *central aphasia*; lesion often located in the posterior portion of the superior temporal gyrus in the left hemisphere (Wernicke's area); in some cases, the angular gyrus, the second temporal gyrus, and the surrounding parietal region also may be involved; use the assessment procedures described under Aphasia and pay special attention to the following:

Major Symptoms

- Good (even excessive) fluency
- Rapid rate, incessant speech in some cases
- Meaningless speech
- Normal (or longer) phrases, articulation, grammar, and prosody
- Paraphasia, neologism, and jargon
- Severe auditory comprehension deficits
- Mild to severe naming difficulties
- Impaired repetition
- Poor reading comprehension and free, copious, and errorful writing

Diagnostic Criteria/Guidelines

- Fluent, apparently grammatically correct speech with little meaning and severe auditory comprehension deficits
- History and etiology consistent with aphasia

Differential Diagnosis

- Impaired repetition skills distinguish Wernicke's aphasia from transcortical sensory aphasia with its intact repetition skills

- Normal or excessive fluency; apparently normal grammar, articulation, and prosody; severe auditory comprehension deficits; and limited communication in spite of copious speech distinguish Wernicke's aphasia from Broca's aphasia
- Normal or excessive fluency and impaired repetition skills distinguish Wernicke's aphasia from transcortical motor aphasia with its dysfluent speech and intact repetition

Recommendations

- Aphasia treatment

For Treatment of all Types of Aphasia:

- See the cited sources and *PGTSLP* for details

Bayles, K. A., & Kaszniak, A. W. (1987). *Communication and cognition in normal aging and dementia.* Austin, TX: Pro-Ed.

Brookshire, R. (1997). *An introduction to neurogenic communication disorders* (5th ed.). St. Louis, MO: Mosby Year Book.

Chapey, R. (Ed.). (1994). *Language intervention strategies in adult aphasia.* Baltimore, MD: Williams & Wilkins.

Collins, M. (1991). *Diagnosis and treatment of global aphasia.* San Diego, CA: Singular Publishing Group.

Darley, F. (1982). *Aphasia.* Philadelphia: W. B. Saunders.

Davis, G. A. (1993). *A survey of adult aphasia* (2nd ed.). Englewood Cliffs, NJ: Prentice-Hall.

Hegde, M. N. (1998). *A coursebook on aphasia and other neurogenic language disorders* (2nd ed.). San Diego, CA: Singular Publishing Group.

Helm-Estabrooks, N., & Albert, M. L. (1991). *Manual of aphasia therapy.* Austin, TX: Pro-Ed.

LaPointe, L. L. (Ed.). (1997). *Aphasia and related neurogenic language disorders* (2nd ed.). New York: Thieme Medical Publishers.

Lubinski, R. (199 1). *Dementia and communication.* Philadelphia: B. C. Decker.

Rosenbek, J. C., LaPointe, L. L., & Wertz, R. T. (1989). *Aphasia: A clinical approach.* Austin, TX: Pro-Ed.

Ripich, D. (Ed.). (1991). *Handbook of geriatric communication disorders.* Austin, TX: Pro-Ed.

Aphonia.   Loss of voice; see <u>Voice Disorder</u>.

Aplasia.   Underdevelopment of an organ or tissue. See also Agenesis and Hypoplasia.

Apraxia.   Disordered volitional movement in the absence of muscle weakness, paralysis, or fatigue.

Apraxia of Speech (AOS) in Adults.   A neurogenic speech disorder with documented neuropathology in the left cerebral hemisphere including such areas as Broca's and supplementary motor; primarily an articulatory (phonologic) disorder characterized by sensorimotor problems in positioning and sequentially moving muscles for the volitional production of speech; unimpaired reflex and automatic acts; associated with prosodic problems; not caused by muscle weakness or neuromuscular slowness; presumed to be a disorder of motor programming for speech; also called, among several names and at various times, aphemia, afferent motor aphasia, anarthria, apraxic dysarthria, cortical dysarthria, oral verbal apraxia, primary verbal apraxia, and pure motor aphasia; frequently Aphasia may be a co-existing disorder; less often, Dysarthria of unilateral upper motor neuron type may be a co-existing disorder; may be an independent problem (speech programming deficit) in some aphasic patients; in its pure form, may not affect language skills; frequently, but not always associated with nonverbal oral apraxia; in some cases, can be the only presenting symptom of neurological disease.

Etiology

- Generally, injury or damage to brain structures in the dominant hemisphere involved in speech programming
- Most commonly, vascular lesions (resulting in strokes) that specifically affect speech programming structures and pathways; single left hemisphere stroke in about 58% of cases; multiple strokes in about 10%; often, frontal and parietal lesions; occasionally, temporal lobe lesions but never alone
- Such degenerative neural diseases as Multiple Sclerosis (MS), Primary Progressive Aphasia and Creutzfeldt-Jakob Disease (CJD) in about 16% of cases

Apraxia of Speech (AOS) in Adults

- Left hemisphere trauma; surgical trauma to the left hemisphere in the process of tumor removal, aneurysm repair, and hemorrhage evacuation in about 15% of cases
- Tumors in the left hemisphere in about 6% of cases
- Undetermined etiology in about 4% of cases
- Seizure disorder and multiple causes in about 1% each

Nonverbal Symptoms

- Impaired oral sensation in some patients, but not a critical diagnostic feature of AOS
- Facial and lingual weakness only when dysarthria is a coexisting problem
- Nonverbal oral apraxia (NVOA) in many patients; NVOA and AOS may be independent of each other
- Right hemiparesis and sensory deficits in some cases; not an invariable symptom
- Limb apraxia in some cases; not an invariable symptom

Auditory Processing Deficits (APDs)

- APDs are not characteristic of AOS
- APDs may be present only when there is a coexisting aphasia
- APDs, when present, may not be causally related to AOS
- APDs, when present, may exacerbate AOS

Verbal (Speech) Symptoms

- General characteristics
  - patients generally aware of their speech problems; sometimes surprised by their mistakes
  - volitional sequencing of movements required for speech most notably affected
  - automatic speech less affected than more spontaneous or volitional speech
  - highly variable speech errors; different kinds of errors on repeated attempts; normal or disordered production of the same word on different occasions
  - compensatory strategy of reduced rate in some but not all patients
- Articulatory problems
  - substitutions, distortions, and omissions of speech sounds

- substitutions more common than other types; some substitutions may be distortions
- the greatest number of substitutions involve place-related productions; manner, voicing, and oral/nasal distinctions involve decreasing frequency of errors in that order
- fewer errors on bilabial and lingual-alveolar consonants
- greater number of errors on affricates and fricatives
- greater number of errors on consonant clusters than on singletons
- vowel errors less frequent than consonant errors
- anticipatory substitutions (a phoneme that occurs later in the word replaces the one that occurs earlier; e.g., "lelo" for "yellow")
- postpositioning errors (a phoneme that occurs earlier replaces the one that occurs later; e.g., "dred" for "dress")
- metathetic errors (switched position of phonemes in words; e.g., "tefalone" for "telephone")
- some consonant substitutions complicate rather than simplify intended productions
- distortions and substitutions closer to intended productions
- frequency of errors increase with increasingly complex productions (e.g., longer words and phrases)
- delayed initiation of speech
- trial-and-error groping and struggling associated with speech attempts
- initial position of sounds may be more difficult than other positions, though sound position may not be a significant variable in most cases
- higher frequency of errors on infrequently occurring sounds
- automatic productions easier than volitional/purposive productions
- nonsense syllables more difficult than meaningful words

- attempts at self-correction
- impaired imitation of modeled words in some cases; in most cases, imitative performance may be comparable to, or better than, spontaneous productions
- Prosodic problems
  - reduced rate of speech
  - difficulty in increasing speech or changing rate when instructed
  - isolated production of words (silent pauses in between words)
  - increased duration of consonants and vowels
  - even stress on syllables
  - limited intonation
  - even loudness of speech or restricted range of intensity
  - restricted range of pitch
  - overall dysprosody
  - characteristics of a foreign accent
- Fluency problems
  - Silent pauses, especially when speech is to be initiated
  - repetitions due to false starts and attempts to correct articulatory errors
- Acoustic and physiologic problems
  - variability in voice onset time (VOT) values
  - overlapping VOT values for voiced and voiceless stops
  - increased consonant and vowel durations
  - inconsistent or delayed coarticulation
  - variations in lip and jaw movement velocity
  - variable movement of articulators
  - longer movement durations involving the lip and the jaw
  - variability in intensity across syllables
  - lack of variability in syllable duration
  - lack of stress patterns
  - production of stops without a complete closure of the vocal tract, resulting in distorted speech due to noise
  - acoustic or EMG indication of repeated or stuttered speech

- discoordination between amplitude and velocity of jaw, lip, tongue, and velar movements

Assessment Objectives/General Guidelines

- To assess articulatory proficiency in volitional speech
- To assess fluency and prosodic aspects of speech
- To assess other communication skills including auditory comprehension, oral language skills, and reading and writing skills
- To make a diagnosis of apraxia in general and AOS in particular
- To distinguish AOS from other motor speech disorders including Dysarthrias, Neurogenic Fluency Disorders, Palilalia, and Aprosodia
- To distinguish AOS from neurogenic language disorders including Aphasia and Dementia
- To describe potential treatment targets and to assess prognosis
- To describe the client's strengths and intact skills
- To suggest potential neuropathology

Case History/Interview Focus

- See **Case History** and **Interview** under Standard/Common Assessment Procedures
- Concentrate on the patient's detailed biographical data and medical data; pay special attention to family communication patterns

Ethnocultural Considerations

- See Ethnocultural Considerations in Assessment

Assessment

Assessment of AOS includes procedures designed to diagnose aphasia as well; the focus of language assessment in AOS is the possibility of a coexisting nonfluent aphasia, often Broca's aphasia.

- Assess language to determine a coexisting aphasia
  - obtain a language sample
  - administer one or more Aphasia tests
  - design client-specific procedures to assess specific language deficits (e.g., naming problems) associated with aphasia

Apraxia of Speech (AOS) in Adults

- Assess auditory comprehension deficits associated with aphasia
  - use the procedures described under <u>Aphasia</u>
- Assess reading and writing problems associated with aphasia
  - use the procedures described under <u>Aphasia</u>
- Assess speech to diagnose AOS
  - devise your own stimulus materials to assess speech production problems or use the following suggestions which are based on *Motor Speech Evaluation* described by Wertz, LaPointe, and Rosenbek (1991)[1]
  - tape record the patient's responses for later scoring, or score as you evoke the responses; transcribe responses phonetically; take note of struggle and groping; self-correction; repetition and other forms of dysfluencies; errors of articulation; delayed reaction; facial grimacing; and other behaviors that suggest apraxia
  - evoke imitative production of a speech sound
    → ask the patient to "say /a/ as long and as evenly as you can"; model the response for the client to imitate
  - evoke the repetitive production of syllables; model all responses for the client to imitate
    → ask the patient to "say pʌ-pʌ-pʌ as long and as evenly as you can"
    → ask the patient to "say tʌ-tʌ-tʌ as long and as evenly as you can"
    → ask the patient to "say kʌ-kʌ-kʌ as long and as evenly as you can"
  - evoke the repetitive production of multiple syllables
    → ask the patient to "say pʌ-tʌ-kʌ as long and as evenly as you can"
  - evoke imitative production of selected words; model the responses for the client

[1]Adapted from R. T. Wertz, L. L. LaPointe, and J. C. Rosenbek (1991). *Apraxia of speech in adults*, San Diego, CA: Singular Publishing Group. Copyright 1991 Singular Publishing Group, Inc. Used by permission.

→ "say *several*"
→ "say *tornado*"
→ "say *artillery*"
→ "say *linoleum*"
→ "say *snowman*"
→ "say *television*"
→ "say *catastrophe*"
→ "say *gingerbread*"
→ "say *probability*"
→ "say *thermometer*"
→ "say *refrigeration*"
→ "say *responsibility*"
→ "say *unequivocally*"
→ "say *parliamentarian*"
→ "say *statistical analysis*"
→ "say *Encyclopedia Britannica*"
→ "say *Boston, Massachusetts*"
→ "say *Minneapolis, Minnesota*"
→ "say *San Francisco, California*"
→ "say *Nuclear Regulatory Commission*"
→ "say *thick*"
→ "say *thicken*"
→ "say *thickening*"
→ "say *love*"
→ "say *loving*"
→ "say *lovingly*"
→ "say *please*"
→ "say *pleasing*"
→ "say *pleasingly*"
→ "say *jab*"
→ "say *jabber*"
→ "say *jabbering*"
→ "say *mom*"
→ "say *judge*"
→ "say *peep*"
→ "say *bib*"
→ "say *nine*"

Apraxia of Speech (AOS) in Adults

→ "say *tote*"
→ "say *dad*"
→ "say *coke*"
→ "say *gag*"
→ "say *fife*"
→ "say *sis*"
→ "say *zoos*"
→ "say *church*"
→ "say *churn*"
→ "say *lull*"
→ "say *shush*"
→ "say *roar*"

- evoke repeated, imitative production of words and phrases; score each production
  → "say *artillery* five times"
  → "say *impossibility* five times"
  → "say *disenfranchised* five times"
  → "say *catastrophically* five times"
  → "say *barometric pressure* five times"
- evoke the imitative production of sentences
  → "say *The valuable watch was missing*"
  → "say *In the summer they sell vegetables*"
  → "say *The shipwreck washed up on the shore*"
  → "say *Please put the groceries in the refrigerator*"
  → "say *Please tell the gardener to fertilize the plants*"
  → "say *I do not understand the reasons for repeating it*"
- evoke counting responses
  → "Please count from one to twenty"
  → "Now Please count backwards, from twenty down to one"
- evoke picture description that lasts at least 1 min; use the "Cookie Thief" picture from the *Boston Diagnostic Aphasia Examination*
  → "Tell me what is happening in this picture"
- assess imitation of sentences the patient produced during the examination; use any four sentences

→ "repeat [a sentence the patient has produced]"
→ "repeat [a second sentence the patient has produced]"
→ "repeat [a third sentence the patient has produced]"
→ "repeat [a fourth sentence the patient has produced]"

- assess oral reading; use the *Grandfather* passage; take note of errors of significance
  → "please read this passage out loud"
- Assess oral, nonverbal movement to evaluate oral apraxia or a coexisting dysarthria in case of significant muscle weakness or paralysis; the following suggestions are from Wertz, LePointe, and Rosenbek (1991)[2]:
  - conduct an **Orofacial Examination** described under Standard/Common Assessment Procedures
  - assess isolated oral movements; ask the patient to listen carefully and perform the action requested:
    → "stick out your tongue"
    → "try to touch your nose with your tongue"
    → "try to touch your chin with your tongue"
    → "bite your lower lip"
    → "pucker your lips"
    → "puff out your cheeks"
    → "show me your teeth"
    → "click your teeth together"
    → "wag your tongue from side to side"
    → "clear your throat"
    → "cough"
    → "whistle"
    → "show that you're cold by making your teeth chatter"
    → "smile"
    → "show me how you would kiss a baby"
    → "lick your lips"
  - assess oral motor sequencing; ask the patient to watch you carefully and perform the actions you demonstrate;

→ touch the upper lip center with the tongue tip; lower and raise the jaw
→ click teeth once; pucker lips
→ lower and raise the jaw; bite lower lip with teeth; show teeth by stretching the lips
→ touch the lower lip center; bite the lower lip; lower and raise the jaw; lick the lips
→ puff out the cheeks; pucker lips; lower and raise the jaw; lick the lips
→ click teeth once; pucker lips; lower and raise the jaw; lick lips; bite the lower lip
→ pucker lips; lick the lips; click teeth once; puff out cheeks; touch upper lip center with tongue tip

• assess limb movements to evaluate limb apraxia; ask the patient to listen carefully and perform the action requested; the following examples are from Wertz, LaPointe, and Rosenbek (1991)[3]; use similar commands
→ "show how an accordion works"
→ "show me how you salute"
→ "wave good-bye"
→ "threaten someone with your hand"
→ "show that you are hungry"
→ "thumb your nose at someone"
→ "snap your fingers"
→ "show how you would play a piano"
→ "indicate that someone is crazy"
→ "make the letter 'O' with your fingers"

• take note of patients' awareness of problems, motivation for treatment, frustration, coping strategies, response to instructions, level of cooperation, and so forth

Standardized Tests

Very few standardized tests of AOS are commercially available. Most procedures come from research clinicians who have described them in their writings. Administration of aphasia standardized tests,

[3]Adapted from R. T. Wertz, L. L. LaPointe, and J. C. Rosenbek (1991). *Apraxia of speech in adults*, San Diego, CA: Singular Publishing Group. Copyright 1991 Singular Publishing Group, Inc. Used by permission.

of which many are available, is typically a part of apraxia assessment.

- Administer selected standardized tests listed under <u>Aphasia</u>
- Administer selected standardized tests listed under <u>Articulation and Phonological Disorders</u>
- Administer one of the following tests of apraxia:

Test	Purpose
Apraxia Battery for Adults (B. L. Dabul)	To measure the presence and severity of limb, oral, and speech apraxia and changes over time
Comprehensive Apraxia Test (F. G. DeSimoni)	To assess nonverbal and verbal apraxia
Test of Oral and Limb Apraxia (N. Helm-Estabrooks)	To assess oral and limb apraxia in developmental or acquired neurologic disorders

Related/Medical Assessment Data

- Obtain medical records as described under **Case History/ Interview Focus**

Standard/Common Assessment Procedures

- Complete the <u>Standard/Common Assessment Procedures</u>

Analysis of Assessment Results

- Analyze the language sample and the results of administered tests of aphasia to diagnose or rule out a possible, coexisting aphasia; follow the assessment procedures described under <u>Aphasia</u>
- Describe language formulation, expression, and comprehension problems associated with aphasia
- Analyze the results of standardized articulation and phonological tests administered and describe and summarize the kinds of errors noted
- Analyze the speech sample and describe and summarize the kinds of articulatory and phonological errors noted

Apraxia of Speech (AOS) in Adults

- Analyze and summarize the results of motor speech evaluation to diagnose AOS
- Analyze and summarize the results of orofacial examination, oral, nonverbal movement evaluation to identify paralysis, paresis, or oral apraxia
- Analyze and summarize the results of limb movement evaluation to assess limb apraxia
- Analyze and describe the reading and writing problems associated with aphasia as assessed by standardized aphasia tests or by client-specific procedures

Diagnostic Criteria
- Pathology in the left hemisphere
- Vascular pathology typically involving the left middle cerebral artery
- Dominant symptoms of speech programming difficulties with inconsistent errors of articulation, groping and struggling, notable difficulties in volitional speech production, and prosodic problems

Subtypes
- Controversial, but possibly based on site of lesion, patterns of articulatory errors, and prosodic problems
- One possible subtype associated with articulatory substitutions and transpositions coupled with less consistently abnormal prosodic features
- Another possible subtype associated with articulatory distortions and more consistently abnormal prosodic features

Differential Diagnosis
- Distinguish apraxia from aphasia, dementia, language of confusion, dysarthrias, neurogenic stuttering, and palilalia
- Expect the greatest difficulty in distinguishing a coexisting AOS and aphasia in the same patient; while aphasia often exists without AOS, AOS often exists with aphasia; aphasia associated with AOS often is the nonfluent variety
- Distinguish apraxia from other relevant disorders based on the characteristics listed in each of the 6 grids that follow (adapted from Hegde, 1998):

APRAXIA OF SPEECH OR APHASIA?

Apraxia of Speech	Aphasia
Neurogenic speech problem	Neurogenic language problem
Without aphasia, more often or more strongly associated with posterior, frontal, or insular lesions	Without AOS, aphasia more often associated with temporal or temporoparietal lesions
Patient complains of speech production problem (articulation)	Patient complains of word retrieval and related language problem
Trial and error, groping articulatory movements are significant	Trial and error, groping articulatory movements are not significant
Misarticulations more variable, more inconsistent	Misarticulations less variable, more consistent
Generally, no impairment in auditory comprehension	Some impairment in auditory comprehension
Prosodic problems dominant	Prosodic problems not dominant, especially in fluent aphasias
Difficulty in initiating utterances is more obvious or due to difficulty in positioning the articulators	Difficulty in initiating utterances is less obvious or due to naming and language formulation problems
Attempts at self-correction	Lack of attempts at self-correction, especially by patients with fluent aphasia
Articulatory errors more frequent on initial sounds	Articulatory errors more frequent on final sounds
No significant tendency to omit function words	Omission of function words
No word-finding problems	Word-finding problems
Limb or oral apraxia or both may be dominant	Limb or oral apraxia not dominant

(continued)

(continued)

Apraxia of Speech	Aphasia
No reading comprehension deficits	Reading comprehension deficits
AOS typically does not mask aphasia	If severe, aphasia can mask AOS
AOS with or without aphasia may be associated with unilateral upper motor neuron dysarthria.	Aphasia without AOS is less likely to be associated with unilateral upper motor neuron dysarthria
Phonologic problems are predictable and approximations of the intended word	Phonologic problems of fluently aphasic patients are unpredictable, idiosyncratic, and off-target

Note: AOS and aphasia share similar neuropathology (vascular etiology and gross neuropathology); AOS in its pure form is uncommon; AOS and Broca's aphasia often coexist, but not AOS and fluent aphasias; phonologic problems associated with AOS may be confused with similar problems found in fluent aphasias.

APRAXIA OF SPEECH OR DEMENTIA?

Apraxia of Speech	Dementia
Sudden onset	Slow onset in many cases
Unilateral brain damage	Bilateral brain damage
CVA, trauma, or surgery more typical causes	Degenerative neurological diseases more typical causes
More localized brain damage	Diffuse brain damage in most cases
Intact language and mental functions	Impaired language and mental functions
Relatively intact intellectual functions	Progressively deteriorating intellectual functions
More errors of fluency and syntax	Fewer errors of fluency and syntax

(continued)

(continued)

Apraxia of Speech	Dementia
Better preserved reading comprehension	Disturbed reading comprehension
Intact semantic and syntactic skills	Semantic and syntactic errors in the initial sages
Predominant errors of articulation	Errors of articulation not predominant; such errors appear only in later stages
Moodiness, withdrawal, and agitation not a frequent characteristic	May be moody, withdrawn, and agitated
Cognition better preserved	Cognition is mildly or severely impaired, but better language skills until later stages
General behavior is relevant, socially appropriate, and organized	Behavior often is irrelevant, socially inappropriate, and disorganized
Except for the initial acute stage, alert and oriented to time and space	Confused and disoriented to time and space
Well-oriented to self	Disorientation to self in later stages
Often less fluent, especially when Broca's aphasia coexists	Fluent until dementia becomes worse

Caution: Note that degenerative CNS pathology may cause AOS in about 16% of cases. In such cases, dementia and AOS may coexist.

APRAXIA OF SPEECH OR THE LANGUAGE OF CONFUSION?

Apraxia of Speech	Language of Confusion
Unilateral, focal damage	Bilateral, diffuse damage
Vascular pathology and neurosurgical trauma in most cases	Traumatic brain injury and toxic and metabolic disturbance in most cases *(continued)*

(continued)

Apraxia of Speech	Language of Confusion
Speech is relevant	Speech is typically irrelevant
Attention deficits are not characteristics	Attentional deficits are the most striking
Symptoms relatively persistent	Symptoms are more transient
Dominant fluency problems	Relatively intact fluency
Dominant errors of articulation	Few errors of articulation
More syntactic errors	Fewer errors of syntax
Fewer writing problems than speech production problems	Writing problems often greater than speaking problems
No confabulation	Confabulation
No disorientation	Disoriented to time, place, and persons
No significant behavior changes	Significant behavior change

APRAXIA OF SPEECH OR DYSARTHRIAS?

Apraxia of Speech	Dysarthrias
The cause is motor programming deficit, not muscle weakness	The cause is muscle weakness
Lesions often in the <u>Supratentorial Level</u> of the brain	Lesions in supratentorial and other areas (including posterior fossa, spinal structures, or peripheral nerves)
Supratentorial lesions producing apraxia tend to be cortical	Supratentorial lesions producing dysarthria tend to be subcortical
Huntington's chorea, Parkinsonism, Pick's disease, and ALS are *not* associated with apraxia	Huntington's chorea, Parkinsonism, Pick's disease, and ALS *are* associated with dysarthrias

(continued)

(continued)

Apraxia of Speech	Dysarthrias
Can be associated with normal orofacial mechanism and function (except for NVOA)	Often associated with abnormalities of orofacial mechanism and function
NVOA may be associated with AOS	NVOA not typically associated with dysarthrias
Absence of dysphagia	Presence of dysphagia (but usually not in ataxic dysarthria)
Variable misarticulations	Consistent misarticulations (except for ataxic dysarthria which shows irregular articulatory breakdowns)
Better production of automatic utterances than propositional productions	The same problems with automatic and propositional productions
Word length, meaningfulness, frequency of occurrence are significant variables	Word length (with a possible exception of ataxic dysarthria), meaningfulness, frequency of occurrence are *not* significant variables
Besides distortions, complications of speech gestures may be noticeable	Distortions and simplification of speech gestures are dominant
More frequent and variable dysfluencies	Less frequent and less variable dysfluencies
Frequent articulatory groping	Articulatory groping not characteristic
Many attempts at self-correction	Few, if any, attempts at self-correction
Respiratory, phonatory, and resonance problems not as significant as articulatory and prosodic problems	Respiratory, phonatory, and resonance problems as significant as articulatory and prosodic problems
Frequently associated with aphasia	Infrequently associated with aphasia

Note: Both AOS and dysarthrias are neurogenic speech disorders. The two are not confused in most cases. Some symptoms are common to AOS and spastic, hyperkinetic, and ataxic dysarthrias; however, it is more difficult to distinguish AOS from ataxic dysarthria. See Dysarthrias for differential diagnosis between AOS and specific types of dysarthrias.

APRAXIA OF SPEECH OR NEUROGENIC STUTTERING?

Apraxia of Speech	Neurogenic Stuttering
Lesions typically in the left hemisphere	Varied site of lesion including brainstem, basal ganglia, cerebellum, and all cortical lobes except for the occipital lobe
Generally, dysfluencies due to articulatory groping, attempts at self-correction, articulatory revision, and searching	Generally, dysfluencies unrelated to articulatory problems found in AOS
Dysfluencies on the off-target sounds or in an effort to revise them	Repetitions and prolongations of target sounds

APRAXIA OF SPEECH OR PALILALIA?

Apraxia of Speech	Palilalia
Lesions typically in the left hemisphere	Bilateral lesions typically in the basal ganglia
Mechanism of dysfluencies not clear	Mechanism of dysfluencies is neuromuscular problems
Sound, syllable, and word repetitions; sound prolongations	Mostly word and phrase repetitions
Less commonly associated with hypokinetic dysarthria	More commonly associated with hypokinetic dysarthria
Progressive increase in speech rate not evident	The speech rate may increase progressively
Slower speech rate	Not necessarily slower speech rate

(continued)

(continued)

Apraxia of Speech	Palilalia
Dysfluencies may be accompanied by effort and groping	Easy and effortless repetition of word and phrase

Prognosis

Clinically proven, strong, generally applicable, and universally agreed-on variables that clearly predict prognosis are few or nonexistent; however, clinical experience suggests the following:

- Good prognosis for improvement in speech with systematic treatment
- In a few cases, complete or nearly complete recovery in a matter of few days
- Less favorable prognosis for severe, persistent AOS
- More favorable prognosis with better physical health and lack of sensory deficits
- Less favorable prognosis with larger lesions
- More favorable prognosis with a single, small lesion confined to Broca's area
- Less favorable prognosis with multiple strokes
- More favorable prognosis if treatment is initiated within a month postonset than if the treatment is much delayed
- More favorable prognosis in the absence of serious nonverbal, oral apraxia
- More favorable prognosis with coexisting aphasia that is less severe

Recommendations

- Treatment to improve communication
- See the cited sources and *PGTSLP* for details

Brookshire, R. H. (1997). *An introduction to neurogenic communication disorders* (5th ed.). St. Louis, MO: Mosby Year Book.

Duffy, J. R. (1995). *Motor speech disorders: Substrates, differential diagnosis, and management.* St. Louis, MO: C. V. Mosby.

Freed, D. (2000). *Motor speech disorders: Diagnosis and treatment.* San Diego: Singular Publishing Group.

Rosenbek, John, C. (1984). Stuttering secondary to nervous system damage. In R. F. Curlee & W. H. Perkins (Eds.), *Nature and treatment of stuttering: New directions* (pp. 31–48). San Diego, CA: College-Hill Press.

Wertz, R. T., LaPointe, L. L., & Rosenbek, J. C. (1991). *Apraxia of speech.* San Diego: Singular Publishing Group.

Aprosodia. Prosodic disturbance; speech without much intonation; robotlike speech; often found in patients with right hemisphere syndrome.

Arteriosclerosis. Disease of the arteries in which the walls of the arteries thicken and lose their elasticity; has several varieties including cerebral arteriosclerosis (a major cause of strokes and thus aphasia); and coronary arteriosclerosis (disease of the arteries of the heart).

Arthropathy. Disease of joints; a symptom in some genetic syndromes including Stickler Syndrome (see <u>Syndromes Associated With Communicative Disorders</u>).

Articulation and Phonological Disorders. Disorders of speech characterized by difficulty in producing speech sounds correctly; sounds may be omitted, distorted, or substituted; a distinction some experts make between the two terms is that the difficulty in producing single or a few sounds with no pattern or derivable rule is an articulation disorder and multiple errors that can be grouped on some principle and thus form patterns and severely affect intelligibility are <u>Phonological Disorders</u>; other experts do not make such a distinction and consider both terms as referring to a group of speech disorders that are not due to structural deviations or neuromotor control problems, a practice that is becoming more prevalent; the same as functional articulation disorders; a common diagnostic category especially in school-age children; constitute roughly 32% of all disorders of communication; frequently associated with language disorders; articulation disorders due to documented central or peripheral nervous system pathology and are associated with problems in respiratory, phonatory, resonatory, and prosodic problems are known as <u>Dysarthria</u>; articulation problems that are due to central nervous system pathology causing motor programming problems in the absence of weakness or paralysis of the speech muscles are described as <u>Apraxia of Speech</u>; although functional articulation disorders may persist into adulthood in some cases, and some have argued that the children with functional articulation disorders may have subtle neuromotor problems, much of the information presented in this section pertains to children's articulation disorders that cannot be explained on the basis of clear and convincing evidence of organic deficits.

Factors Related to Articulation and Phonological Disorders

- No specific cause or causes explain articulation and phonological (Ar-Ph) disorders
- Research has suggested only that factors may coexist, hence be correlated with, Ar-Ph disorders; such correlations do not suggest causation
- Research also has suggested differences between those who do and those who do not have Ar-Ph disorders on specific variables; such differences, too, do not suggest causation
- Age
  - articulatory performance improves until 8 years of age
- Gender
  - girls may be slightly ahead of boys in phonological acquisition
  - more boys than girls have Ar-Ph disorders
- Socioeconomic status
  - a greater number of children from lower socioeconomic groups have Ar-Ph disorders than those from higher socioeconomic groups
  - nonetheless, most experts conclude that socioeconomic status is not a significant variable
- Familial and genetic factors
  - possibility of familial and genetic influence has emerged in recent research; more research is needed

- older and only children have better articulatory skills than children whose siblings are only slightly older
- Personality, emotional disorders
  - children with Ar-Ph disorders are not distinguished by unique personality or emotional disorders
- Intelligence
  - within normal limits, intelligence is not associated with Ar-Ph disorders
  - many children with Ar-Ph disorders have normal intelligence
  - children who are mentally retarded tend to exhibit Ar-Ph disorders
  - Ar-Ph skills of children with mental retardation resemble those of younger children without mental retardation
- Academic performance
  - Ar-Ph disorders may be independent of academic performance in most cases
  - severe Ar-Ph disorders associated with significant language delay may run the risk of poor academic performance including reading and spelling problems
- Structural variations in the speech production mechanism
  - generally, variations within the normal range may not be necessarily associated with Ar-Ph disorders
  - extreme deviations are more likely to be associated with Ar-Ph disorders (e.g., extreme degrees of malocclusions, velopharyngeal incompetence, tongue deformities)
  - some individuals with notable deviations may still learn to produce the speech sounds correctly
  - significant Ar-Ph disorders may be found in the absence of structural anomalies; therefore, such anomalies do not account for Ar- Ph disorders in most children
- Oral sensory factors
  - the relationship between oral sensory perception (e.g., oral tactile sensitivity and oral form recognition) and articulation skills is not clear

- Hearing loss
  - hearing loss (significant degree of loss at all ages and even mild loss during the period of speech sound acquisition) is associated with Ar-Ph disorders
  - many children with Ar-Ph disorders have normal hearing; thus hearing loss does not explain their disorder
- Motor skills
  - no significant deficits in general motor skills of children with Ar-Ph disorders
  - the diadochokinetic rate of children with Ar-Ph disorders may be slightly below normal
  - many children with Ar-Ph disorders may perform as well as or even better than those without such disorders on diadochokinetic tests
- Tongue thrust
  - anterior tongue resting position may be associated with lisping in some children
- Auditory speech sound discrimination skills
  - children with Ar-Ph disorders may have speech sound discrimination problems, although the issue still is controversial because of varied research findings
- Language skills
  - mild to moderate Ar-Ph disorders may not be associated with significant language problems
  - severe Ar-Ph disorders tend to be associated with significant language disorders

Description of Articulatory Errors

- Omissions or deletions
  - absence of a required sound in a word; one of the more common errors of articulation
- Substitutions
  - sound replacements; a wrong sound is produced instead of a right sound
- Distortions
  - inaccurate production of sounds
- Addition

- intrusion of a sound that does not belong to the target word
- Devoicing
  - production of voiced sounds without vocal fold vibrations or with limited vibrations
- Frontal lisp
  - production of sibilant consonants with tongue tip placed too far forward (against the teeth or between the teeth); most common lisps involve /s/ and /z/
- Lateral lisp
  - production of sibilant sound with air flowing over the sides of the tongue
- Labialization
  - production of sounds with excessive lip rounding
- Nasalization
  - inappropriate nasal resonance in the production on oral sounds, especially oral stops
- Pharyngeal fricative
  - fricatives produced in the pharyngeal area
- Stridency deletion
  - omission of a strident
- Unaspirated
  - production of an aspirated sound without aspiration
- Initial position error
  - error in the production of a beginning sound of a word
- Medial position error
  - error in the production of a middle sound of a word
- Final position error
  - error in the production of a final sound of a word
- Intervocalic error
  - error in producing a consonant that is preceded and succeeded by a vowel

Description of Phonological Error Patterns
The number and specific descriptions of error patterns vary across writers; some of the more commonly described patterns, as described

by Bernthal and Bankson (1998) and Peña-Brooks and Hegde (2000) include the following:

- Affrication: Production of an affricate in place of a fricative or stop
  - *chun* for *sun*
  - *chu* for *shoe*
- Backing: Production of more posteriorly placed consonants instead of more anteriorly placed consonants (velar consonants in place of alveolar consonants)
  - *boak* for *boat*
  - *hoop* for *soup*
- Cluster reduction or cluster simplification: Omission (deletion) of one or more consonants in a cluster of consonants
  - *bes* for *best*
  - *seep* for *sleep*
- Deaffrication: Production of a fricative in place of an affricate
  - *pez* for *page*
  - *ship* for *chip*
- Depalatalization: Production of an alveolar fricative in place of a palatal fricative or affricate
  - *su* for *shoe*
  - *wats* for *watch*
- Diminutization: Addition of [i] or a consonant and [i]:
  - *eggi* for *egg*
  - *nodi* for *no*
- Denasalization: Production of an oral sound with a similar place of articulation (homorganic sound) in place of a nasal
  - *by* for *my*
  - *dame* for *name*
- Epenthesis: Insertion of a vowel (an error of addition); often between two consonants in a consonantal cluster
  - *bəlu* for *blue*
  - *səmile* for *smile*
- Final consonant deletion: Omission of a consonant at the end of a word or syllable

- *kæ* for *cat*
- *pu* for *pool*
- Final consonant devoicing: Production of an unvoiced final consonant in place of a voiced final consonant
  - *bet* for *bed*
  - *bik* for *big*
- Fronting: Production of more anteriorly placed consonants in place of more posteriorly placed consonants (e.g., alveolar consonants instead of velar consonants)
  - *tee* for *key*
  - *su* for *shoe*
- Gliding: Production of a glide (w, j) in place of a liquid (1, r)
  - *pwey* for *play*
  - *yewo* for *yellow*
- Glottal replacement: Production of a glottal stop (ʔ) in place of other consonants
  - *tuʔ* for *tooth*
  - *baʔə* for *bottle*
- Labial assimilation: Production of a labial consonant in place of a nonlabial consonant in a word that contains another labial
  - *beab* for *bead*
  - *bop* for *top*
- Metathesis: Production of sounds in a word in reversed order
  - *peek* for *keep*
  - *likstip* for *lipstick*
- Nasal Assimilation: Production of a nasal consonant in place of an oral consonant in a word that contains a nasal
  - *nam* for *lamb*
  - *nun* for *fun*
- Prevocalic voicing: Voiced production of voiceless consonants when they precede a vowel (prevocalic position)
  - *bea* for *pea*
  - *Dom* for *Tom*

- Reduplication (doubling): Repetition of a syllable
  - *wawa* for *water*
  - *kaka* for *cat*
- Stopping: Production of stop consonants in place of other sounds (often fricatives)
  - *teat* for *seat*
  - *doup* for *soup*
- Syllable deletion (weak syllable deletion): Omission of a syllable, usually an unstressed syllable
  - *nana* for *banana*
  - *tephone* for *telephone*
- Velar assimilation: Production of a velar consonant in place of a nonvelar in a word that contains a velar
  - *keak* for *teak*
  - *guck* for *duck*
- Vocalization (vowelization): Production of vowels in place of liquids or nasals
  - *fawo* for *flower*
  - *dippo* for *zipper*

Assessment Objectives/General Guidelines

- To assess the articulatory performance of the client in single word positions and in conversational speech
- To assess the presence of phonological processes that may help establish patterns in misarticulations
- To evaluate a child's performance in light of developmental norms
- To evaluate stimulability of speech sounds that are misarticulated
- To identify potential treatment targets
- To evaluate treatment effects by repeated measurement

Case History/Interview Focus

- See **Case History** and **Interview** under <u>Standard/Common Assessment Procedures</u>
- Pay special attention to articulation disorders as described by the parents; speech-language acquisition and such

other clinical conditions as hearing loss and mental retardation

Ethnocultural Considerations

- See <u>Ethnocultural Considerations in Assessment</u> for general guidelines
- See <u>Assessment of Articulation and Phonological Disorders in African American Children</u> at the end of this main entry
- See <u>Assessment of Articulation and Phonological Disorders in Bilingual Children</u> at the end of this main entry

Screening

- When an articulation disorder is not obvious, screen articulation to determine if a more detailed assessment is needed
  - evoke a brief conversation from the child and take note of articulatory errors
  - ask a few questions about the child, names of family members, friends and their names, interests, hobbies, school activities, favorite television shows, teachers, sport activities, recent vacations, and so forth; ask the child to count to 20, recite days of the week, months of the year, and so forth
  - take a brief conversational speech sample from an adult and evaluate speech sound productions
  - have an adult read the *Rainbow Passage* or the *Grandfather Passage* and evaluate speech sound productions

Use Standardized Screening Instruments

- Administer one of the following standardized screening tests or measures:

Test	Purpose
Denver Articulation Screening Exam (A. F. Drumright)	To screen production of 30 sounds in initial and final word positions
	(continued)

Articulation and Phonological Disorders

(continued)

Test	Purpose
Fluharty Speech and Language Screening Test for Preschool Children (N. B. Fluharty) (administer the speech screening portion)	To screen production of speech sounds with object stimuli
McDonald Screening Deep Test (E. T. McDonald)	To screen production of frequently misarticulated sounds in 10 coarticulatory contexts
Predictive Screening Test (C. Van Riper & R. L. Erickson)	To screen production of sounds to predict articulatory skills by the end of second grade
Quick Screen of Phonology (N. W. Bankson & J. E. Bernthal)	To screen 10 phonological processes
Templin-Darley Screening Test (M. C. Templin & F. L. Darley)	To screen production of sounds with color and black-and-white pictures

Assessment of Articulation and Phonological Disorders

- Take a representative sample of connected speech; use the general procedures of obtaining a Speech and Language Sample described under Standard/Common Assessment Procedures
  - in the case of younger children, have the mother and child interact with each other; let them interact in their usual manner; supply toys and picture books the mother and the child prefer; tape record the interactions; observe and take notes
  - engage the child in conversational speech

- use a quiet room and avoid noisy stimulus materials; use a table cloth or any soft material to dampen noise; sit on carpeted floor
- use large pictures, storybooks, and soft toys; consider the child's interests and ethnocultural background in selecting stimulus materials
- tape record the entire speech sample for later analysis
- record in stereo for a more dynamic range
- when possible, transcribe on the spot
- talk less, do not interrupt the child, and listen carefully
- echo what you think the child said when you are not sure what the child said
- do not ask yes/no questions, ask open-ended questions
- use the following to evoke conversation; modify them as necessary to make them appropriate for individual child; (use the questions/suggestions within the parentheses for follow-up):
  → tell me about your favorite TV show
  → tell me about the shows you watch on Saturday mornings (tell me what happens in _____ show or _____ show)
  → tell me about your favorite video game (tell me how to play it; what are some of your other favorite video games?)
  → what did you do last weekend? (what do you plan to do next weekend?)
  → tell me about your favorite vacation (tell me about your other vacations)
  → tell me the story of Cinderella (did you see the movie? did you like it?)
  → tell me the story of [a recent children's movie] (did you see the movie? did you like it?)
  → tell me the story of the "Three Little Pigs"
  → tell me the names of your friends (describe them for me; how much time do you spend with them? do you play with them on weekends? what do you play with them?)

→ who is your best friend (why?)
→ tell me about your favorite baby-sitter (why is she your favorite?)
→ tell me how to make popcorn
→ tell me how to make hot dogs
→ tell me how your mom makes cookies (do you help mom when she bakes cookies? how do you help her?)
→ pretend I have never had pizza before and describe it to me (have you ever helped your mom make pizza at home? how did you help her?)
→ who is your favorite teacher (and why?)
→ what subjects do you like the most (and why?)

- show large picture cards that depict a variety of activities and ask the child to tell a story; when the response is sparse, ask such follow-up questions as the following while you point to different aspects of the picture:
  → what about this?
  → what about that?
  → what is going on here?
  → what is he doing here?
  → why is she doing that?
  → what is she (he, they) doing over there?
  → what is happening here? why?
- show funny and incongruous pictures and ask such questions as the following:
  → what is funny about this?
  → what is wrong here?
- ask the child to narrate a story; prompt the child to say more; direct the child's attention to aspects of the story he or she ignores
- tell a story and ask the child to retell it; prompt the child about details not given
- tell a story about a picture and then ask the child to retell it as he or she looks at the picture

- pretend to go on a shopping trip to a store; have a toy cash register, plastic food items, and some play money; let the child do the shopping and talking
- use hand puppets to carry on a conversation and to tell stories to each other
- misname objects, toys, or pictures and let the child correct you
- show the child only parts of a disassembled toy (e.g., Mr. Potato Head); let the child ask for missing parts
- role-play a daily activities (cooking, shopping, planning a picnic)
- create a play or toy farm and ask questions about the animals, farm activities
- use a doll house to engage the child in conversation and description of stimuli
- ask the child to explain a game (e.g., hide and seek)
- have the child play teacher and talk to the kids or teach words to the kids
- obtain a sample of oral reading from children who can read; but note that fewer errors are revealed in reading tasks than in connected speech tasks
- Take a sample of single word productions
  - use a standardized test that samples single-word productions
  - make your own stimulus material to test sounds in the initial, medial, and final positions; minimally, include the most frequently misarticulated speech sounds: /s, z, θ, ð, ʃ, tʃ, dʒ, v, r/
  - select attractive and unambiguous pictures to evoke single-word responses
  - use a combination of pictures and objects (especially toys with young children) to introduce variety
  - ask the child to name the picture
  - record the response for later analysis; preferably, write down the response in the phonetic alphabet
  - if the child does not seem to know the name of a picture or object, name it and move on to the next stimulus

- after a while, re-present the stimulus you had named earlier
- with a client-specific procedure (not a standardized test), ask for repetition of an unclear response that is difficult to score (note that standardized tests may not allow this)
- ask the child to repeat given responses if it appears that oral-motor problems are creating inconsistent responses
- note that articulatory performance in single-word productions may not totally reflect the problems the child may have in connected speech; however, by single-word production tasks you can be sure of sampling all sounds in all positions; do not use single-word performance data exclusively unless the child's connected speech is extremely limited or unintelligible
- compare single-word performance data with connected speech performance data; the two sets of data may diverge especially in the case of oral-motor problems

Assess Stimulability of Misarticulated Sounds

- Select the sounds the child misarticulates and assess their stimulability
  - ask the child to watch, listen carefully, and say what you say; do not give special instructions on the correct production (e.g., about the placement of the articulators or voicing)
  - model the production of selected phonemes and ask the child to imitate
  - model them initially in isolated sound levels
  - model the sounds in words; if preferred, model them in nonsense syllables
  - take note of the percent success rate to determine the stimulability for each sound
  - note the limitations of stimulability tests; although popular, their value in predicting improvement either with or without therapy is questionable; lack of stim-

ulability does not suggest poor prognosis for treatment; treatment is recommended regardless of stimulability scores; poor stimulability should discourage neither the clinician nor the client

Make a Structured Contextual Assessment

- Use a deep test (see the next section) to assess the production of sounds in different phonetic contexts; note that although conversational speech provides contextual information, structured assessment of contextual influence is valuable in identifying contexts in which a misarticulated sound is correctly produced; such contexts may be used in treatment; structured assessment will systematically alter the phonetic context in ways that may not naturally occur in conversational speech
- Assess consistency of misarticulations by sampling in varied phonetic contexts
  - analyze phonetic contexts of conversational speech in which each of the misarticulated phonemes is produced correctly

Standardized Tests of Articulation

- Administer one or more of the following standardized tests:

Test	Purpose
Arizona Articulation Proficiency Scale (J. B. Fudala & W. B. Reynolds)	To assess primarily single phoneme productions with black-and-white picture stimuli; a few sentences
Fisher-Logemann Test of Articulation Competence (H. Fisher & J. Logemann)	To assess single phonemes with color pictures and sentence productions; includes a screening component
Goldman-Fristoe Test of Articulation (R. Goldman & M. Fristoe)	To assess single phonemes with color pictures and sentence productions *(continued)*

(continued)

Test	Purpose
Iowa Pressure Test (H. L. Morris, D. D. Spriestersbach, & F. L. Darley)	To assess mostly fricatives and plosives and indirectly assess the adequacy of velopharyngeal closure; items from the *Templin-Darley Test of Articulation*
McDonald Deep Test of Articulation (E. T. McDonald)	To assess contextual production of phonemes (two-word combinations and in sentences)
Photo Articulation Test (K. Pendergast, S. F. Dickey, J. W. Selmar, & A. L. Soder)	To assess single phoneme productions with color pictures of objects
Templin-Darley Test of Articulation (M. C. Templin & F. L. Darley)	To assess sound production in words, sentences, and in sentence completion formats

Measures of Phonological Processes

- Use one of the following to make a phonological analysis of misarticulations:

Test	Purpose
Assessment of Link Between Phonology and Articulation—Revised (R. J. Lowe)	To assess 15 phonological processes through short sentences and with picture stimuli
Assessment of Phonological Processes—Revised (B. W. Hodson)	To assess 40 phonological processes in seven categories with objects, pictures, and body parts
Bankson-Bernthal Test of Phonology (N. W. Bankson & J. E. Bernthal)	To assess consonant productions, phonological error patterns, and intelligibility
Compton-Hutton Phonological Assessment (A. J. Compton J. S. Hutton)	To assess sound productions in initial and final word positions to identify phonological error patterns

(continued)

(continued)

Test	Purpose
Computerized Profiling (S. Long & M. Fey)	To assess phonological processes with an IBM compatible or Macintosh computer
The Khan-Lewis Phonological Analysis (L. Khan & N. Lewis)	To assess 15 phonological processes with 44 words from the *Goldman-Fristoe Test of Articulation*
The Macintosh Interactive System for Phonological Analysis (J. Masterson & F. Pagan)	To assess 27 phonological processes or rules with a Macintosh computer
Natural Process Analysis (L. Schriberg & J. Kwiatkowski)	To assess 8 natural phonological processes with a 90-word spontaneous speech sample
Phonological Process Analysis (F. Weiner)	To assess 16 phonological processes with 136 picture stimuli

Measure of Phonological Knowledge
- An approach to articulation assessment and treatment that seeks to evaluate a child's phonological knowledge; knowledge is assessed by the consistency with which a child misarticulates sounds; an approach that has strong treatment implications; see Phonological Knowledge for procedures

Related Assessment Data
- Obtain results of intellectual and behavioral assessment in cases of children with mental retardation and behavioral disorders
- Obtain information on academic and language performance with school-age children
- Obtain information on physical or neurological disabilities and dental abnormalities
- Obtain information on audiological assessment if relevant

- Obtain information on other sensory impairments if relevant

Standard/Common Assessment Procedures

- Complete the Standard/Common Assessment Procedures with an emphasis on the orofacial examination

Scoring and Analysis of Assessment Data

- Transcribe the speech sample to determine the errors of articulation
- Use the International Phonetic Alphabet to transcribe the speech of the child
- If practical, use diacritics to make a narrower transcription (close transcription system) to obtain a more specific and detailed description of errors especially for children with cleft palate or bilingual backgrounds
- Take note of the consistency with which errors are produced; calculate the percentage of misarticulation for each phoneme in error (e.g., /s/ misarticulated in 100% of the sampled contexts; /p/ misarticulated 70% of the sampled contexts, etc.)
- List the phonetic contexts in which any of the misarticulated sounds were correctly produced
- Calculate the percent correct production of misarticulated sounds that the child correctly imitated on stimulability trials
- Analyze the results of standardized tests according to the test manuals
- Make a phonological analysis if the child has multiple misarticulations and it appears that a pattern analysis will be worthwhile
- Analyze the results of phonological assessment instruments according to the prescribed procedures
- Integrate information from different sources (case history, speech samples, standardized tests, phonological assessment instruments, reports from other specialists that bear upon the diagnosis, etc.)
- List the sounds in error; classify them according to an acceptable format (e.g., omissions, substitutions, and

distortions; errors in the initial, medial, and final positions; etc.); compare the child's performance to Developmental Norms for Phonemes
- List the <u>Phonological Processes</u> that were identified in your phonological analysis
- List the child's phonological processes in the order of early disappearing to late disappearing processes; use the following guidelines given by Stoel-Gammon and Dunn (1985) to evaluate the processes that should have disappeared in the assessed child:

Processes Disappearing by Age 3 Years	Processes Persisting After Age 3 Years
Unstressed syllable deletion	Cluster reduction
Final consonant deletion	Epenthesis
Consonant assimilation	Gliding
Reduplication	Vocalization
Velar fronting	Stopping
Diminutization	Depalatization
Prevocalic voicing	Final devoicing

- Take note that processes that may persist the longest include gliding of liquids, stopping, cluster simplification, vocalization, and final consonant deletion; significant decrease in the use of processes between the ages of 2.5 and 4 years (Bernthal & Bankson, 1998)
- If preferred, list the <u>Distinctive Features</u> that are missed or misused; organize the errors according to the missing distinctive features
- Calculate the percent intelligibility based on the number of words or utterances understood with or without the knowledge of context; if preferred, rate severity on a 3- or 5-point rating scale

Diagnostic Criteria
- Errors of speech sound production when the child is expected to be producing them correctly

- Multiple errors that fall into patterns that suggest one or more phonological processes
- The child's continued use of phonological processes when his or her peers no longer use them
- Clinically significant problem of unintelligible speech
- The number of phonemes in error that suggest a cutoff score for services as established in given clinical service settings (e.g., public schools)
- Take note of individual variability in speech sound acquisition; be aware that norms predict acquisition in a group of children and such predictions may not hold for individual children
- Consider alternatives to strictly normative approaches in making assessment and recommending treatment; use the Client-Specific Assessment Procedures to determine the effects of misarticulation on the child's social, communicative, and academic demands and recommend treatment on this basis

Differential Diagnosis

- Distinguish Ar-Ph disorders from Developmental Apraxia of Speech (DAS); characteristic oral apraxia, motor incoordination, poor imitative skills for articulation, inconsistent and variable errors, groping and silent articulatory postures, speech sound sequencing problems distinguish DAS by their presence and Ar-Ph disorders by their absence
- Distinguish Ar-Ph from dysarthria associated with Cerebral Palsy; the characteristics of a history of cerebral damage to the immature nervous system, obvious neuromuscular problems, and associated respiratory, resonance, phonatory, and prosodic problems distinguish cerebral palsy by their presence and Ar-Ph disorders by their absence
- Distinguish functional Ar-Ph disorders from those associated with hearing impairment; a confirmed audiological diagnosis of hearing impairment, and characteristics of hypo- and hypernasality, reduced rate of speech, pauses, slower articulatory transitions, disturbed stress patterns, disorders

of vocal pitch (too high or too low), disturbed prosodic features, hoarse or breathy voice quality, predominance of voiced-voiceless and oral-nasal confusion, and imprecise or distorted vowel production distinguish hearing impairment by their presence and Ar-Ph disorders by their absence

- Describe such associated conditions as mental retardation and emotional disorders and suggest additional or more intensive evaluation when needed

Prognosis

- Generally good for children with Ar-Ph disorders; most children's articulation skills improve with systematic treatment
- The presence of such additional variables as hearing impairment, mental retardation, physical disabilities, negative environmental factors, and sensory deficits may affect the rate of improvement and the final outcome

Recommendations

- Detailed assessment for the client who has failed the screening evaluation
- Treatment for the client who is diagnosed as having an Ar-Ph disorder
- See the cited sources and *PGTSLP* for details

Bernthal, J. E., & Bankson, N. W. (1998). *Articulation and phonological disorders* (4th ed.). Boston: Allyn & Bacon.

Bleile, K. M. (1995). *Manual of articulation and phonological disorders.* San Diego, CA: Singular Publishing Group.

Creaghead, N. A., Newman, P. W., & Secord, W. A. (1989). *Assessment and remediation of articulatory and phonological disorders* (2nd ed.). Columbus, OH: Merril Publishing Company.

Elbert, M., & Gierut, J. (1986). *Handbook of clinical phonology.* San Diego, CA: College-Hill Press.

Lowe, R. J. (1994). *Phonology: Assessment and intervention applications in speech pathology.* Baltimore, MD: Williams & Wilkins.

Peña-Brooks, A., & Hegde, M. N. (2000). *Assessment and treatment of articulation and phonological disorders in children.* Austin, TX: Pro-Ed.

Stoel-Gammon, C., & Dunn, C. (1985). *Normal and disordered phonology in children.* Austin, TX: Pro-Ed.

Articulation and Phonological Disorders in African American Children. Disorders of speech sound production in children who speak African American English (AAE); these children are more likely to use both AAE and a variety of Standard American English (SAE); not all African American children speak AAE and, therefore, clinicians should not stereotypically assume that all African American children need to be assessed for AAE; many African American children who speak AAE also speak SAE competently; among those who speak AAE, the degree of proficiency may vary greatly; an articulation disorder may be evident in one or both the forms of English; assessment presents challenges to clinicians who do not know the phonological properties of AAE; inappropriate assessment practices to be avoided are essentially two: (1) a mistaken diagnosis of an articulation disorder in SAE when the sound productions simply reflect the influence of AAE, and (2) overdiagnosis or underdiagnosis of an articulation disorder in AAE; both can be avoided with (1) a good knowledge of the phonological system of AAE, and (2) a general understanding that AAE is a product of unique historical and cultural forces; that it is a recognized form of English with its own phonologic, syntactic, semantic, and pragmatic rules and conventions; see Ethnocultural Considerations in Assessment for general guidelines; see also, Articulation and Phonological Disorders for a general description that apply to most children who misarticulate speech sounds.

Factors Related to Articulation and Phonological Disorders

- No unique factors that cause articulation and phonological (Ar-Ph) disorders in African American children have been convincingly demonstrated
- Factors that are associated with Ar-Ph disorders in other children also may be associated with such disorders in African American children; see under Articulation and Phonological Disorders for a summary of such factors

Articulation and Phonological Disorders

Description of Articulatory Errors in African American Children

- Note that, for the most part, African American children exhibit the same error patterns as monolingual children (e.g., omissions, deletions, substitutions, and specific phonological processes)
- Note also that the issue is not whether African American children exhibit unique patterns of errors; it is whether a given pattern of production should or should not be diagnosed as Ar-Ph disorders in light of the phonological system of AAE
- See under <u>Articulation and Phonological Disorders</u> for a summary of common error patterns found in children who misarticulate speech sounds

Assessment Objectives/General Guidelines

- To analyze errors of speech sound production and phonological processes in use in AAE and in SAE if a child speaks both the forms; note that this requires knowledge of the phonological characteristics of AAE
- To analyze errors in SAE that are *not* due to the influence of AAE; note that such errors do constitute a true articulation disorder; note, too, that this task requires knowledge of the phonological system of AAE
- To analyze patterns of SAE speech sound productions that vary from those of SAE but are a function of AAE patterns; note that such variations are not a basis to diagnose an articulation disorder; this analysis is done to achieve a comprehensive understanding of a child's phonological skills; however, treatment may be offered if the child, the family, or both wish to minimize variations in SAE articulation
- To identify potential treatment targets that are ethnoculturally appropriate for the child and are consistent with the wishes and needs of the child and his or her family

Case History/Interview Focus

- See **Case History** and **Interview** under Standard/Common Assessment Procedures
- Ask questions designed to obtain information on the family communication patterns; for instance:
  - do the family members speak only AAE at home?
  - do the family members also speak SAE at home?
  - how is the talking time roughly distributed across the two forms of English?
  - what is the level of SAE proficiency of family members?
  - what is the level of AAE proficiency of family members?
  - do they all effectively code-switch depending on communicative situations?
  - what are the parents' expectation regarding clinical services? Are they concerned about proficiency in SAE and SAE phonological patterns?
  - what kinds of educational demands are made on the child?
  - does the child's classroom teacher accept AAE?
  - how is the child doing in the classroom?
  - is there an indication of poor performance due to limited SAE proficiency, limited AAE proficiency, or both?
  - are there any associated clinical conditions that might affect treatment prognosis (e.g., developmental disabilities, hearing loss, neurological impairment, genetic syndromes)?
  - what are the recommendations of the child's teachers?
  - what are the educational and career goals of the client or as envisioned by the parents?

Assessment of Articulation and Phonological Disorders in African American Children

- Few satisfactorily standardized tests are available to evaluate articulatory proficiency in African American children; currently, use of nonstandardized, systematic, client-specific procedures with a good background in AAE is the best diagnostic approach

- Note that most standardized tests of articulation and phonology may not have adequately sampled African American children in their standardization process
- SAE speech sound errors need to be assessed even if no diagnosis of a disorder is made solely on this basis; because the parents and the child may opt for articulation treatment geared toward standard English productions, it is essential to make a thorough analysis of errors in both the forms of English
- Take extended, representative samples of connected speech in both English and the primary language of any bilingual child; use the general procedures for obtaining a speech and language sample described under Standard/Common Assessment Procedures; note that when one form of English is more dominant than the other, the samples will differ in their extent
- Use the procedures described under Articulation and Phonological Disorders to structure and evoke speech from the child; however, in selecting stimulus materials to evoke speech, consider the child's family and cultural background; let the parents guide the selection of materials that are familiar to their child
- Let the parents interact with the child as you tape record the conversational interaction; assist the parents in manipulating the stimulus materials to evoke a variety of speech productions to sample all speech sounds
- Take a sample of single word productions; use the procedures described under Articulation and Phonological Disorders

Assess Stimulability of Misarticulated Sounds

- Select the sounds the child misarticulates in both the forms of English and assess their stimulability
- Use procedures described under Articulation and Phonological Disorders

Related Assessment Data

- Obtain results of intellectual and behavioral assessment of children with mental retardation and behavioral disorders

- Obtain information on academic and language performance with school-age children
- Obtain information on physical or neurological disabilities and dental abnormalities
- Obtain information on audiological assessment
- Obtain information on other sensory impairments

Standard/Common Assessment Procedures

- Complete the Standard/Common Assessment Procedures with an emphasis on the orofacial examination

Scoring and Analysis of Assessment Data

- Use the procedures described under Articulation and Phonological Disorders
- Obtain the help of an African American SLP or one with a good knowledge of AAE
- Analyze errors in AAE in light of the AAE phonological patterns; only productions that are inconsistent with AAE phonological patterns are a basis to diagnose an articulation disorder in AAE
- Analyze variations in SAE phoneme productions that may be a function of the phonological patterns of AAE; these variations are *not* a basis to diagnose an articulation disorder
- Analyze errors in SAE that are independent of the phonological patterns of AAE; these errors are a basis to diagnose an articulation disorder in SAE

Diagnostic Criteria

- Note that the phoneme inventory of children speaking AAE will match that of SAE; a majority of phonemes are used in the same way in both AAE and SAE; only some phonemes will be used differently, substituted for other phonemes, or omitted in certain contexts
- Assess which AAE phonemic usages that differ from those of SAE are indeed characteristics of AAE; in making this assessment, consider the following phonological patterns that are accepted in AAE and hence are *not* a basis to diagnose an articulation disorder:

- /l/ lessening or omission (e.g., *too'* for *tool*; *a'ways* for *always*)
- /r/ lessening or omission (e.g., *doah* for *door*; *mudah* for *mother*)
- /θ/ substitution for /f/ in word final or medial positions (e. g., *teef* for *teeth*, *nofin'* for *nothing*)
- /t/ substitution for /θ/ in word initial positions (e.g., *tink* for *think*)
- /d/ substitution for /ð/ in word initial and medial positions (e.g., *dis* for *this* and *broder* for *brother*)
- /v/ substitution for /ð/ at word final positions (e.g., *smoov* for *smooth*)
- omission of consonants in clusters in word initial and final positions (e.g., *thow* for *throw* and *des'* for *desk*)
- consonant substitutions within clusters (e.g., *skrike* for *strike*)
- unique syllable stress patterns (e.g., **gui** tar for *guitar* and **Ju** ly for *July*)
- modification of verbs ending in /k/ (e.g., *li-id* for *liked* and *wah-tid* for *walked*)
- metathetic productions (e.g., *aks* for *ask*)
- devoicing of final voiced consonants (e.g., *bet* for *bed* and *ruk* for *rug*)
- deletion of final consonants (e.g., *ba'* for *bad* and *goo'* for *good*)
- /i/ substitution for /e/ (e.g., *pin* for *pen* and *tin* for *ten*)
- /b/ substitution for /v/ (e.g., *balentine* for *valentine* and *bes'* for *vest*)
- diphthong reduction or ungliding (e.g., *fahnd* for *find* and *ol* for *oil*)
- /n/ substitution for /g/ (e.g., *walkin'* for *walking* and *thin'* for *thing*)
- unstressed syllable deletion (e.g., *bout* for *about* and *member* for *remember*)
- Note that a diagnosable articulation disorder for a child who speaks AAE is a disorder in the context of AAE (and SAE), not in the sole context of SAE

Articulation and Phonological Disorders

Differential Diagnosis
- Use all the guidelines for differential diagnosis summarized under Articulation and Phonological Disorders
- Note that the most critical task of differential diagnosis is to separate articulatory errors in AAE and those in SAE that are not a function of AAE phonological patterns; take note of all variations in SAE; however, diagnose a disorder in SAE only if the errors are not due to the phonological patterns of SAE
- Diagnose articulatory errors in AAE only when they are inconsistent with AAE phonological patterns

Prognosis
- No systematic evidence suggests that prognosis for improved articulation in African American children is any different from that in other children
- Most if not all children may be expected to improve with systematic treatment
- The presence of such additional variables as developmental disabilities, genetic syndromes, and sensory disabilities (e.g., hearing loss) may affect the rate of improvement

Recommendations
- Recommend treatment for articulation disorders in AAE; recommend treatment targets that are consistent with AAE
- Recommend treatment for articulatory variations in SAE only if the client or the family members request such treatment because of the advantage standard English offers in educational, social, and occupational settings
- Recommend treatment on a priority basis for errors in phonemes that are common to AAE and SAE

Peña-Brooks, A., & Hegde, M. N. (2000). *Assessment and treatment of articulation and phonological disorders in children.* Austin, TX: Pro-Ed.

Roseberry-McKibbin, C. (1995). *Multicultural students with special needs.* Oceanside, CA: Academic Communication Associates.

Stockman, I. (1996). Phonological development and disorders in African American children. In A. G. Kamhi, K. E. Pollock, & J. L.

Harris (Eds.), *Communication development and disorders in African American children* (pp. 117–153). Baltimore: Paul H. Brookes.

Articulation and Phonological Disorders in Bilingual Children. Disorders of speech sound production in children who speak two (or more) languages; the disorder may be evident in one or both the languages spoken by a large and varied group of children in the United States; for the most part, these children include those whose primary language is Spanish, an Asian language, or a Native American language; may include children of European background who speak a language other than English; present assessment challenges because of the variety of primary languages that influence the secondary English spoken in the United States; see <u>Ethnocultural Considerations in Assessment</u> for general guidelines; see also, Articulation and Phonological <u>Disorders</u> for a general description that applies to most children who misarticulate speech sounds.

Factors Related to Articulation and Phonological Disorders

- No unique factors that cause articulation and phonological (Ar-Ph) disorders in bilingual children have been convincingly demonstrated
- Factors that are associated with Ar-Ph disorders in monolingual children also may be associated with such disorders in bilingual children; see under Articulation and Phonolog<u>ical Disorders</u> for a summary of these factors

Description of Articulatory Errors in Bilingual Children

- Note that, for the most part, bilingual children exhibit the same error patterns as monolingual children (e.g., omissions, deletions, substitutions, and specific phonological processes)
- The issue is not whether bilingual children exhibit unique patterns of errors; it is whether a given pattern of production should or should not be diagnosed as Ar-Ph disorders in light of bilingual children's first language

Articulation and Phonological Disorders

- See under <u>Articulation and Phonological Disorders</u> for a summary of common error patterns found in children who misarticulate speech sounds

Assessment Objectives/General Guidelines

- To analyze errors of speech sound production and phonological processes in use in the primary language of the child; note that this requires knowledge of the primary language's phonological characteristics; in the absence of such knowledge, refer the child to a speech-language pathologist (SLP) who has the knowledge or use a qualified interpreter
- To analyze errors in English that are *not* due to the influence of the primary language; note that this task, too, requires knowledge of a bilingual child's primary language
- To analyze English sound productions that vary from those in Standard or a regional American English; such an analysis need not result in a diagnosis of an articulation disorder and a recommendation for treatment; this analysis is done to achieve a comprehensive understanding of a child's phonological skills; however, treatment may be offered if the child, the family, or both wish to minimize the English articulatory variations
- To identify potential treatment targets that are ethnoculturally appropriate for the child and are consistent with the wishes and needs of the child and his or her family

Case History/Interview Focus

- See **Case History** and **Interview** under <u>Standard/ Common Assessment Procedures</u>
- Ask questions designed to obtain information on the family communication patterns; for instance:
  - what percentage of the time do family members speak the primary language, such as Spanish or Hmong, at home?
  - what is the level of English proficiency of family members?
  - what is the level of primary language proficiency of family members?
  - what is the specific variety of primary language spoken at home (e.g., Mexican Spanish or Puerto Rican Spanish)?

- do they speak English, and if so, what percentage of the time or in what kinds of communicative situations?
- is one or the other language dominant in certain speaking situations?
- what are the parents' expectation regarding clinical services? Are they concerned about proficiency in SAE and English speech sound production?
- what kinds of educational demands are made on the child? Is the child in a regular classroom or in a special bilingual program?
- how is the child doing in the classroom? Is there an indication of poor performance due to English language deficiency, primary language deficiency, or deficiency in both the languages?
- are there any associated clinical conditions that might affect prognosis (e.g., developmental disabilities, hearing loss, neurological impairment, genetic syndromes)?
- what are the recommendations of the child's teachers?
- what are the educational and career goals of the client or as envisioned by the parents?

Assessment of Articulation and Phonological Disorders in Bilingual Children

- Note that few satisfactorily standardized tests are available to evaluate articulatory proficiency in bilingual children; a few tests of Spanish language may be available, but for bilingual children who speak an Asian language, standardized tests are more limited or nonexistent
- Make sure that an available Spanish test of articulation samples the specific variety of Spanish (e.g., Mexican Spanish or Cuban Spanish) the child and the family members speak
- Note that English speech sound errors need to be assessed even if no diagnosis of a disorder is made solely on this basis; because the parents and the child may opt for articulation treatment geared toward standard English productions, it is essential to make a thorough analysis of errors in both languages

Articulation and Phonological Disorders

- Take extended, representative samples of connected speech in both English and the primary language of a bilingual child; use the general procedures for obtaining a speech and language sample described under Standard/Common Assessment Procedures; note that when one language is more dominant than the other, the samples will differ in their extent
- Use the procedures described under Articulation and Phonological Disorders to structure and evoke speech from the child; however, in selecting stimulus materials to evoke speech, consider the child's family and cultural background; let the parents guide the selection of materials that are familiar to their child
- Let the patents interact with the child as you tape record the conversational interaction; assist the parents in manipulating the stimulus materials to evoke a variety of speech productions to sample all speech sounds
- Take a sample of single word productions; use the procedures described under Articulation and Phonological Disorders

Assess Stimulability of Misarticulated Sounds
- Select the sounds the child misarticulates in both the languages and assess their stimulability
- Use procedures described under Articulation and Phonological Disorders

Related Assessment Data
- Obtain results of intellectual and behavioral assessment in cases of children with mental retardation and behavioral disorders
- Obtain information on academic and language performance and academic demands made on the child
- Obtain information on physical, medical, and neurological disabilities and dental abnormalities
- Obtain information on audiological assessment
- Obtain information on other sensory impairments if relevant

Articulation and Phonological Disorders

Standard/Common Assessment Procedures
* Complete the Standard/Common Assessment Procedures with an emphasis on the orofacial examination

Scoring and Analysis of Assessment Data
* Use the procedures described under Articulation and Phonological Disorders
* Obtain the help of a bilingual speech-language pathologist who knows the child's primary language
* Analyze errors separately in the primary language and the secondary English
* Analyze errors in English that may be a function of the primary language; in this case, the errors are variations and not a basis to diagnose an articulation disorder

Diagnostic Criteria
* Use the following characteristics of **Spanish-influenced English** in diagnosing articulation and phonological disorders in a child whose primary language is Spanish; note that these characteristics, when they influence the production of English as second language, are not the bases to diagnose an articulation and phonological disorder in English:
    * Spanish has only 5 vowels (as against 15 in English)
    * the English consonants /v/, /θ/, /ð/, /z/, and /ʒ/ are not in Spanish; while speaking English, some of these may be produced as allophonic variations of phonemes present in Spanish
    * some Spanish consonants, although similar to certain consonants in English, may be produced differently
    * Spanish has only a few consonants in word final positions (only /s/, /n/, /r/, /l/, and /d/)
    * Spanish consonantal clusters are fewer and simpler; the /s/ cluster, most common in English, does not occur in Spanish; final clusters are rare in Spanish
    * English /t/, /d/, and /n/ tend to be dentalized
    * final consonants may be devoiced (e.g, *dose* for *doze*)
    * /b/ may be substituted for /v/ (e.g., *bery* for *very*)

- weak or deaspirated stops, giving the impression of omission of stop sounds
- / tʃ / may be substituted for /ʃ/ (e.g., *Chirley* for *Shirley*)
- /d/ or /z/ may be substituted for /ð/, which does not exist in Spanish (e.g., *dis* for *this* or *zat* for *that*)
- schwa may be inserted before word-initial consonant clusters (*eskate* for *skate* or *espend* for *spend*)
- omission of many consonants at word-final positions
- /r/ may be trapped (as in the English word *butter*) or trilled
- word-initial /h/ may be silent (e.g., *old* for *hold* or *it* for *hit*)
- /y/ may be substituted for /dʒ/, an absent sound in Spanish (e.g., *yulie* for *Julie*)
- /s/ may be produced more frontally, giving the impression of a lisp

- In diagnosing articulation and phonological disorders in children whose primary language is an **Asian language**:
  - use the general guidelines already specified for assessing bilingual children
  - note that because of the diversity of Asian languages—they belong to different language families with diverse phonological properties—a general description of phonological characteristics is neither practical nor meaningful
  - note that many descriptions in the literature under the heading of *Asian* children or speakers apply only to the Chinese, not to other Asian languages
  - develop a database of Asian languages spoken in your service area and prepare lists of their phonological characteristics of the kind provided for Spanish in this section
  - make a diagnosis of articulation and phonological disorders based on such characteristics

- In diagnosing articulation and phonological disorders in children whose primary language is a **Native American language**:
  - use the general guidelines already specified for assessing bilingual children

- note that because of the diversity of Native American languages—they belong to different language families with diverse phonological properties—a general description of phonological characteristics is neither practical nor meaningful
- note that many children of Native Americans do not speak their parents' language or have only extremely limited proficiency in it
- note that there are useful websites on American Indian or Native American culture and languages that offer information on certain languages and their properties; use these resources in understanding aspects of Native American languages
- determine first if a Native American child is a bilingual speaker; then follow the guidelines offered in this section
- develop a database of Native American languages spoken in your service area and prepare lists of their phonological characteristics of the kind provided for Spanish in this section

Differential Diagnosis

- Use all the guidelines for differential diagnosis summarized under <u>Articulation and Phonological Disorders</u>
- Note that the most critical task of differential diagnosis is to separate articulatory errors in English from articulatory variations that are caused by the child's primary language; take note of all variations in English; however, diagnose a disorder only if the errors are not due to the phonological patterns of the child's first language
- Differentiate articulatory errors in the primary language in light of the phonological characteristics of that language

Prognosis

- No systematic evidence suggests that prognosis for improved articulation in bilingual children is any different from that for monolingual children
- Most if not all children may be expected to improve with systematic treatment

- The presence of such additional variables as developmental disabilities, genetic syndromes, and sensory disabilities (e.g., hearing loss) may affect the rate of improvement

Recommendations

- Recommend treatment for articulation disorders in the first language that is consistent with the phonological patterns of that language
- Recommend treatment for articulatory variations in standard English only if the client or the family members request such treatment because of the advantage standard English offers in educational, social, and occupational settings
- Recommend treatment for errors in phonemes that are common to the child's primary language and the secondary standard English on a priority basis
- Refer the child to a bilingual clinician who knows the child's primary language

Kayser, H. (1995). *Bilingual speech-language pathology: An Hispanic focus.* San Diego: Singular Publishing Group.

Peña-Brooks, A., & Hegde, M. N. (2000). *Assessment and treatment of articulation and phonological disorders in children.* Austin, TX: Pro-Ed.

Roseberry-McKibbin, C. (1995). *Multicultural students with special needs.* Oceanside, CA: Academic Communication Associates.

Assessment. (a) Description and assessment of a client's existing and nonexisting communicative behaviors, background variables, and associated factors to evaluate or diagnose a communicative problem; (b) clinical measurement of a person's communicative behaviors; (c) evaluation of communicative patterns of a client and his or her family; (d) assessment of strengths, limitations, and needs of a client and his or her family; (e) a clinical activity that precedes treatment, often continues throughout treatment, and is repeated before dismissal and during follow-up; take the following steps to make an assessment:

- Obtain case history
- Interview client (or caregivers of client)
- Conduct an orofacial examination

- Make client-specific judgments on use of standardized or nonstandardized measures
- Use measures appropriate to the client and his or her cultural background
- Screen hearing
- Obtain a speech-language sample
- Analyze results
- Draw conclusions; make a diagnosis; recommend treatment; disseminate information to the client, the family, and the referring professional

Assimilation Processes.   See <u>Phonological Processes</u>.

Assimilative Nasality.   Undesirable nasal resonance on vowels that are adjacent to nasal consonants.

Ataxia.   A neurological disorder characterized by disturbed balance and movement due to injury to the cerebellum.

Ataxic Dysarthria.   See <u>Dysarthria: Specific Types</u>.

Athetosis.   A neurological disorder characterized by slow, writhing, wormlike movements due to injury to the extrapyramidal motor pathways.

Atresia.   Absence or closure of a normally open structure; as in <u>Aural Atresia</u>.

Atrophy.   Wasting away of tissues or organs.

Augmentative and Alternative Communication (AAC). Methods of communication that supplement oral means of communication or provide alternative means of communication for individuals with extremely limited oral communication skills; means of communication that partially or fully compensate for severe, oral-expressive communication deficits; involve a variety of methods to encode, transmit, and in many cases, physically exhibit messages that cannot be vocally produced by the individual; always includes the residual vocal and verbal communication even if they are extremely limited; are always multimodal in that gestures, manual signs, vocal productions, and external devices are all used simultaneously; use of the methods may be temporary or permanent; methods vary widely in their use of technology; may be simple or complex devices including sophisticated computerized voice and speech synthesizers; useful for persons within varied diagnostic categories; some experts believe that all forms of communication described under this entry are augmentative (not alternative) because individuals who use them have some vocal, gestural, or other typical means of communication no matter how limited.

Basic Terms of AAC

- *AAC system:* A group of components, symbols, aids, and strategies all integrated into a functional unit
- *AAC user:* The individual who has limited oral communication skills and thus needs to use a form of AAC
- *Access:* Means by which a communicator composes a message and manipulates (controls) the device
- *Aid or device:* Physical objects or instruments that transmit or receive messages; include a note pad, a message book, message boards, charts, mechanical equipment, or such electronic equipment as a microcomputer
- *Aided and unaided:* AAC strategies that either use some external device or equipment (aided; e.g., use of a communication board, symbol systems, computer-generated communication) or those that do not use such devices or equipment (unaided; e.g., gestures, sign languages)
- *Alternative:* Technically, a method of communication that replaces the typical oral communication; because this (often is not the case, some experts believe that all communication methods described under AAC are technically augmentative (not alternative)
- *Augmentative:* Methods or devices that enhance or supplement the available means of typical communication (often oral communication); for example, a communication board that enhances or supplements oral communication
- *Communication partner (CP):* Person or persons who interact with the AAC user
- *Direct selection:* Selecting a message by pointing, depressing an electronic key, touching a key pad, touching an

item or object, and other direct means (contrasted with scanning)

- *Display (output):* The means by which a communicator, after having gained access to a system or device, shows the messages to his or her communication partner; includes such low-technology devices as a communication board or such high-technology devices as a computer monitor
- *High-technology device:* An AAC method that uses electronic instruments including computers
- *Iconic and non-iconic symbol:* A picture or a symbol that looks like the object it represents (iconic); a picture or a symbol that does not look like the object it represents (noniconic) and thus are arbitrary symbol whose meaning has to be taught
- *Low-technology device:* An AAC method that does not use electronic instruments; such means as a message board or a note pad
- *Scanning:* Sequential offering of available messages by the communication partner or a mechanical device until the AAC user indicates the right message he or she wishes to convey (contrasted with direct selection)
- *Symbols:* Means of representation; includes drawings, photographs, objects, all kinds of gestures, manual signs, printed words, geometric shapes, Braille, and spoken words

Classiflcation of AAC

Note that the classification of AAC is varied, often unwieldy, and is in need of simplification; the following is simpler of the many available (Silverman, 1995)

- **Gestural (unaided):** Form of AAC in which no instruments are used and communication is achieved through gestures and other patterned movement; may be accompanied by some speech, but the gestures play a major role in message transmission; gestures may convey a letter, a phoneme, or a concept; the following are among the many varieties of gestural-unaided communication:
  - American Sign Language (ASL or AMESLAN): Consists of manual signs for the 26 letters of the alphabet; can sign

words or phrases; recognized as a language by itself; often used with oral speech (total communication)

- American Indian Hand Talk (AMER-IND): A sign language system developed by North American Indians; includes gestures and movements to suggest ideas and concepts; not phonetic; complex ideas are expressed by a series of gestures
- Left-Hand Manual Alphabet: Similar to American Manual Alphabet, but more suitable for persons with right-sided paralysis; consists of concrete gestures that approximate printed letters of the alphabet
- Limited Manual Sign Systems: Several systems with limited number of signs and gestures; useful for patients in medical settings; used to communicate basic needs, self-care needs, and to simply say yes or no; a variety of systems available
- Pantomime: Mostly the use of gestures and dynamic movements often involving the entire body; consists of facial expressions, transparent messages, dramatizations of meanings expressed
- Eye Blink Encoding: Learning to transmit basic messages by specific number of blinks (e.g., one blink means *yes*, two blinks means *no*)
- **Gestural-assisted (aided).** Form of AAC in which gestures or movements are combined with a message display device or instrument; gestures may directly point to or select a message displayed or indirectly generate messages by providing input to an electronic unit resulting in a message display; displays include a board, a screen, or a computer monitor; aided because of the use of a display instrument; the following are among the many varieties of gestural-assisted (aided) communication:
  - symbol sets: Various symbols that stand for messages or symbols that may be associated with messages; include ordinary objects, pictures, and drawings, special set of symbols such as Blissymbols and rebuses; Premack-type plastic tokens; Yerkish language (LANA Lexigrams);

printed letters and words; synthesized speech (messages stored in a device that AAC user activates by touching a symbol or a sequence of symbols); natural sounding digitized speech (natural speech recorded and stored, and activated by the AAC user); Morse code; and Braille alphabet

- Non-electronic gestural-assisted AAC: Three major types: (1) Communication boards which display messages; the AAC user may confirm a message that CP scans; may directly point to a message; may gaze at a message; may select with a head pointer; may point to or otherwise select numbers or symbols that stand for specific messages; (2) symbols that the AAC user arranges or manipulates on a magnetic board to convey messages; and (3) symbols that the AAC user draws or writes to communicate, black board, magic slate, paper, or other device may be used to write or draw on; AAC user may print words of a natural language and draw objects and symbols

- Electronic gestural-assisted AAC: Use of electronic devices to communicate with the help of a switching mechanism the AAC user manipulates; a central unit that processes the signals; and the output device that displays the message; (1) switching mechanisms vary widely and include pushing or touching switches (e.g., key boards, graphic tablets), sliding handles, wobblesticks, joysticks, squeeze bulbs, tip or tilt position switches, pneumatic switches that are blown into, and sound and light controlled switches; (2) display devices that show the message also vary and include noise and light generators, various kinds of matrix displays in which rows and columns contain messages; cathode-ray tube displays; LED and LCD displays; printer displays; typewriters; computer printers; and various speech generators; (3) the central or control units connect the switch to the display, store messages, and help display the selected messages by switch activation.

- **Neuro-assisted (aided).** Form of AAC in which bioelectrical signals (e.g., muscle action potentials) help generate messages on a display device; aided because of the use of instrumentation; useful for severely impaired AAC user whose hand mobility is extremely limited and thus cannot operate a switching mechanism; bioelectrical potentials activate switches and thus the messages; electrodes attached to the user and connected to the instrument help activate switching mechanisms; equipment is more expensive and sophisticated; less developed than the other systems; the method is the same as that of gestural-assisted except for the switching mechanisms which include the following:
    - muscle action potentials: Electrical activity of the muscles associated with their contraction is used to activate switching mechanisms; electrodes attached to the skin pick up electrical discharges which are amplified so that they can activate special kinds of switches called myoswitches or specific displays; the user gets a feedback (e.g., onset of light or sound or changes in their intensity) when a switch or a display is activated and thus learns to use muscle action potentials for activating messages (biofeedback learning)
    - brain waves: Alpha brain waves may be used to generate messages on a computer screen through Morse code patterns; still in the research phase

Assessment Objectives/General Guidelines
- To assess the communicative needs of the potential AAC user
- To assess the educational or occupational demands made on the potential AAC user
- To assess the physical capabilities of the potential AAC user
- To obtain information on the cognitive level of the potential AAC user
- To assess the overall strengths and limitations of the potential AAC user

- To assess the family constellation and its communication strengths and limitations
- To assess the client's sensory capabilities
- To assess the cost of AAC device options that may be appropriate for a client
- To assess candidacy for a particular type of AAC
- To suggest a particular type of AAC for a client

Case History/Interview Focus
- See **Case History** and **Interview** under Standard/Common Assessment Procedures
- Pay special attention to the clients' motor and sensory capabilities that may be needed to use AAC

Ethnocultural Considerations
- See Ethnocultural Considerations in Assessment

Typical AAC Target Population
- Note that in most diagnostic categories that follow, those who are the most severely affected are the typical candidates
  - aphasia, especially global aphasia
  - apraxia in adults and developmental apraxia in child
  - amyotrophic lateral sclerosis
  - autism
  - cerebral palsy
  - deafness
  - dementia (the most severely affected, in the most advanced stage, may not be capable of using any system of AAC)
  - dysarthria
  - glossectomy
  - intubation
  - laryngectomy
  - spinal cord injury
  - tracheostomy
  - traumatic brain injury
  - mental retardation

Assessment: General Strategies

- Assess the current communication skills of the client (speech, writing, typing, gestures, any special skills such as sign language)
- Assess the current communication demands the client faces; describe all daily communicative activities of the client; document activities in home, school, occupational settings, social settings, and so forth
- Assess how others (family members, teachers, peers, colleagues, supervisors) react with the client: gestures, signs, writing, words, connected speech, a combination of several means
- Assess what problems or barriers limit interaction between the client and his or her communication partners (e.g., poor gesturing or signing skills in family members; poor motor control in the client)
- Assess dispositions of significant persons toward communication, the individual with communication disabilities, and new methods that may be appropriate (e.g., family members' negative disposition toward sign language or mechanical instruments; supervisors' negative dispositions toward individuals who need to communicate in unusual ways)
- Assess dispositions of the client to various forms of AAC (e.g., rejection of artificial larynx by a laryngectomee; synthesized speech by a neurologically impaired person); find out the reasons for such dispositions (e.g., a physician's negative comments about electronic larynx)
- Evaluate how well the client and his or her communication partners can learn a new system of communication; their general level of education, sophistication, expressed willingness and enthusiasm, ease with which they understand the information offered, and willingness to put efforts into the venture to make it work
- Evaluate funding sources because AAC methods involving instruments can be expensive (e.g., personal sources,

health insurance, community organizations, government agencies)
- Determine, to the extent possible, the current or maintaining causes of the limited communication skills; take note of the reasons for expressive problems (e.g., paralysis of facial muscles; neurologic diseases; laryngectomy mental retardation, hearing loss, visual problems)
- Assess whether the clinical condition creating the problems is progressive, stable, or temporary
- If and when appropriate, assess Articulation and Phonological Disorders, Language Disorders in Children, Voice Disorders, and Fluency Disorders; assess receptive communication skills; recognize that most of the communication skills will be at the basic level in a potential candidate for AAC
- Note that the final selection of an AAC method or device is a team decision involving the client, family members or other caregivers, educators, physical therapists, psychologists, medical specialists, and social workers
- In consultation with the persons involved, make a preliminary judgment about one or two potential AAC methods or devices that might be useful to the client

Assess the Client's Motor Skills
- Note that the level of motor skills plays the most important role in the use of AAC; hence their assessment is important
- Assess mobility and dexterity of hands first as they are the most important for AAC
- Assess the functional integrity of muscles of the neck and face next
- Assess the functional integrity of legs and feet last as they are important only when the mobility and dexterity of hands, neck, and face are extremely limited
- Assess motor skills in a hierarchical fashion: if the client exhibits a higher skill, there is no need to assess lower skills
- Assess movements of the elbow, hand, wrist, fingers, shoulders, head, and neck; assess movements of the jaw,

forehead muscles, cheek muscles, eyebrow muscles; assess blinking, eye closing and opening; assess movements of thigh, legs, and foot

- Assess motor skills necessary to gain direct access to an AAC instrument, device, or method: (1) assess whether the client can operate various kinds of switches, including cursor movements in a hierarchical fashion (e.g., if not with hands, maybe with head movement or leg or foot movement); assess skills in pressing, holding, and releasing switches; assess whether the client can wait, minimize errors, and be prompt in operating switches

- Assess hand and finger mobility and fine motor skills if a sign language system is being considered

- Take note of difficulties in understanding instructions, need to repeat instructions and suggestions, client's attention span, and apparent speed of learning

- Assess the client's current level of symbolic communication: select 10 to 15 objects or concepts with which the client is familiar; find a variety of symbols (pictures, photographs, line drawings) that represent them; assess the client's understanding of the symbol (e.g., ask the client to point to a particular symbol or give the symbol to you); ask the client to match the object and its symbol; ask the client to sort symbols (all symbols of houses in one pile and those of dogs in another pile)

- Assess word and letter recognition; present a set of simple printed words that are relevant to the client

- Assess paragraph reading comprehension; use a passage relevant to the client

- Assess spelling skills; use a set of simple words relevant to the client

Considerations in Selecting a Gestural (Unaided) AAC

- Hand movement flexibility allows for one of the sign languages (ASL or AMER-IND); the family and other regular communication partners need to learn the system; most

efficient nonverbal communication; AMER-IND is easier for others to understand
- Movement flexibility of both hands allows for most gestural systems
- Movement flexibility in one hand allows for somewhat limited gestural systems (e.g., Manual Shorthand)
- Some facial and hand movement flexibility will allow for mimes and other organized gestural systems
- Only eyeblink or eyebrow movement capability will allow for eyeblink encoding and or gestural Morse code; limited communication potential

Considerations in Selecting a Gestural-Assisted (Aided) AAC

- Pointing gesture capability allows for any symbol set usage, including the use of communication boards
- Limited cognitive functions require concrete symbol sets
- Inability to read or spell requires a system such as Blissymbolics, photographs, and other symbol sets
- Potential for learning to read or the presence of reading skills allows for a combination of printed words and symbol sets
- Limited vision will allow the use of plastic symbols or Braille
- Hand dexterity allows for written communication
- Simplicity, ease of learning to use, cost to obtain and to run will determine the selection of a switching mechanism
- Portability, editing capability, and need for a printer will determine the selection of an electronic-assisted display device

Considerations in Selecting a Neuro-Assisted (Aided) AAC

- Extremely limited movement capability of extremities dictate the use of neuro-assisted devices
- Slight movement capability of a muscle or muscle group allows for the use of neuro-assisted devices (e.g., eye blink, eyebrow movement, facial muscle movement)

Related/Medical Assessment Data

- Obtain available medical and related reports from the client's physician, orthopedic surgeon, neurologist, and physical therapist to evaluate the general medical and physical capabilities and limitations of the client
- Obtain psychological assessment reports that indicate the intellectual and cognitive levels of the client
- Obtain educational assessment reports that suggest strengths, limitations, and needs of the client and the demands the client faces
- Obtain information from the occupational settings to understand the strengths, limitations, and needs of the client and the demands the client faces
- Obtain audiologic and ophthalmologic information on the client's hearing and vision

Standard/Common Assessment Procedures

- Complete the Standard/Common Assessment Procedures

Analysis of Results and Preliminary Selection of AAC

- Integrate information obtained from different sources with your data on assessment of the client's AAC potential
- Select a form of AAC that best suits the client
- Finalize the selection only through a period of intervention; note that the initial selection may not work for the client; initial intervention may suggest modifications in the selected strategy or a different strategy
- Get the client, the family, teachers, supervisors, and other relevant persons involved in making modifications or in selecting a new device

Prognosis

- Highly variable as the population for which AAC is appropriate is extremely heterogeneous
- Clients benefit from a method for which they are good candidates

Recommendations

- A form of AAC for which the client is a good candidate

- Training the client and the family members in making good use of the selected method and in maintaining the instrument selected
- Periodic assessment to ensure continued success or to suggest a different form of AAC
- See the cited sources and *PGTSLP* for details

Beukelman, D. R., & Mirenda, P. (1998). *Augmentative and alternative communication: Management of severe communication disorders in children and adults* (2nd ed.). Baltimore, MD: Paul H. Brookes.

Silverman, F. H. (1995). *Communication for the speechless* (3rd ed.). Boston, MA: Allyn and Bacon.

Auditory Comprehension Deficit. Difficulty in understanding spoken language; a symptom of aphasia in general and Wernicke's aphasia in particular; also a symptom of dementia; see <u>Aphasia</u> for assessment procedures.

Aural Atresia. Closure or absence of the external auditory canal.

Autism: A pervasive developmental disorder that in a majority of clients persists into adulthood; previously considered a psychiatric (emotional) disorder; affects 4 to 5 children in 10,000; more males than females are affected; female cases tend to be more severe; both verbal and nonverbal characteristics help diagnose autism; some children exhibit only autistic-like behavior; often associated with mental retardation; communication disorders are a significant characteristic; lack of interest in people and communication is a dominant characteristic; most of the assessment procedures described under <u>Language Disorders in Children</u> are applicable with the following special considerations:

Etiology
- Unknown (the earlier theory that autism is due to impaired maternal bonding is discredited)
- Influence of genetic factors suggested
- Neurological basis also is suggested
- No theory has been fully supported

Characteristics of Autism
- Onset during infancy and early childhood
- No affectionate or emotional response to people
- Unconcerned about feelings of other people
- Disinterested in mother's or primary caretaker's voice
- Seeking extraordinary level of comfort when ill
- No play or bizarre play
- Disinterest in friends and human contacts
- No interest in imaginative play
- Stereotypic body movements (e.g., endless rocking)
- Preoccupation with objects or body parts
- Insistence on the same living arrangements all the time
- Perseverative involvement with one or a few activities
- Preference for being left alone
- Preference for mechanical voice; disinterested in human voice
- Reluctance to be hugged, held, or touched
- Self-injurious behaviors in some children
- Unusual mathematical or musical talent in some children

Associated Problems
- Some evidence of left cerebral injury in some cases
- Abnormal brain electrical activity
- Seizures in some cases
- Fragile X syndrome in some cases
- Hearing loss
- Hypo- or hypersensitivity to sensory stimuli
- Motor deficits
- Central auditory problems
- Mental retardation in some cases

Communication Disorders Associated With Autism
- Disinterest in communication
- Poor or no response to speech
- Delayed acquisition of speech sounds
- Some articulation disorders
- Better response to pure tones than to speech stimuli
- Not interested in asking questions or pointing to things
- Stereotypic and meaningless speech

Autism

- Slow acquisition of speech
- Easier learning of object names rather than words that express human emotions or expressions
- Easier and faster learning of concrete words than abstract words, although fast acquisition of abstract words in some cases
- Restricted word meanings (lack of generalized meanings)
- Lack of understanding of relational meanings (e.g., inability to relate the words *needle* and *thread*)
- Pronoun reversal
- Production of simpler and shorter sentences
- Wrong syntactic structures including wrong word order
- Omission of grammatic morphemes
- Inappropriate language
- Pragmatic language problems including lack of eye contact, topic maintenance, and turn taking during conversation
- Difficulty in language comprehension
- Meaningless repetition of previously heard speech
- High-pitched, monotonous speech
- Echolalia

Assessment Objectives/General Guidelines
- To assess communication disorders associated with autism
- To assess the strengths and limitations of the child
- To assess the family constellation and support for communication intervention

Case History/Interview Focus
- See **Case History** and **Interview** under Standard/Common Assessment Procedures
- Pay special attention to the listed early signs of autism

Ethnocultural Considerations
- See Ethnocultural Considerations in Assessment

Assessment
- Assess communication disorders
  - take a Speech and Language Sample (see Standard/ Common Assessment Procedures)
  - use the procedures described under Speech and Language Sample and Language Disorders in Children

- pay special attention to echolalia
- take note of occasional wrong word order
- focus on pronoun reversal
- look for meaningless repetition of previously heard speech
- watch for inappropriate language
- document a general lack of interest in communication
- take note of lack of interest in any kind of reciprocal inter-action including such nonverbal interaction as pat-a-cake
- take note of excessive involvement in objects and toys used during assessment
- take note of high-pitched, monotonous speech
- take note of the kinds of words the child uses
- document all other semantic, morphologic, syntactic, and pragmatic language problems listed
- Observe and record associated problems
  - take note of any self-injurious behaviors
  - observe reluctance to be touched
  - record any tendency toward abnormal play
  - document stereotypic body movements
  - observe perseverative movements, postures, and other motor behaviors
  - take note of errors of articulation

Standardized Tests
- Consider one of the tests of language listed under Lan-guage Disorders in Children
- Consider one of the tests of articulation described under Articulation and Phonological Disorders

Related/Medical Assessment Data
- Obtain medical reports of relevance; especially a neuro-logical report
- Obtain psychological reports
- Obtain audiologic reports
- Obtain reports from teachers and special educators

Standard/Common Assessment Procedures
- Complete the Standard/Common Assessment Procedures

Analysis of Results

- Make an analysis of the speech and language sample as described under <u>Language Disorders in Children</u> and <u>Articulation and Phonological Disorders</u>
- Analyze the listed unique features of autism noted during assessment and as evidenced in the speech and language sample
- Integrate the information from different sources
- Relate communication disorders that suggest autism with the behavioral analysis and diagnosis
- Summarize the observed speech and language characteristics

Diagnostic Criteria

- An independent diagnosis of autism supported by behavioral assessment
- Diagnosis of autism supported by communication assessment
- Early signs of autistic behaviors
- Significant disinterest in people and communication

Differential Diagnosis

- Differentiate autism from mental retardation: the unique characteristics of autism that distinguish it from mental retardation include lack of interest in people, feelings, affection, and communication; preoccupation with routines; interest in objects versus people; and some unusual language including pronoun reversal, wrong word order, and echolalia
- Differentiate autism from hearing impairment: autism is differentiated from hearing impairment by the former's unique characteristics as listed; persons with hearing impairment have an independent audiological diagnosis; speech and voice characteristics associated with hearing impairment also help distinguish the two types of disorders
- Differentiate children with autism from those with brain injury: autism is differentiated from brain injury by the former's unique characteristics as listed; the brain injured

have an independent diagnosis of neurological involvement; memory problems, cognitive deficits, and emotional responses of the brain injured also help distinguish the two types of disorders

Prognosis
- Variable depending on the severity of autistic behaviors
- Most children benefit from behavioral and communication intervention

Recommendations
- Early intervention for communication deficits
- Coordination of treatment with general behavioral intervention
- Family counseling and training for home treatment
- Coordination of treatment with academic programs in the case of school-age children
- See the cited sources and *PGTSLP* for details

American Psychiatric Association. (1987). *Diagnostic and statistical manual of mental disorders* (3rd ed., rev.). Washington, DC: Author.

Hegde, M. N. (1996). *A coursebook on language disorders in children* (2nd ed.). San Diego: Singular Publishing Group.

Nelson, N. W. (1993). *Childhood language disorders in context.* New York: Macmillan.

Paul, R. (2001). *Language disorders from infancy through adolescence: Assessment and intervention* (2nd ed.). St. Louis, MO: C. V. Mosby.

Reed, V. (1994). *An introduction to children with language disorders* (2nd ed.). New York: Macmillan.

Autosomal Dominant. Any chromosome apart from the sex chromosome is autosomal; not sex-linked; autosomes are alike in males and females; dominant indicates that the defective gene dominates its normal partner in its phenotypic expression.

Autosomal Recessive. A genetic trait or defect not capable of expression unless coupled with a similar trait or defect by both members of a pair of homologous chromosomes.

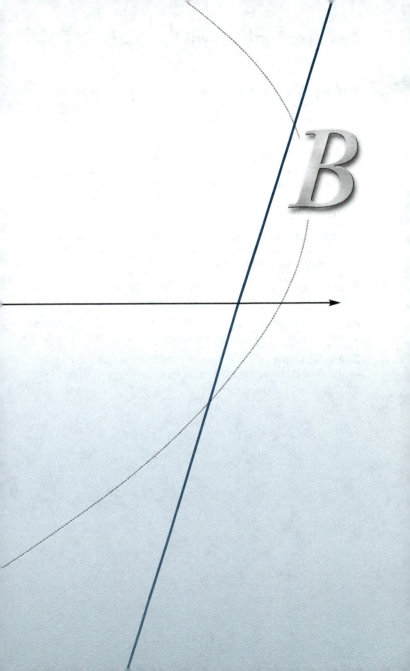

B

Bardet-Biedl Syndrome. The same as Laurence-Moon syndrome (see Syndromes Associated With Communicative Disorders).

B-Mode Carotid Imaging. A noninvasive method used to assess the health of the superficial arteries, especially those of the neck; also known as *echo arteriogram*; a high frequency sound generator is placed over the neck; a computer analyzes the sound deflected by the arteries and thus helps diagnose arterial diseases.

Brachman-de Lange Syndrome. The same as Cornelia de Lange syndrome (see Syndromes Associated With Communicative Disorders).

Brachycephaly. Shortness of head with a cephalic index of 81.0 to 85.4; characteristic of certain genetic syndromes.

Brachydactyly. Shortness of the fingers and toes; characteristic of certain genetic syndromes.

Bradykinesia. Slowness of movements; difficulty in stopping movement once initiated; freezing of movement.

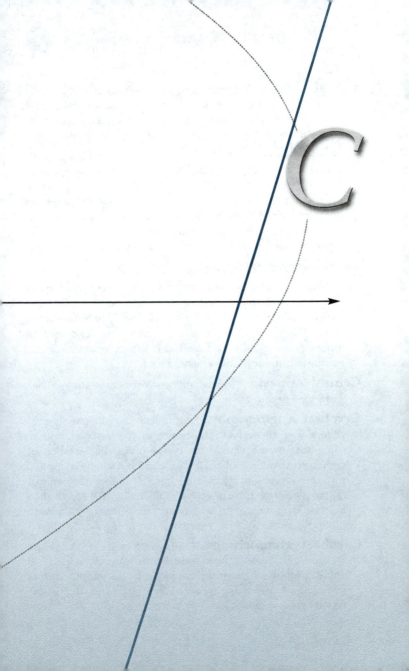

Canthi. The angle the meeting of the lower and upper eyelids form; may be nasal (inner) canthus or temporal (outer) canthus; a wider canthi is a part of several genetic syndromes; see Waardenburg syndrome (see <u>Syndromes Associated With Communicative Disorders</u>).

Carotid Phonoangiography. A noninvasive method used to diagnose the health of the blood vessels by assessing the sound of blood flow; the machine picks up and amplifies the sound of the blood gushing through the arteries; can help diagnose arterial stenosis which creates turbulence as the blood moves through a constricted artery.

Case History. See Standard/Common Assessment Procedures.

Catatonic Motor Behavior. A symptom of schizophrenia, characterized by reduced reactivity to environmental stimuli, catatonic stupor (the person is totally unaware of the surroundings), rigid or bizarre posture, and resistance to movement; may also be found in other disorders including medication-induced movement disorder.

Central Aphasia. The same as Wernicke's aphasia (see <u>Aphasia: Specific Types</u>).

Cerebral Angiography. An invasive, radiographic procedure used to evaluate the health of the vascular system, often that of the carotid artery; involves the insertion of catheter into a femoral artery in the groin, moving it upward into the selected artery, and injecting radio-opaque contrast material through the catheter; a rapid series of X-rays is then taken of the artery or arteries; results may show variations in blood flow that might suggest vascular occlusions.

Cerebral Hemorrhage. Bleeding within the brain because of ruptured blood vessels; an immediate cause of aphasia (of the hemorrhagic type); due to various factors including weakened arterial walls, high and fluctuating blood pressure, and trauma to blood vessels.

Cerebral Palsy.   A nonprogressive neuromotor disorder resulting from damage to a child's brain before, during, or shortly after the birth; often described as congenital, although the damage may occur sometime after birth; generally, damage to still-developing brain (up to age 16 years) resulting in neuromotor control problems qualifies for the term; neuromotor control tends to improve with growth; causes speech disorders in many, but not all cases; incidence is estimated at about 2 in 1000 births; varied symptoms affecting respiration, laryngeal function, general neuromotor control; associated with mental retardation in about 50% of the cases; probably associated with a higher prevalence of hearing impairment; associated with feeding problems in some cases.

Classiflcation of Cerebral Palsy (CP)
* Topographic or orthopedic classification:
  * diplegia: bilateral paralysis of like parts
  * monoplegia: paralysis of one extremity
  * herniplegia: paralysis of one side of the body
  * paraplegia: paralysis of the two lower extremities
  * triplegia: paralysis of three extremities
  * quadriplegia: paralysis of four extremities
* Classification based on the affected neurological system:
  * pyramidal lesions causing spasticity (most cases)
  * extrapyramidal lesions causing athetosis, tremor, or both
  * cerebellar lesions causing ataxia (only about 1% of children with CP)
  * mixed type (lesions in both pyramidal and extrapyramidal regions although lesion in one of the structures may be dominant); in almost 30% of the cases
* Current two-category classification
  * spasticity (60% of children with CP)
  * dyskinesia (20% of children with CP)

Etiology
* Unknown in about 40% of the cases
* Prenatal factors

C

- radiation exposure
- intrauterine infections, including HIV
- exposure to toxic drugs
- exposure to metal toxicity
- fetal anoxia (oxygen deprivation and resulting fetal brain damage)
- damage caused by blood infiltration of the nervous system
- cerebral hemorrhage
- chromosomal abnormalities
- abruptio placenta (premature detachment of the fetus)
- brain growth deficiency
- Perinatal factors
  - birth complications
  - trauma to brain during birth (only in a small percentage of cases)
  - cerebral hemorrhage
- Postnatal factors
  - prematurity
  - asphyxia
  - sepsis (blood toxicity and microorganisms in the blood)
  - cerebral hemorrhage
  - inflammatory diseases of the brain (encephalitis and meningitis)
  - head trauma

Symptoms and Effects of Cerebral Palsy

- Neuromotor symptoms
  - persistence of primitive reflexes in infancy: For example, asymmetric tonic neck reflex, tonic labyrinthine reflex, and the positive support reflex: an early sign of cerebral palsy
  - spasticity and rigidity of muscles: Increased tone or rigidity of muscles; tight or excessively contracted muscles with exaggerated stretch reflex; the most common symptom of CP; injury to the pyramidal motor pathways and the higher cortical centers of motor control

- athetosis: Slow, involuntary, writhing movements; injury to the extrapyramidal motor pathways, especially to the basal ganglia; currently, the term dyskinesia, rather than athetosis, is the preferred term to describe involuntary and excessive movements
- ataxia: Disturbed balance and uncoordinated movement; injury to the cerebellum; currently, an infrequently used diagnostic category
- currently, spasticity and dyskinesia are considered the two primary symptoms of cerebral palsy
- the central problems of inefficient muscular control, not muscle weakness
- Motor development
  - 10 to 24 months of delay in motor development in some cases
  - permanently deficient motor control in severely involved cases
  - delayed attainment of all motor milestones, including head control, sitting, crawling, standing, and walking
  - general slowness in initiating movement
- Mental development
  - normal in nearly 50% of the cases
  - retarded in about 50% of the cases
- Sensory impairments
  - greater prevalence of hearing impairment than in the non-CP population
  - frequent episodes of middle ear pathology resulting in conductive hearing loss
  - spasticity may be more often associated with conductive hearing loss than with other types of loss
  - athetosis may be associated with a greater degree of hearing loss and bilateral loss than with other groups
  - greater prevalence of visual impairment than in the non-CP population
- Perceptual and attentional problems
  - distractibility, short attention span

C

- preference for a rigid schedule (perceptual rigidity)
- disassociation (difficulty in integrating different aspects of the same event)
- disinhibition (random activity)
- Emotional disturbances
  - emotional lability (emotional instability or overreactivity)
  - frequent episodes of emotional upsets
- Educational problems
  - general learning disorders
  - difficulty in learning to read or write
- Communication problems: General considerations
  - communication disorders associated with CP are highly variable
  - some may not have significant communication problems
  - communication disorders may not help clearly distinguish different types of CP
  - the degree of neuromotor impairment will affect the degree of communication impairment
  - measures of intelligibility are best indicators of communication deficits associated with CP
- Speech disorders (Dysarthria)
  - jerky, effortful, labored, and irregular speech of reduced intelligibility
  - more severe articulation problems with athetosis than with spasticity
  - more severe speech problems with herniplegia and quadriplegia than with paraplegia
  - dysarthria as the main symptom: problems in articulation, respiration, voice, and resonance
  - generally inefficient articulation
  - difficulty phonating or prolonging sounds
  - significant difficulty with tongue-tip sounds
  - predominance of omissions over substitutions or distortions
  - greater difficulty with sounds in word-final positions than in other positions

- such <u>Phonological Processes</u> as consonant cluster deletion, stopping, depalatalization, fronting, and gliding,

- Language disorders
  - note that less is known about the language skills of children with CP than about speech
  - generally delayed language development in at least some children
  - significant language disorders due to other, coexisting conditions including mental retardation and hearing impairment
- Fluency problems
  - higher prevalence of stuttering than in the general population
  - lack of smooth flow of speech
  - generally limited fluency skills
- Voice problems
  - weak voice, lack of loudness
  - poor control of loudness resulting in irregular bursts of loudness
  - loss of voice toward the end of sentences and phrases, resulting in whisper
  - monotone
  - high pitch in some cases
  - strained voice quality in some cases due to hyperadduction of vocal folds
  - breathiness in some cases due to hypoadduction of vocal folds
- Prosodic problems
  - dysprosody as a result of the respiratory, articulatory, fluency, and voice problems
- Respiratory problems
  - persistence of rapid breathing rate beyond the first year of infancy (as against normal slow-down of the rate)
  - possibly, excessive diaphragmatic activity and reduced activity of the chest and neck muscles
  - flattening or flaring of the rib cage

- indented (sucked-in) sternum
- air wastage during speech production resulting in short phrases or weak productions of final segments of sentences
- Resonance problems
  - hypernasality due to velopharyngeal dysfunctions
- Oromotor dysfunctions
  - slow or jerky jaw movements
  - impaired or discoordinated tongue movements during speech production
  - retarded diadochokinetic rate

Assessment Objectives/General Guidelines

- To assess the communication deficits associated with CP
- To assess the strengths of the child
- To work closely with other professionals involved in the rehabilitation of the child with CP
- Note that assessment is a team effort
- Note that a child with CP will need the services of many professionals
- Note that a child with CP will need long-term care and thus repeated assessment is necessary
- Adapt all testing and assessment procedures to suit the child's needs (e.g., let the child look at a stimulus instead of pointing to it; let the child tap the table instead of clapping hands)

Case History/Interview Focus

- See **Case History** and **Interview** under Standard/Common Assessment Procedures
- Concentrate on prenatal, perinatal, and postnatal conditions of significance

Ethnocultural Considerations

- See Ethnocultural Considerations in Assessment

Assessment

- Observe and obtain information on neuromotor functions
  - obtain reports from the child's physician or neurologist
  - take note of the listed neurologic symptoms during assessment

Cerebral Palsy

- Observe and obtain information on motor development
  - use a developmental scale or checklist to assess the child's motor and general behavioral development
  - obtain systematic information from the parents
- Obtain information on mental development
  - obtain a copy of the child's psychological report
  - make clinical judgments based on your assessment of speech and language development
- Assess speech disorders and speech intelligibility
  - take an extended Speech and Language Sample (see Standard/Common Assessment Procedures)
  - obtain a speech sample involving the child and the parent or another family member
  - make clinical judgments about speech intelligibility for single words and sentences and with and without contextual cues; make a more detailed analysis of articulation skills when intelligibility is reduced
  - take into consideration any oral structural deviations (e.g., tongue weakness, asymmetries in the tongue and soft palate, abnormalities of the jaw, unusually high palate, malocclusions)
  - take into consideration functional oral-motor problems (e.g., oral apraxia, lateral tongue deviations, sluggish movement of the tongue; uncontrolled movements of facial muscles, chewing, sucking, and swallowing problems)
  - analyze the speech samples for individual sound errors and for patterns of errors suggesting phonologic processes (e.g., final consonant deletion, cluster reduction, fronting); use procedures described under Articulation and Phonological Disorders
- Assess language disorders
  - use the recorded speech and language sample to analyze the child's language skills
  - take note of the language structures the child produces and those the child does not

- use the procedures described under <u>Language Disorders in Children</u>
- Assess fluency problems
  - use the recorded speech and language sample to make a clinical judgment about the presence or absence of a fluency disorder
  - if warranted, make a more detailed analysis of the types and frequency of dysfluencies
  - use the procedures described under <u>Stuttering</u> for procedures, analysis, and diagnostic criteria
- Assess prosodic problems
  - take note of the stress patterns, intonation, rate of speech, and pauses
  - make clinical judgments about prosody
  - list prosodic problems noted
- Assess voice and respiratory problems
  - make clinical judgments about vocal loudness and pitch and their social adequacy and their appropriateness for age and gender of the client
  - judge whether variations in loudness and pitch are smooth and normal or jerky and abnormal
  - take note of voice quality (harshness, hoarseness, breathiness, strained-strangled voice)
  - take note of any difficulty in voicing that may be due to vocal folds that are either too tightly adducted or remain abducted for too long
  - judge the adequacy of breath support for speech
  - take note of the listed breathing abnormalities; see "Make an Aerodynamic Evaluation" under <u>Voice Disorders</u> for additional procedures used in assessing respiratory functions
  - use the assessment procedures described under <u>Voice Disorders</u> including the use of instrumental assessment of voice characteristics
- Assess resonance problems
  - observe presence of hypernasality, hyponasality, and reduced oral resonance

- consider the resonance data along with information on velopharyngeal functioning
- use the assessment procedures described under Voice Disorders including the use of instrumental assessment of nasal resonance
- Assess oromotor dysfunctions
  - complete a detailed Orofacial Examination; see Standard/Common Assessment Procedures
- Assess the need for augmentative and alternative methods of communication
  - assess the child's oral communication potential; if low, assess potential for a variety of alternative and augmentative communication devices the child might use
  - see Augmentative and Alternative Communication (AAC) for assessment methods and selection of an appropriate means of communication
- Observe and obtain information on other areas
  - observe perceptual and attentional problems; obtain the psychological report
  - observe the child's emotional responses during assessment, obtain parents' report on the child's emotional stability and reactivity
  - obtain information from teachers and parents on the child's educational performance and problems
  - screen hearing; refer the child to an audiologist when warranted
  - obtain information on the child's visual problems
  - obtain information from the child's physical therapist

Related Medical Assessment Data
- Obtain reports from other specialists as indicated in earlier sections
- Integrate your assessment data with those offered in the various reports obtained

Standard/Common Assessment Procedures
- Complete the Standard/Common Assessment Procedures

C

Analysis of Assessment Data

- Analyze the speech and language sample as needed to identify language and speech disorders; use the procedures described under <u>Language Disorders in Children</u> and <u>Articulation and Phonological Disorders</u>; list language and speech disorders of the child
- Analyze data relative to voice, resonance, and breathing abnormalities and list the disorders or deviations
- Analyze data relative to fluency and prosody and summarize the problems noted; calculate the percent dysfluency rate; see <u>Stuttering</u> for procedures
- Integrate data from other professional sources and summarize the overall strengths and weaknesses

Diagnostic Criteria

- History consistent with damage to a developing brain
- Neuromotor symptoms, behavioral patterns, and communication problems consistent with damage to a developing brain as listed previously

Prognosis

- Highly variable depending on the severity of neuromotor involvement and associated sensory, perceptual, and intellectual deficits
- Generally, prognosis for improved functioning with systematic and comprehensive rehabilitation is good for most if not all children with CP
- Prognosis for improved oral or augmentative and alternative communication is good for most if not all children with CP

Recommendations

- Communication treatment as part of a comprehensive rehabilitation program
- See the cited sources and *PGTSLP* for details

Hardy, J. C. (1983). *Cerebral palsy.* Englewood Cliffs, NJ: Prentice-Hall
Love, R. J. (1992). *Childhood motor disability.* New York: Macmillan.
Mecham, M. J. (1996). *Cerebral palsy* (2nd ed.). Austin, TX: Pro-Ed.

Cerebrovascular Accidents (Strokes)

Cerebrovascular Accidents (Strokes). The most common cause of aphasia; the third leading cause of death in the U.S.; may be ischemic or hemorrhagic; the basic cause of ischemic strokes is interruption of blood supply to a part of the brain because of arterial thrombosis or embolism; hemorrhagic strokes are due to bleeding in the brain; see Cerebral Hemorrhage.

Choreiform Movements. Jerky, irregular, involuntary, and rapid movements; caused by damage to the caudate and the putamen; major symptom of Huntington's Disease (HD).

Cleft Lip. An opening in the lip, usually the upper lip and very rarely the lower lip; a congenital malformation; often associated with cleft of the palate, although clefts of the palate are often not associated with cleft lip; see Cleft Palate for details and assessment procedures.

Cleft Palate. Various congenital malformations resulting in opening in the hard palate, the soft palate, or both; clefts of the lip may be present, but infrequently; due to disruptions of the embryonic growth processes; due to such disruptions, palatal and lip structures fail to grow and fuse; may be a part of a genetic syndrome with other anomalies; other anomalies more commonly associated with clefts of the palate than clefts of the lip; range of incidence is 1 in 600 to 750 live births; the highest to the lowest incidence rates: North American Indians, Japanese, Chinese, Whites, and African Americans in that order; in the male, higher frequency and greater severity of cleft lip (with or without cleft palate); in the female, higher frequency of palatal clefts (without the cleft lip); nearly half of all cases show cleft of the palate and lip; one quarter show cleft of the lip only; and another quarter show cleft of the palate only; cleft lip with or without palatal involvement is thought to have a different etiology than isolated palatal clefts; may be associated with various communication disorders; less severe clefts that are medically and surgically managed early in life may not pro-

C

duce significant communication disorders; the more severe the malformations and more delayed the surgical and medical intervention, the greater the severity of communication disorders; communication disorders more common in children with clefts that are part of genetic syndromes.

Etiology

- Genetic abnormalities (see <u>Syndromes Associated With Communicative Disorders</u> for all syndromes mentioned in this section)
  - clefts associated with autosomal dominant syndromes (e.g., Apert syndrome, Stickler syndrome, van der Woude syndrome, Waardenburg syndrome, and Treacher Collins syndrome)
  - clefts associated with recessive genetic syndromes (e.g., oro-facial-digital syndrome)
  - clefts associated with X-linked syndromes (e.g., otopalatal-digital syndrome)
  - chromosomal abnormalities (e.g., trisomy 13)
- Environmental teratogenic disorders
  - fetal alcohol syndrome
  - illegal drug use
  - prescription drugs including anticonvulsant drugs and thalidomide (a sedative)
  - rubella
- Mechanical factors
  - intrauterine crowding
  - twinning
  - uterine tumor
  - amniotic ruptures

Types of Clefts

There are several classifications of clefts, each with its limitations; none accepted universally; clefts vary in extent (often measured in thirds (1/3, 2/3, and 3/3) and widths; the major types include the following; the implied classification system (cleft lip through facial clefts) is similar to the one suggested by the American Cleft Palate Association:

- Cleft lip (complete or incomplete; unilateral or bilateral)
- Cleft of alveolar process (unilateral, bilateral, median, and submucous)
- Cleft of prepalate (combination of previous types with or without prepalate protrusion or rotation)
- Clefts of the palate (clefts of the soft palate, clefts of the hard palate, and submucous)
- Clefts of prepalate and palate (any combination of clefts of the prepalate and palate)
- Facial clefts other than prepalate and palate (e.g., such rare forms as horizontal clefts, lower mandibular clefts, lateral oro-ocular clefts, and naso-ocular clefts)
- Microforms (minimal expressions of clefts including hair-line indentation of the lip or just notch on the lip; palatal defects that are revealed only through laminographic examination; submucous clefts may be included here as well)

Congenital Palatopharyngeal Incompetence (CPI)

Not a form of cleft, but a related disorder; of special interest to speech-language pathologists because of its effects on speech production; characteristics include:

- No overt or submucous clefts
- Apparently normal velopharyngeal structures and mobility
- Significant impairment of velopharyngeal functions as revealed by videofluoroscopy or encloscopy (inadequate velopharyngeal closure)
- Causes include:
  - short palate
  - deficient muscular mass of soft palate
  - deep or enlarged larynx
  - wrong insertion of levator muscles (insertion to hard palate instead of the normal insertion to soft palate)
  - a combination of such factors
- Significant problems after adenoidectomy in some cases (a compensated CPI is revealed after surgery)
- Hypernasal speech, ranging from mild to severe

Cleft Palate

Communication Disorders Associated With Clefts

- Articulation and phonologic disorders
  - greater difficulty with unvoiced sounds than with voiced sounds
  - greater difficulty with sounds that require a build-up of intraoral pressure resulting in weak production of pressure consonants (e.g., stops, fricatives, and affricates)
  - apparent substitutions of nasal sounds for non-nasal sounds (may not be true substitutions because the added nasal resonance may be due to VTI)
  - audible or inaudible nasal air emission while producing many sounds
  - some distortion of vowels
  - compensatory errors (errors of place of articulation that are due to organic problems, including VIP); include various types of substitutions that help compensate for the inadequate closure of the velopharyngeal mechanism; generally, substitution of stops, fricatives, and affricates with unusual (often posterior) movements and posture of the tongue to stop the air or to produce friction noise: substitution of glottal stops for stop consonants
    → substitution of laryngeal stops for stop consonants and laryngeal fricatives for fricatives (involving posterior movement of the tongue so as to move the epiglottis toward pharynx back to block the air or to create friction noise)
    → substitution of pharyngeal stop for stop consonants and pharyngeal affricates for affricates (involving posterior movement of the tongue to make contact with pharynx to build up pressure that is suddenly released or to constrict the air to create friction)
    → substitution of posterior nasal fricative for fricative (use of the posterior dorsum of the tongue and the soft palate to create friction sound)
    → substitution of mid-dorsum palatal stop for /t/, /d/, /k/, and /g/ (building pressure by raising the mid-dorsum of the tongue to the hard palate)

Cleft Palate

→ substitution of mid-dorsum palatal fricatives and mid-dorsum palatal affricates for fricatives and affricates (movement of the mid-dorsum toward the hard palate to create friction of pressure buildup)

- reduced speech intelligibility to varying extents
- note that many children may have normal articulation or achieve normal articulation as they grow older
- note that cleft lip alone rarely results in misarticulations
- note that bilateral complete clefts of the hard and soft palates create the most severe speech problems

- Language disorders
  - generally, delayed language development with significant improvement as the child grows older (may attain normal language by age 4 or so)
  - significant language disorders in children whose clefts are a part of genetic syndromes
  - language problems may be more severe or more persistent in children with clefts and significant hearing loss
  - note that not much is known about specific language skills of children with clefts as researchers mostly have concentrated on speech and resonance aspects

- Laryngeal pathologies and phonatory disorders
  - generally, higher prevalence of phonatory (voice) disorders in children with palatal clefts
  - higher frequency of vocal nodules
  - hypertrophy and edema of the vocal folds
  - hoarseness of voice
  - soft voice (inability to increase vocal intensity because of velopharyngeal inadequacy)
  - monotonous voice (limited pitch variation) strangled voice (excessive effort and tension in producing voice to avoid hypernasality)
  - note that most phonatory disorders may be due to velopharyngeal inadequacy (which leads to hyperfunctional voice production)

- Resonance disorders
  - hypernasality on vowels and voiced oral consonants due to inadequate velopharyngeal closure and restricted mouth opening
  - hyponasality (reduced nasal resonance on nasal sounds)
  - denasality (near-absence of nasal resonance on nasal sounds)

Related Problems

- Velopharyngeal incompetence resulting in inadequate closure of the velopharyngeal port
- Hearing
  - middle ear infections
  - hearing loss in about 50% of children with palatal clefts (typically, conductive hearing impairment)

Assessment Objectives/General Guidelines

- To determine communication disorders of the child with clefts
- To make periodic assessments of communication and its potential to generate information that might help plan surgical intervention
- To suggest communication treatment targets

Case History/Interview Focus

- See **Case History** and **Interview** under Standard/Common Assessment Procedures
- Concentrate on the medical and surgical history and speech and language development of the child

Ethnocultural Considerations

- See Ethnocultural Considerations in Assessment

Assessment

- Assessment of Velopharyngeal Incompetence
  - note that clinical judgments about hypernasality and hyponasality described under assessment of resonance disorders later in this section yield indirect information about the velopharyngeal mechanism
  - note that besides posterior and superior movement of the soft palate, lateral movement of the pharyngeal wall is necessary for adequate velopharyngeal closure

- note that different individuals show different patterns of velopharyngeal closures; all or only some of the involved structures may move or move more notably (e.g., primary lateral movement of the pharyngeal walls; primary movement of the soft palate; movements of the soft palate and lateral pharyngeal walls but little or no movement of the posterior pharyngeal wall; and all structures moving to achieve a sphincteric action)
  - → make objective assessment of the velopharyngeal mechanism
  - → make an endoscopic examination of the velopharyngeal mechanism (nasopharyngoscopy); see Endoscopy; follow the procedures prescribed by the manufacturer of the particular instrument used
  - → make a videofluoroscopic examination of the velopharyngeal mechanism; see Videofluoroscopy; follow the procedures prescribed by the manufacturer of the particular instrument used; observe and record the movements of the soft palate, the lateral pharyngeal wall, posterior pharyngeal wall, and the tongue as the client produces consonant-vowel combinations, two voiced and voiceless fricatives, and selected phrases
- Make a complete **Orofacial Examination** (see Standard/Common Assessment Procedures); pay special attention to:
  - → clefts in the lip, the hard palate, and the soft palate
  - → repaired clefts and a judgment about the adequacy of the repair
  - → facial abnormalities that suggest a genetic syndrome (e.g., micrognathia, macrognathia, hypoplasia)
  - → abnormalities of the external ear
  - → abnormalities of the eyes
  - → observations of the velopharyngeal mechanism
- note that movements of the soft palate during the sustained production of /a/ may not always be an indication of soft palate movement in connected speech

Cleft Palate

- Assessment of articulation and phonological disorders
  - record a Speech and Language Sample (see Standard/ Common Assessment Procedures for both speech and language assessment
  - sample production of sounds of special relevance to evaluate the effects of clefts on speech; create words and phrases that contain:
    → stops, fricatives, and affricates (pressure consonants)
    → have the child produce the stimulus materials
  - administer the *Iowa Pressure Articulation Test* (a subtest of the *Templin Darley Test of Articulation*; see Articulation and Phonological Disorders
  - administer one of the articulation and phonological tests; see Articulation and Phonological Disorders
  - see Articulation and Phonological Disorders for a description of assessment procedures
  - analyze individual sounds that are in error and a phono- logical pattern analysis if warranted; see Articulation and Phonological Disorders for a description of procedures
- Assessment of language disorders
  - use the recorded speech and language sample to analyze comprehension and production of various semantic, mor- phologic, syntactic, and pragmatic language structures
  - use procedures of language assessment described under Language Disorders in Children or use procedures described under Language Disorders in Infants and Tod- dlers, depending on the age of the client
  - administer selected language tests described under Lan- guage Disorders in Children or those described under Language Disorders in Infants and Toddlers, depending on the age of the client; assess infants and toddlers at risk for developing speech and language delay
  - note that assessment of language functions in children with clefts does not significantly differ from assessment in children without clefts

- list language structures the child produces and those the child does not produce
- Assessment of phonatory disorders
  - listen to the speech and determine if a detailed voice assessment is needed
  - use procedures described under Voice Disorders to assess vocal quality deviations (e.g., hoarseness, harshness, breathiness); assess vocally abusive behaviors
  - evaluate pitch and loudness of voice; see Voice Disorders for procedures; use clinical judgment and rating; if necessary, use instruments to measure pitch and loudness
- Assessment of resonance disorders
  - assess hypernasality; make clinical judgments as you listen to the client's speech about the presence of excessive nasality
  - have two or more clinicians judge and rate hypernasality of connected speech
  - use procedures described under Voice Disorders including instrumental assessment
  - assess hyponasality; use procedures described under Voice Disorders including instrumental assessment
  - note that reliability and validity of resonance ratings are questionable; train observers and constantly monitor reliability and validity; use more than one judge (clinician) whenever possible

Related/Medical Assessment Data

- Obtain medical and surgical reports
- Integrate communication assessment data with medical assessment data
- Make assessment or diagnostic decisions as a member of the cleft palate team
- Integrate information about the child's academic performance with communication assessment data
- Obtain psychological assessment data if available and integrate them with your assessment data

Standard Common Assessment Procedures. *Complete the* <u>*Standard/Common Assessment Procedures;*</u> *pay special attention to* **Orofacial Examination** *to assess all aspects of oral-facial structures and functions*

Analysis of Assessment Data

- Analyze and summarize the child's articulation disorders and phonological pattern, if any
- Analyze and summarize the language structures the child uses and those that the child does not
- Analyze and summarize the phonatory and resonatory problems and supplement clinical observations and ratings with results of instrumental measures
- Analyze and summarize the results of instrumental observations of the velopharyngeal mechanism

Prognosis

- Varies across children; presence of multiple handicaps and severe expression of genetic syndromes affect prognosis negatively
- Generally good for improved communication skills in cases of children who have only clefts that are repaired early in life
- Most children benefit from systematic treatment

Recommendations

- Early language stimulation if there is evidence of language delay
- Treatment of articulation and phonologic disorders
- Treatment of behaviorally persistent hypernasality after velopharyngeal function is surgically restored or improved
- Repeated assessments before and after various surgical procedures
- See the cited sources and *PGTSLP* for details

Moller, K. T., & Starr, C. D. (1993). *Cleft palate: Interdisciplinary issues and treatment.* Austin, TX: Pro-Ed.

McWilliams, B. J., Morris, H. L., & Shelton, R. L. (1990). *Cleft palate speech* (2nd ed.). Philadelphia: B. C. Decker.

Client-Specific Assessment Procedures

Peterson-Falzone, S. J., Hardin-Jones, M. A., & Kernell, M. P. (2001). *Cleft palate speech*. St. Louis, MO: Mosby.

Shprintzen, R. J., & Bardach, J. (1995). *Cleft palate speech management: A multidisciplinary approach*. St. Louis, MO: Mosby.

Client-Specific Assessment Procedures. Assessment tools or procedures that are designed for a given client; needed when standard, standardized, or readily available procedures are judged not appropriate or found to be ineffective with a given client; both individual uniqueness and diverse ethnocultural background may necessitate such procedures; consider the following in designing client-specific procedures:

- See Ethnocultural Considerations in Assessment
- Use the case history information to understand the cultural background, bilingual/multilingual status, education, occupation, and general level of sophistication of the client and the family
- Make initial judgments about potential assessment tools, standardized tests, and the need for client-specific procedures based on the case history information
- During the interview, ask questions about the client's interests, hobbies, social activities, and literacy; in the case of children, ask questions about favorite toys, books, and activities
- Select assessment stimulus items that are used in the home, familiar in the culture, accepted by the client or the family; avoid using stimuli that are culture-bound and are irrelevant to the client's cultural background
- Instead of selecting standardized tests, design client-specific procedures:
  - select target behaviors or skills to be assessed (e.g., a certain number of grammatic morphemes, specific syntactic structures, specific speech sounds, naming skills, drawing, writing a paragraph, copying geometric shapes, recalling events, narrating experiences, and so forth)

C

- write words, phrases, sentences, or identify gestures or signs that will be useful in evaluating the target behaviors or skills (e.g., words that include the target phonemes, words and phrases that include the target grammatic morphemes, sentences that typify syntactic structures, names to be recalled, geometric shapes to be copied, pictures to be drawn; any exemplar of a target skill)
- identify stimulus items that help evoke the behaviors or skills (e.g., pictures that help evoke language structures or target phonemes)
- select the stimulus items from everyday sources including, especially, the client's home environment; create your own collection of stimuli by cutting out colorful pictures from magazines; include three-dimensional, naturalistic pictures; select toys and objects; before their administration, assess their familiarity to the client
- design multiple stimulus items or exemplars for each target (e.g., four items that evoke the same sound in the same position, the same grammatic feature)
- freely substitute for stimuli that are found to be inappropriate for the client
- include additional exemplars of target behavior to be assessed if time permits
- note that the flexibility involved in client-specific procedures is typically absent in the use of standardized tests (e.g., you cannot expand exemplars or substitute stimulus items)
- analyze and interpret the results of client-specific assessment procedures the way you would the outcome of Criterion-Referenced Testing

Closed-Head Injury. The same as Nonpenetrating Head Injury. See Traumatic Brain Injury.

Cluttering. A disorder predominantly affecting speech but also may involve language and thought processes; primarily a disorder of fluency but additional features are significant; a fluency disorder related to, but different from, Stuttering; may co-exist with stuttering; characterized by rapid and irregular speech rate and indistinct articulation; generally hurried speech even under normal circumstances; also known as tachyphemia; possibly underdiagnosed in the U.S.; prevalence rate not well established in the U.S.; most stuttering assessment procedures appropriate for cluttering.

Etiology

Etiology is mostly unknown; the following often are discussed as possible etiologic factors:

- Heredity: most investigators believe genetic factors are important in cluttering; however, no genetic basis has been identified; there are no systematic familial incidence data
- Neurophysiological abnormalities as suggested by deviant electroencephalographic (EEG) findings; however, only about 50% of clutterers show EEG abnormalities

Description of Cluttering

- Excessively fast rate of speech
- Progressively faster rate of speech (festinating)
- Errors of articulation, possibly due to hurried speech:
  - omission of sounds, syllables, and even words
  - sound transpositions within words
  - inversion of the order of sounds
  - syllable telescoping
- Reduced speech intelligibility due to errors of articulation
- Dysrhythmic respiration in some cases
- Motor incoordination in some cases
- Disorganized thought processes in some cases
- Language difficulties including poor syntactic structures, run-on sentences, and incorrect use of prepositions and pronouns in some cases
- Reading and writing problems including poor spelling in writing
- Monotonous speech in some cases
- Various kinds of dysfluencies including

Cluttering

- repetition of initial sounds and syllables
- repetition of words
- repetition of phrases
- revisions
- interjections
- sound prolongations
- Worsening of dysfluencies when relaxed, when reading a familiar text
- Improved fluency when attention is drawn to dysfluencies, giving short answers, talking in foreign language, speaking after interruption, and when speaking under stress
- Academic problems and learning disabilities in some cases
- Unaware of, less aware of, or unconcerned about the speech problem and its effects on listeners

Assessment Objectives/General Guidelines
- To assess behaviors that suggest cluttering
- To assess any co-existing stuttering
- To suggest treatment options
- Note that cluttering and stuttering assessments use similar methods

Case History/Interview Focus
- See **Case History** and **Interview** under Standard/Common Assessment Procedures

Ethnocultural Considerations
- See Ethnocultural Considerations in Assessment

Assessment
Generally, use the methods described under Stuttering; take note of some unique procedures highlighted here.
- Assess the types and frequency of dysfluencies; obtain a conversational speech sample; see Stuttering for details
- Assess articulatory performance
  - screen articulation to assess or rule out misarticulations; note that clutterer's articulation problems may not be revealed in isolated word productions; however, a clut-

terer may have an independent articulation disorder as well

- evaluate articulation in conversational speech and oral reading when the client used his or her typical rate of speech
- have the client repeat progressively longer words (*love, loving, lovingly; thick, thicken, thickening*); take note of deterioration in articulation as the word length increases
- ask the client to speak slowly for a period of time; make sure the rate is actually reduced
- take note of improved articulation when the rate is slowed down

• Assess rate of speech
- assess both the overall rate of speech and the articulatory rate; see <u>Stuttering</u> for procedures
- assess intelligibility in relation to rate; ask the client to slow down the rate for a period of time; take note of improvement in intelligibility at slower rates
- take note of progressively faster speech
- take note of fast and short bursts of speech
- take note of rate variations and irregular rates

• Assess language skills
- use the conversational speech sample to assess the use of various morphologic, syntactic, and pragmatic structures; see <u>Language Disorders in Children</u> for language assessment; use similar methods but with suitable modifications in the case of older clients
- take note of fluency and rate breakdowns as the complexity of language tasks increases
- administer selected language tests if necessary; see <u>Language Disorders in Children</u>

• Assess oral reading skills
- select fairly easy material; in the case of children, select material that is at least one grade below their academic level
- take note of word omissions, sound distortions, sound telescoping, sound transpositions, and so forth

Cluttering

- Obtain a writing sample
  - ask the client to write two short paragraphs to dictation
  - take note of the errors including spelling errors, letter formation, organization of paragraphs, margins, punctuation, and so forth
- Assess voice and resonance
  - during the interview, informally assess voice and resonance qualities
  - take note of any voice quality deviations and any resonance problems
  - if warranted, make a more complete assessment of voice and resonance; use procedures described under Voice Disorders

Related/Medical Assessment Data
- Obtain any available neurologic and medical assessment reports; take note of any allergies
- Obtain psychological and neuropsychological assessment reports
- Obtain reports from teachers about academic performance

Standard/Common Assessment Procedures
- Complete the Standard/Common Assessment Procedures

Analysis of Assessment Data
- Analyze the types and frequency of dysfluencies; calculate the percent dysfluency rate; see Stuttering
- Analyze the speech rate data; calculate the speech rate and articulatory rate
- Analyze articulation assessment data; make a list of errors of articulation
- Analyze improvement or deterioration in articulation depending on the rate of speech and articulatory rate
- Analyze errors of articulation that may be independent of the rate problem (errors in slower speech; errors in single word productions)
- Analyze language skills; take note of morphologic, syntactic, and pragmatic problems; take note of any indica-

tion of language formulation problems and disorganized thought processes

- Analyze the reading and writing problems; relate them to teacher's reports and data from educational assessment (e.g., learning disabilities)
- Summarize voice and resonance problems, if any

Diagnostic Criteria

- Excessively fast rate associated with sound omissions substitutions, transpositions, and word telescoping resulting in reduced intelligibility of speech
- Excessive dysfluencies
- Other listed symptoms that may be present in some cases

Differential Diagnosis

- Differentiate between cluttering and stuttering; see Stuttering for guidelines
- Note that cluttering and stuttering often co-exist

Prognosis

- No hard data to predict prognosis; generally more difficult to treat than clients with stuttering; greater clinical effort needed to promote self-monitoring skills

Recommendations

- Treatment designed to induce slower rate of speech, careful formulation of language expression when warranted, and procedures to increase awareness and self-monitoring
- See the cited sources and *PGTSLP* for details

Daly, D. A. (1986). The clutterer. In K. O. St. Louis (Ed.), *The atypical stutterer: Principles and practices of rehabilitation* (pp. 155–192). Orlando, FL: Academic Press.

Myers, F. L., & St. Louis, K. O. (1992). *Cluttering: A clinical perspective*. Kibworth, England: Far Communications.

Clinodactyly.   Fingers that are medially or laterally deflected (bent); a genetic defect, characteristic of certain syndromes.

Coloboma.   A defect in which portions of a structure, especially the eye, are missing; a characteristic of Treacher-Collins syndrome (see Syndromes Associated With Communicative Disorders)

Computerized Axial Tomography. A radiographic imaging procedure; a camera that rotates around a structure (scans) and takes pictures of sections of that structure; previously known as CAT scan and currently known as CT (for computed tomography) scan; the machine scans tissue density; a computer analyzes the images generated by the scanning machine and produces pictures of the scanned structure; can show internal structures, hemorrhages, lesions, tumors, and other pathologies; often used in the diagnosis of neuropathology associated with strokes.

Concordance Rate. The frequency with which a clinical condition found in one member of an identical or fraternal twin pair also is found in the other twin member; higher concordance rate of such disorders as stuttering, for example, has been used to support genetic etiology.

Concurrent Validity. See Validity.

Confrontation Naming. Naming stimulus items when asked to; naming in response to "What is this?"; a difficult task for most patients with aphasia; see Aphasia for details and assessment procedures.

Congenital. Any condition noticed at the time of birth or soon thereafter; may be genetic or acquired.

Congenital Abducens-Facial Paralysis. The same as Moebius syndrome (see Syndromes Associated With Communicative Disorders).

Congenital Apoculofacial Paralysis. The same as Moebius syndrome (see Syndromes Associated With Communicative Disorders).

Congenital Facial Diplegia. The same as Moebius syndrome (see Syndromes Associated With Communicative Disorders).

Congenital Palatopharyngeal Incompetence. An inadequate velopharyngeal mechanism that cannot close the velopharyngeal port for the production of non-nasal speech sounds; not due to clefts; hard palate may be too short or the nasopharynx may be too deep; speech is hypernasal; depending on the degree of incompetence, resonance (voice) therapy may be ineffective without surgical or prosthetic help.

Consistency Effect.   Stuttering on the same words or same loci when a printed passage is orally read repeatedly; contrasts with the Adaptation Effect; may be assessed through five repeated readings of a brief passage; suggests that the greater the consistency effect, the stronger the stimulus control of stuttering; see Stuttering for assessment procedure.

Constructional Apraxia.   The same as Constructional Impairment.

Constructional Impairment.   Difficulty in visuospatial tasks; includes problems in constructing block designs, copying or drawing geometric figures, reproducing stick figures; often found in patients with Right Hemisphere Syndrome; also called Constructional Apraxia.

Construct Validity.   See Validity.

Craniocerebral Trauma.   The same as Traumatic Brain Injury.

Creutzfeldt-Jakob Disease (CJD).   A degenerative, rare, fatal encephalopathy; involves partial degeneration of pyramidal and extrapyramidal systems; associated with dementia and dysarthria.

Criterion-Referenced Testing.   A form of assessment the results of which are not compared against norms derived from the performance of a representative sample; an approach in which the examiner selects target behaviors to be assessed and prepared stimulus materials that are effective; more similar to the Client-Specific Assessment Procedures than to standardized testing; the results are described

C

more in terms of the skills that are present, mastered, not mastered yet, absent, and so forth; there is not explicit evaluation against age-based norms; may include aspects or skills that standardized tests do not include; may assess skills in greater depth than standardized tests do; also helps assess progress under treatment.

Cultural Diversity and Assessment Procedures. See Ethnocultural Considerations in Assessment.

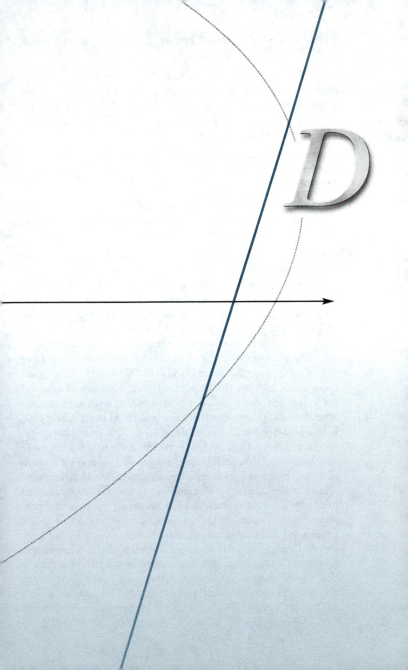

D

Deaf. A person whose hearing impairment is severe enough to prevent normal oral language acquisition, production, and comprehension with the help of audition; profound hearing loss that exceeds 90 dB HL.

de Lange Syndrome. The same as Cornelia de Lange syndrome (see Syndromes Associated With Communicative Disorders).

Deletion Processes. A set of phonological processes that affects the structure of syllables; see Syllable Structure Processes under Phonological Processes.

Dementia. An acquired neurological syndrome associated with deterioration in intellectual and communicative functions and general behavior; sustained over a period of months or years; varied etiologic factors, but often associated with such neurologic diseases as Alzheimer's Disease (AD), Huntington's Disease (HD), and Parkinson's Disease (PD); the most frequently occurring form is associated with Alzheimer's disease (50% of the cases); also frequently associated with vascular diseases (15 to 20% of the cases); affects about 10% of the population over 65 years of age; onset in late life, but incidence rate increases with each decade after the 60s; progressive and irreversible in most cases; static in a few cases and reversible in 10 to 20% of the cases; reversible dementia may leave residual symptoms or some may develop more serious and progressive dementia later in life; may be classified as primary degenerative, multi-infarct, and all other; also may be classified as cortical (degeneration primarily in neocortical association areas) with better preserved motor speech skills, subcortical (degeneration in the basal ganglia, thalamus, and brainstem) with better preserved language skills, and mixed; much of the information presented here about the neuropathology and communication disorders associated with dementia is based on research on progressive dementias, especially on dementia of Alzheimer's type (DAT); for specific information on dementia associated with Parkinson's Disease (PD), Huntington's Disease (HD), Pick's Disease, Wilson's Disease, and Progressive Supranuclear Palsy (PS), see their respective alphabetical main entries.

Etiology of Progressive Dementia

- Cortical disorders including Alzheimer's disease and Pick's disease
- Subcortical disorders including Parkinson's disease (PD), Huntington's disease (HD), Wilson's disease (WD), and Progressive Supranuclear Palsy
- Vascular diseases resulting in repeated large vessel strokes and small arterial ruptures (lacunar state)
- Demyelinating disorders including multiple sclerosis
- Traumatic conditions including posttraumatic encephalopathy, subdural hematoma
- Toxic conditions including alcohol-related syndromes and multiple drug abuse; and toxicity due to various prescription drugs including anticonvulsive and antihypertensive drugs
- Infection-related conditions including human immunodeficiency virus encephalopathy, syphilis, and Creutzfeldt-Jakob disease
- Combination of two or more diseases (e.g., Alzheimer's disease and multiple strokes)

Etiology of Reversible Dementia

- Drug abuse and drug interactions, and other toxicity that receives timely and effective medical management
- Depression and is successfully treated
- Some metabolic disorders (e.g., encephalopathies from kidney or liver diseases that are successfully treated)
- Vitamin deficiencies (e.g., thiamine deficiency that is medically managed)
- Some endocrine disorders (e.g., thyroid deficiencies) that are successfully treated
- Head trauma that produces transient symptoms
- Normal pressure hydrocephalus

- Certain brain tumors that are surgically or medically treated without undue effects
- Some infections (e.g., meningitis and encephalitis that are medically managed)
- Inflammation

Neuropathological and Neurophysiological Factors Associated With Dementia

- Neuropathology varies somewhat with specific forms of dementia; generally, there are brain atrophy and neurochemical deficiencies; some variations in the localization of atrophy, depending on the specific form of dementia
- Neurofibrillary tangles, which are twisted and tangled structures of dendrites and axons (especially in DAT)
- Neuritic (senile) plaques, which are small areas of cortical and subcortical degeneration (especially in DAT)
- Granulovacuolar degeneration, which are degeneration of nerve cells because of the formation of small fluid-filled cavities containing granular debris (especially in (DAT)
- Reduced gray and white matter of the brain mainly because of loss of large neurons in the frontal and temporal regions of the brain; about 10% loss of brain weight
- Decreased dendritic connections
- Neurochemical deficiencies in the brain that affect neurotransmission, especially cholinergic and dopamine deficiency along with deficient neuropeptides
- Decreased cerebral metabolism
- Reduced cerebral blood flow
- Enlarged ventricles and widened sulci
- Bilateral brain damage due to repeated CVA
- Damaged subcortical structures due to multiple infarcts (Binswanger's disease)

Early and Intermediate-Stage Symptoms Including Communication Disorders

- Typically mild and often ignored or missed mild symptoms as the onset is slow and gradual
- Subtle memory problems

- Reasoning problems and poor judgment
- Brief, subtle, or transitory problems of disorientation
- Mild depression, other mood changes
- Mild naming problems which becomes progressively worse
- Verbal paraphasia
- Subtle language comprehension problems, especially comprehension of meanings, implied meanings, and humor; more obvious difficulty as the disease progresses
- Impaired picture description
- Beginning of progressive decrease in vocabulary
- Inadequate use of pronouns
- Impaired pantomime recognition and expression
- Pragmatic language problems including difficulty in topic maintenance
- Impaired interaction during conversation (e.g., failure to ask for clarification when encountering ambiguous questions or requests or clarifying a statement when a listener requests it)
- Repetitious speech
- Intact automatic speech
- Intact articulation and phonological skills
- Intact syntactic skills

Advanced Symptoms Including Communication Disorders

- Severely impaired memory
- Pronounced and generalized intellectual deterioration eventually resulting in profound intellectual deterioration
- Restlessness and agitation
- Emotional lability
- Profound disorientation to time, place, and person
- Aimless wandering
- Periodic incontinence (urinary control problems) worsening to complete incontinence
- Motor problems, especially spasticity
- Diurnal rhythm disturbance in some cases
- Delusions and hallucinations in some cases

Dementia

- Violent outbursts in some cases
- Continued decrease in vocabulary
- Literal paraphasias
- Circumlocution
- Empty speech (expression of fewer ideas even when the number of words produced do not decline much)
- Jargon and stereotypic expressions
- Incoherent, irrelevant speech
- Rapid rate of speech
- Echolalic speech
- Palilalia (compulsive repetition of one's own speech, often with accelerating rate and decelerating loudness)
- Slowness or difficulty in initiating conversation
- Inattention to social conventions (greetings, thanking, farewell)
- Eventually, no meaningful speech
- Complete disorientation to time, space, and person
- Disorientation to self

Assessment Objectives/General Guidelines

- To assess language, cognitive, memory, and visuospatial skills
- To assess changes in behavior and personality
- To identify the strengths and weaknesses of the patient with a view to developing an intervention or management plan for the patient and the family
- Note that identifying advanced stage dementia is not as challenging as identifying early and mild forms of dementia
- Note that such automatic tasks as pointing to named pictures and reciting alphabets and days of the week are not especially diagnostic of mild dementia
- Note that syntactic disturbances are not evident in mild dementia; hence they need not be assessed in great detail (except in case of multi-infarct dementia and dementia associated with Pick's disease)
- Note that articulation and phonological skills are not diagnostic of early dementia as they are retained until the advanced stage when dementia is obvious

- Note that sentence repetition skills are not diagnostic of early dementia as they are preserved even when the patient cannot comprehend the meaning of repeated sentences
- Note that creative thinking and abstract reasoning tasks are of especial diagnostic value (e.g., verbal description, story telling, verbal fluency)
- Note that language assessment alone will not determine the diagnosis; deterioration in memory, visuospatial skills, and general intellect also should be demonstrated

Case History/Interview Focus

- See **Case History** and **Interview** under Standard/Common Assessment Procedures
- Concentrate on detailed history of the patient's health, changes over time, major illnesses, and behavioral changes over time

Ethnocultural Considerations

- See Ethnocultural Considerations in Assessment

Assessment

Use the following procedures, most of which have been described by Bayles and Kasznaik (1987) and Ripich (1991); several tasks are included in some of the standardized tests of dementia:

- Assess language and communication skills
  - assess vocabulary
    - → take a conversational speech sample
    - → use verbal description data to assess use of words
    - → assess the variety and specificity of words used in a conversational speech sample and verbal description task
    - → use a standardized measure such as the Peabody Picture Vocabulary Test (PPVT)
    - → note that PPVT is sensitive to early phases of dementia
  - assess verbal description skills
    - → present a few common objects to the patient

- → ask the patient to describe each of them
- → if necessary, model a complete description of an object (such as a pencil)
- → tape record the descriptions and transcribe them later
- → take note of the number of meaningful and relevant pieces of information the patient offers
- → note that verbal description tasks can identify early phases of dementia
- assess story telling skills
  - → ask the patient to listen carefully to the story you are about to tell
  - → tell the patient that he or she will have to retell the story soon after and at the end of the testing session
  - → tell a short story
  - → ask the nonexpressive patient to rearrange picture cards to retell the story
  - → take note of significant reduction in the number of story elements remembered
- assess verbal fluency or generative naming task
  - → ask the patient to say as many words as possible that begin with a specific alphabet; sample responses for at least three letters
  - → allow 1 minute of response time for each letter
  - → note that generative naming measures help identify early phases of dementia
  - → assess appropriate or expected responses in structured conversations
  - → ask an ambiguous question or make an ambiguous request to see of the patient requests more information or clarification
  - → ask for clarifications when the patient's statements are not clear
  - → compliment the patient to see if he or she makes a relevant response

- → judge the presence or appropriateness of responses when you say "I enjoyed meeting you."
- → judge meaningfulness and relevance of sentences produced; consider contexts of utterances
- → analyze stories or descriptions of patients for contextual and setting information; most patients with dementia omit information on context and setting
- assess pantomime expression
  - → show common objects or pictures of objects and ask the patient to demonstrate their use by gestures
  - → note that pantomime expression tasks can help identify mild dementia
- judge syntactic skills in conversational speech; assess syntactic skills in detail if necessary
  - → note that syntactic skills are intact in early phases of dementia
  - → make an informal analysis of sentence types, lengths, and variety and take note of any deviations or deficiencies
- Assess reading comprehension
  - have the patient match printed words with pictures
  - have the patient silently read a story and answer your questions
  - note that dementia patients are likely to have much more difficulty in comprehending sentences and paragraphs than single words
- Assess pragmatic language skills
  - take a discourse sample
  - observe conversational turn taking
  - observe topic maintenance
  - observe conversational repair
  - observe topic initiation
- Assess articulation and phonological skills
  - note that articulation and phonological skills are intact in early phases of dementia

- use the conversational speech sample to analyze speech sound productions; take note of any problems
- Assess cognitive functions
  - make a mental status examination
    - → ask questions about general awareness and about time and space orientation, ("Where are you now?" "What time is it?" "What is today's date?")
    - → administer a standardized test
  - assess reasoning and event planning skills (knowledge of schemata) by asking the patient to describe how he or she would
    - → plan a birthday party
    - → plan a summer vacation, a camping trip, or a picnic
    - → get an airline ticket
    - → obtain a doctor's appointment
  - assess memory skills
    - → use the delayed story telling procedure in which you tell a short story and have the patient recall it after 1 hour
    - → administer a memory test
  - assess drawing skills
    - → ask the patient to draw some common pictures (e.g., a clock, a circle, a triangle)
    - → note that patients with even mild dementia perform poorly on this visuospatial task
  - obtain a measure of general intellectual functioning
    - → obtain reports from a psychologist about intelligence testing
  - assess abstract reasoning
    - → ask the patient to specify the meaning of a few selected proverbs (e.g., "what is meant by the saying a stitch in time saves nine")
    - → assess whether the patient gives a literal or abstract interpretation of such statements

Standardized Tests
- Administer one or more of the following tests:

Test	Purpose
Arizona Battery for Communication Disorders of Dementia (K. A. Bayles & C. Tomoeda)	To assess dementia through 14 subtests and screen it with four subtests
Benton Revised Visual Retention Test (A. L. Benton)	To assess visual memory with figural recall
Brief Cognitive Rating Scale (B. Reisberg)	To assess cognitive decline due to any reason
Clinical Dementia Rating Scale (C. P. Hughes and associates)	To rate dementia on 5-point rating scale; does not assess communication skills
Discourse Abilities Profile (B. Terrel & D. Ripich)	To assess various forms of discourse during conversation with the patient and conversation between the patient and family members/caregivers
Global Deterioration Scale (B. Reisberg and associates)	To rate dementia on a 7-point rating scale
Mini-Mental State Examination (M. F. Folstein, S. E. Folstein, & P. R. McHugh)	To assess the mental status with 11 items
Wechsler Memory Scale—Revised (F. W. Russell)	To assess various memory functions

- Administer a test of aphasia as found appropriate (see Aphasia

Related/Medical Assessment Data

- Obtain copies of medical reports
- Ascertain diagnoses of neurological and other diseases of the patient
- Obtain brain imaging and other special diagnostic data
- Obtain copies of social service reports
- Obtain psychological assessment data
- Obtain any other family service information available on the patient

Dementia

Standard/Common Assessment Procedures
- Complete the Standard/Common Assessment Procedures
- Analysis of Assessment Data
- Analyze the results of the communication assessment
- Analyze the results of cognition and memory assessment
- Integrate the results of communication, cognition-memory, medical, social service, and psychological assessment procedures
- Make a summary statement of the significant findings
- Obtain a total picture of the patient and his or her strengths and weaknesses
- Integrate the clinical assessment data with those of case history information

Diagnostic Criteria
- Generally, impairment should be documented in (1) language; (2) memory; (3) visuospatial skills; (4) emotion or personality; (5) cognition
- Minimally, three out of the five listed functions should show impairment to diagnose dementia (Cummings & Benson, 1983)

Differential Diagnosis
- Definite diagnosis is possible only with autopsic or biopsic evidence of histopathology
- Differentiate dementia from aphasia
- Differentiate dementia from the language of confusion
- Differentiate dementia from depression (pseudodementia) and other psychiatric conditions
- Differentiate dementia from right hemisphere syndrome
- Distinguish among cortical dementias caused by Alzheimer's Disease or Pick's Disease.
- Distinguish among mixed dementias caused by Korsakoff's disease (or syndrome, which is currently considered a form of amnestic disorder); Creutzfeldt ease, or Multi Infarct Dementia.
- Distinguish among subcortical dementias (and possibly dysarthria as well) caused by Huntington's Disease, Parkinson's Disease, Wilson's Disease, or Progressive Supranuclear Palsy.

Dementia

- Note that generative naming problem is a more sensitive early sign of dementia than is confrontation naming
- Note that early stage dementia is characterized by relatively intact phonological and syntactic skills
- Use the following four grids to distinguish dementia from the other potentially confusing disorders

Dementia or Aphasia?

Dementia	Aphasia
Onset mostly is slow	Onset mostly is sudden
Bilateral brain damage	Damage in the left hemisphere
Diffuse brain damage in most cases	Focal brain lesions in most cases
May be moody, withdrawn, and agitated	Mood usually is appropriate, though depressed or frustrated at times
Cognition is mildly or severely impaired, but better language skills until later stages	Impaired language, but generally intact cognition
Memory is impaired to various degrees, often severely	Memory typically is intact
Behavior often is irrelevant, socially inappropriate, and disorganized	Behavior generally is relevant, socially appropriate, and organized
Mentally confused and disoriented to time and space	Mentally alert and oriented to time and space
Disorientation to self in later stages	No disorientation to self
Progression of deterioration from semantic to syntactic to phonologic performance	Semantic, syntactic, and phonologic performance simultaneously impaired
Fluent until dementia becomes worse	Fluent or nonfluent

(continued)

(continued)

Dementia	Aphasia
Relatively poor performance on spatial and verbal recognition tasks	Relatively better performance on spatial and verbal recognition tasks
Relatively poor story retelling skills	Relatively better story retelling skills
Relatively poor description of common objects	Relatively better description of common objects
Relatively poor silent reading comprehension	Relatively better silent reading comprehension
Relatively poor pantomimic expression	Relatively better pantomimic expression
Relatively poor drawing skills	Relatively better drawing skills

Caution: (a) Patients with fluent aphasia are more likely to be confused with dementia than are those with fluent aphasia; (b) aphasia and dementia may coexist; (c) an aphasic patient may develop a neurological disease resulting in dementia (Alzheimer's disease); (d) a patient with dementia may suffer a stroke, resulting in aphasia.

Dementia or the Language of Confusion?

Dementia	Confusion
Degenerative diseases more common causes	Traumatic brain injury and toxic and metabolic disturbances are the most common causes
Reduced range and variety of word usage	No significant problems in word usage
Slow onset	Generally more abrupt onset
Disorientation to time, place, and person only in more advanced stages	Disoriented to time, place, and persons
Progressive worsening of symptoms	More rapid, positive changes in symptoms

Dementia

Dementia or Depression (Pseudodementia)?

Dementia	Pseudodementia
Imprecise onset date	More precise onset date
Family members often do not know about the symptoms	Family members know about the symptoms
Slow progression of symptoms	Rapid progression of symptoms
No or rare history of psychiatric problems	History of psychiatric problems
Patients do not complain of cognitive problems in detail	Patients complain of cognitive problems
Patients try to conceal their problems	Patients highlight their disability, failure, sense of distress
Patients struggle to perform	Patients make no or little effort to perform even simple tasks
Social skills often preserved until the later stages	Loss of social skills
Attentional deficits and poor concentration	No attentional deficits, good concentration
Patient's response to orientation tests is confusion	Patient's response to orientation tests is "don't know"
More severe loss for recent events, more severe than that for remote events	The same degree of memory loss for both recent and remote events
Generalized memory problems	Selective memory problems
Consistent difficulty in performing the same task	Variability in performing the same task

Note: Pseudodementia is dementia-like symptoms associated with depression; the differentiating characteristics summarized here are based on Wells (1980).

Dementia

Dementia or Right Hemisphere Problems?

Dementia	Right Hemisphere Problems
Significant problems in naming, especially generative naming	Only mild problems in naming, reading, and writing
Significant problems in auditory comprehension	Mild problems in auditory comprehension
Left-sided neglect not a diagnostic feature	Left-sided neglect a diagnostic feature
Prosodic defects less severe	Significant prosodic defect
	Inappropriate humor
May retell stories without context or location	May retell only nonessential, isolated details of stories (no integration)
Pragmatic impairments less striking until the latter stages	Pragmatic impairments more striking (eye contact, topic maintenance, etc.)
Significant linguistic deficits except for syntactic and phonological skills which also decline in later stages	Pure linguistic deficits are not dominant

Cortical Dementias:
Dementia of Alzheimer's Disease or of Pick's Disease?

Alzheimer's Disease	Pick's Disease
Gradual onset of the disease	Gradual onset of the disease
Diffuse damage associated with senile plaques, neurofibrillary tangles, granulovascular degeneration, neuronal loss, astrocytic gliosis, and amyloid angiopathy	Atrophy in the frontal and temporal regions; Pick bodies (filamentous intracytoplasmic inclusions in neurons)

(continued)

180

(continued)

Alzheimer's Disease	Pick's Disease
Impairment of semantic and pragmatic language functions in early stages; syntactic and phonological skills preserved until later stages; speech impairment in very late stages	Impaired rate and prosody characterized by slow and deliberate speech; naming problems; syntactic difficulties; auditory comprehension problems
Impaired memory, but worse for remote events	Impaired memory, but worse for recent events
Willing to perform, tries to perform	Apathetic, shows emotional lability
Generally normal motor functions	Impaired motor functions in later stages

Mixed Dementias: Dementia of Korsakoff's Disease, Creutzfeldt-Jakob Disease, or Multi-Infarct Dementia?

Korsakoff's Disease	Creutzfeldt-Jakob Disease	Multi-Infarct Dementia
Onset is gradual	Onset gradual or sudden	Onset is sudden
Alcohol abuse resulting in cortical atrophy	Viral infection; resulting cortical degeneration and encephalopathy	Vascular pathology; generalized cortical damage resulting from multiple strokes
Somewhat stable	Rapidly progressive	Stepwise in progression
Language deterioration is controversial or not well understood except for confabulation possibly due to memory problems	Aphasia, apraxia, agnosia, and eventually mutism	Aphasia and varied symptom complex depending on the extent and location of neuropathology

(continued)

Dementia

(continued)

Korsakoff's Disease	Creutzfeldt-Jakob Disease	Multi-Infarct Dementia
Amnesia and other memory problems	Forgetfulness depending on the neuropathology	Varied impairment
Emotional liability	Apathy	Variable emotional responses
May be associated with physical problems	Rigidity, myoclonus, tremor, impaired cerebellar functions, cranial nerve palsies, and sensory and visual impairments	May have physical symptoms depending on the neuropathology

Subcortical Dementias: Dementia of Huntington's Disease, Parkinson's Disease, Wilson's Disease, or Supranuclear Palsy?

Huntington's Disease	Parkinson's Disease	Wilson's Disease	Supranuclear Palsy
Sporadic onset	Insidious onset	Gradual onset	Gradual onset
Genetic and nongenetic causes; involvement of substantia niegra	Degenerative disease of the CNS; loss of Golgi cells in corpus striatum	Involvement of the basal ganglia; excessive amount of copper in the brain and liver	Involvement of reticular formation, thalamus, or hypothalamus
Neuromotor symptoms of shuffling and jerky gait, chorea	Neuromotor symptoms of tremor, rigidity, slowness, bradykinesia, postural instability	Neuromotor symptoms of tremor, rigidity, slowness, bradykinesia, ataxia, dysphagia, masklike face	Neuromotor symptoms of pseudobulbar palsy, dystonia, rigidity of head and neck, and retracted head position
			(continued)

(continued)

Huntington's Disease	Parkinson's Disease	Wilson's Disease	Supranuclear Palsy
Depression and significant language impairment even in the early stages; dysarthria; intervals of inappropriate silence	Speech impairment greater than language impairment; weak, breathy voice; dysarthria; abnormal pitch and loudness	Dysarthria; irregular articulatory breakdown; hypernasality; intervals of inappropriate silence	Inaudible speech; harsh sounds; dysarthria

Prognosis
- Generally, more favorable for reversible than irreversible dementia; generally not favorable for significant improvement in the case of dementia associated with progressive diseases

Recommendations
- Communication treatment for patients in the early stages of all dementia
- Treatment directed toward management of problems (including compensatory strategies) in patients with more advanced stages of irreversible dementia
- Counseling for the family members and family-oriented treatment for all patients, especially for those in the advanced stages of irreversible dementia
- See the cited sources and *PGTSLP* for details

Bayles, K. A., & Kaszniak, A. W. (1987). *Communication and cognition in normal aging and dementia.* Austin, TX: Pro-Ed.

Cummings, J. L., & Benson, D. F. (1983). *Dementia: A clinical approach.* Boston: Butterworth.

Brookshire, R. H. (1997). *An introduction to neurogenic communication disorders* (5th ed.). St. Louis, MO: Mosby Year Book.

Lubinski, R. (1991). *Dementia and communication.* Philadelphia: B. C. Decker.

Ripich, D. N. (1991). *Geriatric communication disorders*. Austin, TX: Pro-Ed.

Wells, C. E. (1980). The differential diagnosis of psychiatric disorders in the elderly. In J. Cole & J. Barrett (Eds.), *Psychopathology in the aged* (pp. 19–29). New York: Raven Press.

Denasality (Hyponasality).   Lack of nasal resonance on nasal sounds; a disorder of resonance; see Voice Disorders for assessment procedures.

Developmental Apraxia of Speech (DAS).   A speech disorder in children characterized by sensorimotor problems in positioning and sequentially moving muscles for the volitional production of speech; associated with prosodic problems; not caused by muscle weakness or neuromuscular slowness; presumed to be a disorder of motor programming for speech; unlike in Apraxia of Speech (AOS) in Adults, no demonstrated neuropathology, hence controversial; some believe that language disorders, especially problems in syntax, are a part of the syndrome; those who believe this to be such a syndrome prefer the term developmental verbal apraxia; others believe that it is strictly a disorder of motor speech control, although independent language and other problems may coexist with it; historically, also known as developmental motor aphasia, executive aphasia, articulatory apraxia, and phonologic programming deficit syndrome; some currently believe that the term does not necessarily suggest neuropathology, but only describes specific speech motor control problem as exhibited by some children.

Etiology
- Etiology is mostly theoretical because of the absence of demonstrated neuropathology that underlies AOS in adults; both the closed loop and open loop models of speech production have been used to explain DAS; suggestions include faulty speech programming, faulty sensory feedback mechanism, faulty sequencing of movements, faulty hierarchical movements involved in speech production, faulty schema of speech production, and problems in developing timing control; no theory fully supported; no explanation of DAS complete

184

Developmental Apraxia of Speech (DAS)

- A higher familial incidence of speech and language disorders associated with DAS; suggestive of a genetic basis
- Association of DAS with certain syndromes, including Down syndrome and Fragile X syndrome (see Syndromes Associated With Communicative Disorders; also suggestive of a genetic basis
- Association of DAS with inborn errors of metabolism; also suggestive of a genetic basis
- More prevalent in boys than in girls
- No significant and consistent evidence of brain lesions
- General clumsiness and lack of coordination reported in some children with DAS
- Oral apraxia, suggestive of a more general, nonverbal, oral motor control problem, may or may not be associated with DAS
- Possibly, multiple etiologic factors
- No particular personality or behavioral pattern associated with DAS

General Considerations
- Children who exhibit DAS are a heterogeneous group; the older hypothesis that DAS is found only in children who are otherwise normal may be due to subject selection biases
- DAS may be found in children with several associated disabilities including sensorineural hearing loss, mental retardation, ataxic cerebral palsy and generalized hypotonia, developmental delay, attention deficit disorders
- DAS is not necessarily the most severe form of articulation disorder due to presumed motor programming deficit; the severity may range from mild to severe, like any other disorder

Speech Disorders
- Moderate to severe speech intelligibility problems
- Most frequent errors on consonant clusters followed by fricatives, affricates, stops, and nasals; errors on fricatives and affricates may persist longer
- Articulatory groping and silent articulatory postures

Developmental Apraxia of Speech (DAS)

- Inconsistency and variability in errors when the same word is produced on repeated trials
- Unusual errors of articulation; errors typically not found in children with functional articulation disorder or found less frequently; predominantly, phonemic sequencing errors; include the following kinds:
  - metathetic errors (transposition or reversal of phoneme sequences; e.g., "maks" for *masks* or "soun" for *snow*)
  - addition of phonemes (e.g., *applesaks* for "applesauce" or *clat* for "cat")
  - prolongation of speech sounds
  - repetition of sounds and syllables, even the final sounds or syllables
  - nonphonemic productions that cannot be transcribed
- Usual errors of articulation
  - more frequent occurrence of omissions and substitutions
  - more prevalent distortions in some older children
  - varied simplification of consonant blends (e.g., omission of one sound, substitution for another sound, correct production of one element, substitution of one sound for the entire cluster)
  - voicing and devoicing errors
  - vowel and diphthong errors (distorted vowels and diphthong reduction)
- Delayed speech development
  - speech production skills lag behind language comprehension skills
  - speech production skills lag behind cognitive skills
- Resonance problems
  - hypernasality, hyponasality, or nasal emission in some or most children
  - resonance problems variable and inconsistent
  - possibly, resonance problems due to poor velopharyngeal control and not a phonological problem
- Prosodic problems
  - abnormal prosody in some cases
  - some children's speech may be aprosodic (flat prosody)

- other children's speech may be dysprosodic (presence of variation in frequency and duration, but inappropriate expression of them)
- inappropriate use of stress patterns

- Fluency problems increased frequency of dysfluencies although information on specific types and their frequencies are not available

Associated Problems

- Language disorders; delayed language development, associated with delayed speech development
- Hearing impairment in some cases
- Mental retardation in some cases
- Neuromuscular disorders (e.g., cerebral palsy) in some cases
- Gross and fine visual and motor skill deficits (e.g., problems of coordination in hand writing and typing)
- Learning disabilities

Assessment Objectives/General Guidelines

- To assess speech production skills and speech intelligibility
- To assess language skills
- To assess other aspects of communication (voice, fluency)
- To describe the nature of a client's speech production problems
- To make a diagnosis of DAS
- To rate or evaluate the severity of DAS
- To identify the child's strengths and limitations
- To assess treatment potential and prognosis
- To identify initial treatment targets

Case History/Interview Focus

- See **Case History** and **Interview** under Standard/ Common Assessment Procedures

Ethnocultural Considerations

- See Ethnocultural Considerations in Assessment

Assessment

- Assess language skills
  - take a conversational speech sample

187

D

- in case of very young children, estimate the size of the vocabulary from parental reports
- assess language comprehension by giving increasingly complex verbal commands to be followed by the child
- ask the child to narrate a story
- tell a story and ask the child to retell it
- Assess literacy skills
  - tape record a reading sample
  - obtain handwriting sample
  - give a brief and simple spelling test
  - test preschool printing and alphabet recognition in case of younger children
- Conduct a detailed orofacial examination (see Standard/ Common Assessment Procedures)
- Assess nonimitative speech production skills
  - obtain speech sample of 75 to 100 utterances
  - record nonimitative production of a set of single words that sample all phonemes; use a standardized test of articulation if appropriate for the child
  - use object or picture naming tasks to evoke nonimitative productions; select age-appropriate stimulus materials
  - evoke productions of progressively longer words (e.g., love, loving, lovingly)
  - evoke production of shorter and longer sentences
  - phonetically transcribe the utterances and speech sound errors; make whole-word transcriptions
  - observe and record signs of speech motor programming problems (e.g., groping, dysfluencies)
  - observe and record speech production problems as the length of words increases
  - use stimulus materials described in Apraxia of Speech (AOS) in Adults in adults and modify the materials to suit the child or use parallel stimulus items selected from child vocabulary
- Assess imitative speech production skills

Developmental Apraxia of Speech (DAS)

- model individual sounds and syllables and ask the child to imitate
- initially, hide your oral movements; if the child cannot imitate, show the normal movements
- model a series of shorter and longer words and ask the child to imitate
- model shorter and longer sentences and ask the child to imitate
- Assess consistency and variability of errors
  - sample speech productions in varied phonetic contexts
  - sample speech production at different complexity levels
  - sample speech production in imitative and spontaneous modes
  - sample production of the same phoneme (in the same word) in multiple trials
- Assess intelligibility of speech
  - assess intelligibility with already collected assessment data
  - assess intelligibility at different levels (syllables, words, phrases, and sentences)
  - rate intelligibility on a 5- or 7-point rating scale if desired
  - note that severity of DAS may range from mild to severe
- Assess resonance problems
  - assess hypernasality, hyponasality, and nasal emission by clinical judgment
  - use a nasal mirror to judge nasal emission in the production of non-nasal sounds
  - visually inspect the velopharyngeal mechanism as a part of the orofacial examination
  - when found necessary or feasible, use mechanical instruments to diagnose resonance problems (see Instruments for Resonance Assessment)
- Assess prosodic problems
  - clinically evaluate the appropriateness of pitch and loudness variation
  - clinically evaluate the stress patterns
- Assess fluency and dysfluencies

- count the frequency of each dysfluency type exhibited in the speech sample
- count the frequency of each dysfluency type exhibited in an oral reading sample

Standardized Tests

- Administer selected tests of articulation described under
- <u>Articulation and Phonological Disorders</u> to sample speech sound productions
- Use the Verbal-Motor Production Assessment of Children (Hayden, 1994)

Medical, Psychological, and Educational Assessment Data

- Obtain any available medical data including the results of brain imaging techniques or neurological examinations
- Obtain psychological data including the results of intelligence testing and cognitive functioning
- Obtain data on the child's educational achievement and assessment that might suggest learning disabilities

Standard/Common Assessment Procedures

- Complete the <u>Standard/Common Assessment Procedures</u>

Analysis of Assessment Data

- Analyze the assessment data
- Analyze the language samples and summarize morphologic, semantic, syntactic, and pragmatic problems noted
- Analyze and summarize the reading, writing, and other literacy skill levels
- Summarize the orofacial examination data
- Calculate the percent dysfluency rate based on the number of words spoken or read orally
- Describe groping, struggle and related problems
- Analyze the phonetically transcribed non-imitative word productions and describe the kinds of articulatory and sequencing errors exhibited; identify the locus of breakdown (e.g., syllables, monosyllabic words, and multisyllabic words)

Developmental Apraxia of Speech (DAS)

- Analyze and summarize the kinds of errors noted on imitative speech tasks
- Analyze and summarize consistency and variability in error patterns
- Calculate the percentage of spoken or orally read words that are intelligible
- Determine the presence or absence of resonance problems
- Analyze and summarize the noted prosodic problems
- Consider medical, psychological, and educational assessment data
- Make a summary statement

Diagnostic Criteria

- Deficiency in sequenced speech movements that are not attributable to other factors
- Problems of speech intelligibility
- Prosodic problems
- Articulatory groping and other characteristics of disordered speech motor control

Differential Diagnosis

- Distinguish DAS from functional articulation disorder by applying the diagnostic criteria
- Rule out paralysis, paresis, and weakness that are attributable to neurological disorders or diseases
- When other problems such as sensory or intellectual impairment are documented in children who otherwise qualify for the diagnosis of DAS, consider them as coexisting problems

Prognosis

- Generally, more treatment time and effort are needed to produce significant changes; several years of treatment in many cases
- Some errors may persist in spite of best efforts
- Intensive and competent treatment can produce functionally adequate speech in many children; expectation of normal speech may be unrealistic in severe cases

D

- Augmentative and alternative communication may be needed in patients with extremely severe DAS who do not respond to intensive and competent oral communication treatment

Recommendations
- Intensive and prolonged treatment
- Counseling the family about the need for such treatment
- Augmentative or alternative communication when found necessary and appropriate
- See the cited sources and *PGTSLP* for details

Hall, P. K., Jordan, L. S., & Robin, D. A. (1993). *Developmental apraxia of speech: Theory and clinical practice.* Austin, TX: Pro-Ed.

Hayden, D. A. (1994). Differential diagnosis of motor speech dysfunction in children. *Clinics in Communication Disorders, 4*(2), 119–141.

Hodge, M. M. (1994). Assessment of children with developmental apraxia of speech: A rationale. *Clinics in Communication Disorders, 4*(2), 91–101.

Hodge, M. M., & Hancock, H. R. (1994). Assessment of children with developmental apraxia of speech: A procedure. *Clinics in Communication Disorders, 4*(2), 102–118.

Developmental Norms for Phonemes. Ages at which different phonemes are acquired or mastered by children speaking normally; often used to evaluate whether a child has an articulation disorder; the child who does not produce a sound at an age when others of the same age produce the sound correctly is said to have an articulation disorder; researched and reported by several investigators; wide discrepancies across studies in reported ages at which specific sounds are mastered; some or most of the differences may be due to methodological variations across studies; definitions of mastery across investigators vary: (a) correct production in all positions by 75% of the children tested, (b) 51% of tested children to derive a customary age of acquisition, (c) correct articulation only in initial and medial word positions, or (d) correct production in all positions; because data are averaged across children, the normative ages provide only broad guidelines but fail to predict performance of any indi-

Developmental Norms for Phonemes

vidual child; significant individual differences in the age of acquisition of speech sounds; most norms are based on white, monolingual, English speaking, middle class children; caution to be exercised in using group means in evaluating an individual child's performance, especially if the child belongs to an ethnocultural minority group; use the norms in the context of accepted practice in your clinical setting to determine the need for treatment; the most commonly reported normative data follow:

Phonemes	Wellman (1934)	Poole (1934)	Templin (1957)	Sander (1972)	Prather (1975)	Arlt (1976)
m	3	3–6	3	before 2	2	3
n	3	4–6	3	before 2	2	3
h	3	3–6	3	before 2	2	3
n	3	4–6	3	before 2	2	3
h	3	3–6	3	before 2	2	3
p	4	3–6	3	before 2	2	3
f	3	5–6	3	3	2–4	3
w	3	3–6	3	before 2	2–8	3
b	3	3–6	4	before 2	2–8	3
ŋ (ng)	–	4–6	3	2	2	3
j	4	4–6	1	3–6	3	2–4
k	4	4–6	4	2	2–4	3
g	4	4–6	4	2	2–4	3
l	4	6–6	6	3	2–4	4
d	5	4–6	4	2	2–4	3
t	5	4–6	6	2	2–8	3
s	5	7–6	4–6	3	3	4
r	5	7–6	4	3	3–4	5

(continued)

Developmental Norms for Phonemes

(continued)

Phonemes	Wellman (1934)	Poole (1934)	Templin (1957)	Sander (1972)	Prather (1975)	Arlt (1976)
tʃ (ch)	5	–	4–6	4	3–8	4
v	5	6–6	6	4	4+	3–6
z	5	7–6	7	4	4+	4
ʒ	6	6–6	7	6	4	4
θ	–	7–6	6	5	4+	5
dʒ	–	–	7	4	4+	4
ʃ	–	6–6	4	4	3–8	4–6
ð	–	6–6	7	5	4	5

Note: + sound not mastered by 75% of tested children
   – sound not tested or reported

Arlt, P. B., & Goodban, M. T. (1976). A comparative study of articulation acquisition as based on a study of 240 normals, aged three to six. *Language, Speech, and Hearing Services in Schools, 7,* 173–180. (Criterion: 75% of children tested in all three word positions.)

Poole, I. (1934). Genetic development of consonant sounds in English. *Elementary English Review, 11,* 159–161. (Criterion: 100% of children tested in all three word positions.)

Prather, E. M., Hedrick, E. L., & Kerin, C. A. (1975). Articulation development in children aged two to four years. *Journal of Speech and Hearing Disorders, 40,* 179–191. (Criterion: 75% of children tested; average for initial and final word positions.)

Sander, E. K. (1972). When are speech sounds learned? *Journal of Speech and Hearing Disorders, 37,* 55–63. (Reanalysis of Templin and Wellman et al.'s data with a criterion of 51%.)

Templin, M. C. (1957). *Certain language skills in children. Institute of Child Welfare Monograph Series No. 26.* Minneapolis, MN: University of Minnesota Press. (Criterion: 75% of children tested in all three word positions.)

Wellman, B., Case, L, Mengert, I., & Bradbury, D. (1931). Speech sounds of young children. *State University of Iowa Studies in Child Welfare, 5*(2). (Criterion: 75% of children tested in all three word positions.)

Diadachokinetic Rate. The same as Alternating Motion Rates (AMRs).

Diagnosis. A clinical activity designed to find causes of diseases or disorders, especially in medicine and medical speech-language pathology; in communicative disorders for which there are no known physical or neurological cause, diagnosis often is aimed at describing and assessing the degree of severity of disorders; requires precise and reliable measurement of communicative behaviors; sometimes means the same as Assessment.

- Take a case history
- Interview the client
- Screen hearing
- Conduct an orofacial examination
- Administer standardized tests that are culturally and linguistically appropriate for the client
- Design and use client-specific procedures
- Take a comprehensive speech-language sample
- Analyze the results and make a clinical judgment
- Write a diagnostic report which includes recommendations

Differential Diagnosis. Distinguishing disorders that present some common or similar symptoms; usually done with the help of a symptom complex and, whenever possible, by identifying different underlying factors or causes.

Diplophonia. Double voice resulting from differential vibration of the two folds or vibration of both the true and false vocal folds.

Distinctive Features. Unique characteristics of phonemes that distinguish one phoneme from the other; each feature is scored as + (for its presence) or − (for its absence); may be used in economically describing errors of articulation and their changes in treatment; Chomsky and Halle's major distinctive features as applied to consonants are shown in the matrix and the definition of the features follow:

Distinctive Features

	Con	Son	Hi	Bck	Rnd	Ant	Cor	Voi	Cnt	Nas	Str
p	+	−	−	−	−	+	−	−	−	−	−
b	+	−	−	−	−	+	−	+	−	−	−
t	+	−	−	−	−	+	+	−	−	−	−
d	+	−	−	−	−	+	+	+	−	−	−
k	+	−	+	+	−	−	−	−	−	−	−
g	+	−	+	+	−	−	−	+	−	−	−
f	+	−	−	−	−	+	−	−	+	−	+
v	+	−	−	−	−	+	−	+	+	−	+
θ	+	−	−	−	−	+	+	−	+	−	−
ð	+	−	−	−	−	+	+	+	+	−	−
s	+	−	−	−	−	+	+	−	+	−	+
z	+	−	−	−	−	+	+	+	+	−	+
ʃ	+	−	+	−	−	−	+	−	+	−	+
tʃ	+	−	+	−	−	−	+	−	−	−	+
dʒ	+	−	+	−	−	−	+	+	−	−	+
j	−	+	+	−	−	−	−	+	+	−	−
r	+	+	−	−	−	−	+	+	+	−	−
l	+	+	−	−	−	+	+	+	+	−	−
w	−	+	+	+	+	−	−	+	+	−	−
m	+	+	−	−	−	+	−	+	−	+	−
n	+	+	−	−	−	+	+	+	−	+	−
ŋ	+	+	−	+	−	−	−	+	−	+	−
h	−	−	−	−	−	−	−	−	−	−	−

Con: Consonant (sounds characterized by vocal tract constriction)

Son: Sonorant (sounds with spontaneous voicing because of unobstructed flow of air)

Hi: High (sounds produced with elevated tongue position)

Bck: Back (sounds produced with the tongue retracted)

Rnd: Rounded (sounds made with lip rounding)

Ant: Anterior (sounds produced with point of constriction being relatively anterior; sounds made in the front of the mouth)

Cor: Coronal (sounds produced with raised tongue blade)

Voi: Voiced sounds (sounds produced with vocal fold vibration)

Cnt: Continuant (sounds produced with partial obstruction of airflow; sounds that can be produced in a continuous manner)

Nas: Nasal (sounds produced with nasal resonance)

Str: Strident (sounds produced by forcing airstream through a small opening)

Distinctive Features

Analysis of Distinctive Features of Articulatory Errors
- Record a representative, continuous speech sample; follow the procedures described under <u>Articulation and Phonological Disorders</u>
- Transcribe the speech; list all the errors
- For each error, score the distinctive features using the features listed in the matrix; score features that are correctly used for each sound and those that are misused (voicing a voiceless sound is a misuse of the voicing feature)
- Score all features that characterize omitted sounds as incorrect
- Summarize the missing and misused features
- Target the sounds that contain missing or misused features for treatment

Limitations of the Distinctive Feature Approach
- Scoring all features of omitted sounds as incorrect may not be appropriate because the sounds are not even attempted
- Distinctive features based on acoustic analysis may or may not be directly related to articulatory productions which are physiological events
- Errors of sound productions often are not binary events (presence or absence); but are quantitatively varied
- Distinctive features do not account for sound distortions
- Scoring according to the Chomsky and Halle system is extremely time consuming and complex
- Phonological analysis seems to be preferred over distinctive feature analysis
- Note that, as you make a phonological analysis, distinctive features that are missing or help group errors may be accomplished to obtain a different view of the error patterns

Bernthal, J. E., & Bankson, N. W. (1998). *Articulation and phonological disorders* (4th ed.). Englewood Cliffs, NJ: Prentice-Hall.

Bleile, K. M. (1995). *Manual of articulation and phonological disorders.* San Diego, CA: Singular Publishing Group.

Creaghead, N. A., Newman, P. W., & Secord, W. A. (1989). *Assessment and remediation of articulatory and phonological disorders* (2nd ed.). Columbus, OH: Merrill Publishing Company.

Dynamic Aphasia

Elbert, M., & Gierut, J. (1986). *Handbook of clinical phonology.* San Diego, CA: College-Hill Press.

Lowe, R. J. (1994). *Phonology: Assessment and intervention applications in speech pathology.* Baltimore, MD: Williams & Wilkins.

Stoel-Gammon, C., & Dunn, C. (1985). *Normal and disordered phonology in children.* Austin, TX: Pro-Ed.

Dynamic Aphasia. The same as transcortical motor aphasia (see Aphasia: Specific Types).

Dysarthrias. A group of motor speech disorders resulting from disturbed muscular control of the speech mechanism due to damage of the peripheral or central nervous system; oral communication problems due to weakness, incoordination, or paralysis of speech musculature; physiologic characteristics include abnormal or disturbed strength, speed, range, steadiness, tone, and accuracy of muscle movements; communication characteristics include disturbed pitch, loudness, voice quality, resonance, respiratory support for speech, prosody, and articulation; may be congenital or acquired, although much of the information presented here is most relevant to acquired disorders in adults; may be chronic, improving, progressive, or exacerbating-remitting; associated with the diagnosis of a neurological condition or disease; the most frequently occurring disorder among the neurogenic communication disorders; classified into types including ataxic dysarthria, flaccid dysarthria, hyperkinetic dysarthria, hypokinetic dysarthria, mixed dysarthria, spastic dysarthria, and unilateral upper motor neuron dysarthria; use this section to make a general assessment of dysarthria and see Dysarthria: Specific Types to distinguish among them.

Etiology
- Varied etiologies, including vascular, traumatic, infectious, neoplastic, metabolic, toxic, and other factors creating neuropathology
- The site of lesion may be the central nervous system, the peripheral nervous system, or both
- Variation in the etiological factors results in different types of dysarthria

Dysarthrias

- The effects of the varied etiological factors are the problems in the motor control of speech
- The basic etiological factors include
  - degenerative neurological diseases including Parkinson's disease, Wilson's disease, progressive supranuclear palsy, dystonia, Huntington's disease, amyotrophic lateral sclerosis (ALS), multiple sclerosis, myasthenia gravis, and Friedreich's ataxia
  - nonprogressive neurological conditions including stroke
  - infections
  - traumatic brain injury
  - surgical trauma
  - congenital conditions including cerebral palsy and Moebius syndrome
  - encephalitis
  - toxic effects from alcohol, drugs, and so forth

Common Sites of Lesions
- Lower motor neuron
- Unilateral or bilateral upper motor neuron
- Cerebellum
- Basal ganglia (extrapyramidal)

Pathophysiology
- Weakness
- Spasticity
- Incoordination
- Rigidity and reduced range of movement
- Involuntary movements

Neuromuscular Effects
- Reduced strength of movement
- Reduced or variable speed of movement
- Reduced or variable range of movement
- Unsteady movement
- Increased, decreased, or variable tone
- Inaccurate movement

Communication Disorders
- Respiratory problems
  - forced inspirations that interrupt speech

D

- forced expirations that interrupt speech
- audible or breathy inspiration
- grunt at end of expiration
- Phonatory disorders
  - pitch too high or too low for the individual
  - abrupt variations in pitch resulting in pitch breaks
  - lack of variations in pitch resulting in monopitch and lack of inflection
  - shaky or tremulous voice
  - diplophonia, simultaneous production of both a lower and a higher pitch
  - too soft or too loud speech
  - lack of variation in loudness, resulting in monoloudness
  - sudden and excessive variation in loudness resulting in too loud or too soft speech
  - loudness decay or progressive decrease in loudness resulting in too soft speech toward the end of utterances
  - alternating changes in loudness
  - harsh, rough, gravely voice
  - hoarse and "wet" voice which is "liquid sounding" hoarseness
  - continuously breathy voice
  - intermittently breathy voice
  - strained-strangled, effortful phonation
  - sudden and uncontrolled cessation of voice
- Articulation disorders
  - imprecise production of consonants
  - prolongation of phonemes
  - repetition of phonemes
  - irregular breakdowns in articulation
  - distortion of vowels
  - weak pressure consonants
- Prosodic disorders
  - slower than the normal rate of speech
  - excessively rapid rate of speech
  - an overall fast rate
  - progressive increase in rate in certain segments of speech

D

- variable rate of speech
- shorter phrase lengths
- reduced stress on stressed syllables
- equal stress on stressed and unstressed syllables
- excessive stress on unstressed syllables
- prolongation of intervals between words or syllables
- inappropriate pauses (silent intervals) in speech
- short rushes of speech
- Resonance disorders
  - hypernasality
  - hyponasality
  - nasal emission
- Other characteristics
  - slow diadochokinetic rate or alternating motion rate (AMRs)
  - fast diadochokinetic rate or AMRs
  - irregular diadochokinetic rate or AMRs
  - palilalia (compulsive repetition of one's own utterances with increasing rate and decreasing loudness)
- Global characteristics of communication
  - decreased intelligibility of speech
  - bizarreness of speech because of its unusualness or peculiarity

Assessment Objectives/General Guidelines
- To determine whether dysarthria is the diagnosis
- To determine the specific respiratory, phonatory, articulatory, and prosodic characteristics of speech
- To judge the severity of the disorder
- To judge whether further assessment to specify the type of dysarthria is necessary
- To make a differential diagnosis
- To determine potential treatment targets
- To suggest prognosis

Case History/Interview Focus
- See **Case History** and **Interview** under Standard/Common Assessment Procedures

D

- Concentrate on a detailed health history; onset of the diseases and change in its course; behavioral changes and signs of neurologic disorder

Ethnocultural Considerations
- See Ethnocultural Considerations in Assessment

Assessment
- Take a conversational speech sample; take note of the manner and content of speech as you interview the client
- Record a reading sample; have the client read the *Grandfather Passage*
- Use a variety of speech tasks including imitation of syllables, words, phrases, and sentences; production of modeled syllables, words, phrases, and sentences, sustained phonation (vowel prolongation)
- Assess the Diadochokinetic Rate or Alternating Motion Rates (ARMs) and Sequential Motion Rates (SMRs)
- Assess the speech production mechanism during non-speech activities
  - observe the face at rest; take note of symmetry, tone, signs of tension, droopiness, expressive or mask-like, and the presence of involuntary movements and tremors
  - observe the movements of the facial structures by asking the patient to puff the cheeks; retract and round the lips; bite the lower lip; blow; smack the lips; open and close the mouth; maintain an opened posture of the mouth; and so forth
  - observe the patient's emotional expressions
  - take note of the patient's jaw at rest; its range of movement and tone; its deviation to one or the other side during movement; resistance offered as you try to close it or open it
  - observe the tongue as you ask the patient to protrude, move it from side to side as fast as possible; lick the lips; push the cheeks out with it; resist your attempts to push the protruded tongue back; and so forth
  - observe the velopharyngeal mechanism as the patient says "ah"; take note of movement, its symmetry, range,

and adequacy; assess nasal airflow by holding a mirror at the nares as the patient prolongs the vowel /i/
- assess laryngeal functions by asking the patient to cough; take note of weak cough associated with weak adduction of the folds, inadequate breath support, or both

• Assess respiratory problems
- observe the patient's posture that might affect breathing; take note of erect or slouched posture
- observe the patient's breathing habits during quiet and speech; take note of rapid, shallow, or effortful breathing, signs of shortness of breath, and irregularity of inhalation and exhalation, and so forth

• Assess phonatory disorders
- have the patient to say "ah" after taking a deep breath; ask the patient to sustain it as steadily and for as long as the air supply lasts; if the patient's pitch or loudness changes, request a more normal repetition of the task; specify whether the patient should try to lower or raise the pitch or loudness; see Maximum Phonation Duration for normative values
- during interview and conversational speech, take note of the patient's pitch level; judge or rate its appropriateness to the patient
- take note of pitch breaks and abrupt variations in pitch
- judge whether pitch variations are normal or absent resulting in monopitch
- take note of voice tremors as the patient speaks
- assess the presence of diplophonia
- judge the appropriateness of vocal loudness; take note of too soft or too loud voice; take note of loudness that is highly variable
- take note of loudness decay and alternating changes in loudness
- judge the quality of voice; take note of hoarseness, harshness, and breathiness; take note of their severity and consistency
- judge whether the voice production is strained or effortful

- take note of sudden cessations of voice
- Assess articulation disorders
  - use the speech sample and standardized test results
  - rate or evaluate consonant productions; judge the precision with which they are produced
  - evaluate the duration of speech sounds; take note of prolongation of phonemes
  - record phoneme repetitions
  - take note of irregular breakdowns in articulation
  - assess the precision with which vowels are produced; take note of distortions
  - judge the adequacy of pressure consonantal productions
- Assess prosodic disorders
  - measure the rate of speech; judge whether the rate is normal, slower than the normal, or excessively fast
  - judge whether the speech rate is highly variable; take note of progressive increase in rate in segments of speech
  - measure phrase lengths in selected portions of speech; judge their adequacy
  - evaluate stress patterns in speech; take note of inappropriate stress patterns including even stress, lack of stress, and undue stress on normally unstressed syllables
  - take note of pauses in speech; judge whether they are at appropriate or inappropriate junctures and whether they are too long
  - take note of any short rushes of speech
- Assess resonance disorders
  - make clinical judgments as you listen to the client's speech or make an instrumental analysis; see Voice Disorders
  - take note of hypernasality, hyponasality, and nasal emission
- Assess other characteristics
  - take note of palilalia; evaluate the rate at which repetitions occur; observe whether loudness of such repetitions decrease as the rate increases

Dysarthrias

- Assess the global characteristics of communication
  - assess speech intelligibility; note that intelligibility may not always be negatively affected in dysarthria
  - make a clinical judgment of intelligibility, which may be adequate in many cases; estimate the percentage of words or phrases that you understand
  - use a rating scale to more formally evaluate intelligibility in cases where this is warranted

Standardized Tests
- Administer one of the following tests

Test	Purpose
Assessment of Intelligibility of Dysarthria Speakers (K. M. Yorkston & D. Beukelman)	To assess single-word and sentence intelligibility and rate of speech
Dysarthria Examination Battery (S. S. Drummond)	To assess severity of dysarthria and functional communication
Frenchay Dysarthria Assessment (P. M. Enderby)	To assess speech related structures and function in dysarthric speakers and to distinguish different types of dysarthria

Related/Medical Assessment Data
- Patient's medical-neurological diagnosis
- Current medication and their side effects
- Current and future medical treatment plans for the patient
- Medical prognosis
- Radiologic and brain imaging data that might be integrated or correlated with speech diagnosis
- Physical rehabilitation plans that might affect communication treatment
- Audiologic findings that might be integrated with communication assessment

Standard/Common Assessment Procedures
- Complete the <u>Standard/Common Assessment Procedures</u>

Dysarthrias

Analysis of Assessment Data

- Analyze and summarize the assessment data to determine the nature of physiologic (speech movement related), respiratory, articulatory, prosodic, phonatory, and resonance disorders
- Integrate the findings with medical-neurologic assessment data to obtain a comprehensive profile of the patient's physiologic, neurologic, and behavioral (including communication) performance
- Rate the severity of the disturbances noted; use the rating scale described in Duffy (1995)

Diagnostic Criteria

- Clear evidence of peripheral or central nervous system damage
- An associated medical-neurological diagnosis with clear evidence of disturbed strength, speed, range, steadiness, tone, and accuracy of movement patterns
- Speech characteristics that support a diagnosis of dysarthria, including disturbed phonation, articulation, prosody, and resonance and supplemented by disturbed respiratory support for speech

Differential Diagnosis

- Initially, determine if the diagnosis is dysarthria
- If dysarthria, then proceed to make further assessment to determine the type of dysarthria (see <u>Dysarthria: Specific Types</u>); consider the overall picture of the client, but generally speaking:
  - if neuromotor weakness, hypotonia, and diminished reflexes are the dominant neuromotor symptoms and hypernasality, continuous breathiness, nasal emission, audible inspiration, and short phrases are the dominant communication problems, consider flaccid dysarthria
  - if spasticity is the dominant neuromotor sign and imprecise consonants, harshness of voice, low pitch, slow rate, short phrases, and pitch breaks are the dominant communication problems, consider spastic dysarthria

206

- if incoordination is the dominant neuromotor sign and excess and equal stress, irregular articulatory breakdowns, distorted vowels, prolonged phonemes, and excess loudness variations are the dominant communication problems, consider ataxic dysarthria
- if rigidity and reduced range of movement are the dominant neuromotor sign and monopitch, monoloudness, reduced stress, inappropriate silences, short rushes of speech, variable or increased rate, and repetitions of phonemes are the dominant communication problems, consider hypokinetic dysarthria
- if involuntary movements are the dominant neuromotor sign and prolonged intervals, variable rate, inappropriate silences, excess loudness variations, prolonged phonemes, sudden forced inspiration or expiration, voice stoppages, and transient breathiness are the dominant communication problems, consider hyperkinetic dysarthria
- if a combination of weakness and spasticity seems to be the dominant neuromotor symptom and imprecise articulation, slow diadochokinetic rate, and harshness are the dominant communication problems, and the brain imaging data suggest unilateral lesions involving the upper motor neurons, consider unilateral upper motor neuron dysarthria
- if multiple neuromotor characteristics and a heterogeneous cluster of communication disorders are evident, consider mixed dysarthria
- see the separate alphabetical entries for different types of dysarthria for assessment procedures
- Distinguish dysarthria from apraxia of speech and other neurogenic speech disorders
- Distinguish dysarthria from aphasia
- Distinguish dysarthria from dementia
- Distinguish dysarthria from language of confusion
- Distinguish dysarthria from other relevant disorders based on the characteristics listed in the following grids (adapted from Hegde, 1998):

Dysarthrias

Dysarthria or Apraxia of Speech?

Dysarthria	Apraxia of Speech
The cause is muscle weakness, paralysis, or incoordination	The cause is motor programming deficit, not muscle weakness
Lesions in supratentorial and other areas (including posterior fossa, spinal structures, or peripheral nerves)	Lesions often in the Supratentorial Level of the brain
Huntington's chorea, Parkinsonism, Pick's disease, and ALS *are* associated with dysarthrias	Huntington's chorea, Parkinsonism, Pick's disease, and ALS *are* not associated with apraxia
Often associated with abnormalities of orofacial mechanism and function	Can be associated with normal orofacial mechanism and function (except for NVOA)
NVOA not typically associated with dysarthrias	NVOA may be associated with AOS
Presence of dysphagia	Absence of dysphagia
Consistent misarticulations (except for ataxic dysarthria in which articulatory breakdowns are irregular)	Variable misarticulations
The same problems with automatic and propositional productions	Better production of automatic utterances than propositional productions
Word length (except for an ataxic dysarthria), meaningfulness, frequency of occurrence are not significant variables	Word length, meaningfulness frequency of occurrence are significant variables
Distortions and simplification of speech gestures are dominant	Besides distortions, complications of speech gestures may be noticeable
Less frequent and less variable dysfluencies	More frequent and variable dysfluencies
	(continued)

(continued)

Dysarthria	Apraxia of Speech
Articulatory groping not characteristic	Frequent articulatory groping
Few, if any attempts at self-correction	Many attempts at self-correction
Respiratory, phonatory, and resonance problems as significant as articulatory and prosodic problems	Respiratory, phonatory, and resonance problems not as significant as articulatory and prosodic problems
Most forms (except for UUMN dysarthria) infrequently associated with aphasia	Frequently associated with aphasia

Dysarthria or Aphasia?

Dysarthria	Aphasia
Neurogenic speech disorder	Neurogenic language disorder
Lesions in the central nervous system, peripheral nervous system, or both	Lesions in the dominant or the left hemisphere language areas and related subcortical structures
Weakness, paralysis, incoordination of orofacial muscles are a distinguishing characteristic	Except in cases of facial paralysis, normal oral mechanism
Does not affect auditory comprehension and reading	Affects auditory comprehension and reading
No significant word-finding problems	Word retrieval and related language problem
No problems in language formulation or interpretation	Significant problems in language formulation and interpretation
Prosodic problems are characteristic	Prosodic problems not dominant, especially in fluent aphasias

Dysarthrias

Dysarthria or the Language of Dementia?

Dysarthria	Dementia
A neurogenic speech disorder	A neurogenic language/cognitive disorder
Motor system affected from the beginning	Motor system is spared until the final stages of the disease
Many patients with dysarthria. do not exhibit dementia	Many patients with dementia may exhibit dysarthria, especially in the later stages
Impaired speech functions	Impaired language
Intact cognition	Impaired cognition
Intact reading comprehension	Disturbed reading comprehension
Intact semantic and syntactic functions	Semantic and syntactic errors in the initial stages
Errors of articulation prominent from the beginning	Errors of articulation not predominant; such errors appear only in later stages
Behavior is relevant, socially appropriate, and not disorganized	Behavior often is irrelevant, socially inappropriate, and disorganized
Mentally not confused and not disoriented to time and space	Mentally confused and disoriented to time and space
No disorientation to self	Disorientation to self in later stages

Caution: There is less information on the relationshiop between dysarthria and dementia. In later stages, patients with dementia exhibit motor speech disorders; dysarthria in such cases may be of the mixed variety. Early stages of subcortical dementias may be associated with dysarthria.

Dysarthrias

Dysarthria or the Language of Confusion?

Dysarthria	Language of Confusion
A neurogenic speech disorder	A neurogenic language disorder
More varied etiology including traumatic brain injury and toxic and metabolic disturbances	Traumatic brain injury and toxic and metabolic disturbances in most cases
Typically relevant	Typically irrelevant
Attentional deficits not the most striking	Attentional deficits are the most striking
Symptoms are more stable	Symptoms are more transient
Greater number of articulation problems	Fewer articulation problems
Speaking problems dominant; no significant writing problems	Writing problems often greater than speaking problems
No confabulation	Confabulation
No disorientation	Disoriented to time, place, and persons
Normal behavior	Significant behavioral change

Note: In cases of dementing dysarthrias, disorientation and behavioral changes may be present; in cases of traumatic head injury, dysarthria and language of confusion may coexist. However, dysarthria due to head injury may have a better chance of improvement.

Dysarthria or Neurogenic Stuttering?

Dysarthria	Neurogenic Stuttering
Dysfluencies occur mostly on initial sounds and syllables	Dysfluencies can occur on final and medial sounds and syllables as well

(continued)

Dysarthria or Neurogenic Stuttering? *(continued)*

Dysarthria	Neurogenic Stuttering
Dysfluencies consistent with other symptoms of dysarthria (e.g., reduced range of movement, rapid rate)	Dysfluencies may not be consistent with other symptoms of dysarthria
Dysfluent productions are characterized by imprecise articulation	Imprecise articulation may not be a characteristic of neurogenic stuttering in the absence of dysarthria

Note: Both dysarthria and neurogenic stuttering are speech disorders. Dysfluencies are often present in hypokinetic dysarthria; they are not characteristic of flaccid dysarthria. Information on different varieties of neurogenic stuttering and characteristics of dysfluencies in dysarthria is limited.

Dysarthria or Palilalia?

Dysarthria	Palilalia
Varied sites of lesions in the central and the peripheral nervous systems	Bilateral lesions typically in the basal ganglia
Typically, sound and syllable dysfluencies without necessarily increasing rate and decreasing loudness	Typically, word and phrase repetitions with increasing rate and decreasing loudness
Dysfluencies at the beginning of utterances	Dysfluencies at the end of utterances

Note: Palilalia is more commonly associated with hypokinetic dysarthria than any other type. In such cases, make a dual diagnosis of dysarthria and palilalia. Dysarthric speakers may have dysfluencies that do not suggest palilalia; just describe those dysfluencies.

Prognosis
- Highly variable, depending on the underlying neuropathology, its severity, course, general health, and med-

ical and rehabilitative treatment potential of individual patients

- Potential to maintain, improve, augment, or supplement communication skills is good enough in most cases to recommend treatment

Recommendations

- Communication treatment based on the individual patient's needs and strengths
- See the cited sources and *PGTSLP* for details

Darley, F. L., Aronson, A. E., & Brown, J. R. (1975). *Motor speech disorders*. Philadelphia: W. B. Saunders.

Duffy, J. R. (1995). *Motor speech disorders*. St. Louis, MO: C. V. Mosby.

Freed, D. (2001). *Motor speech disorders: Diagnosis and treatment*. San Diego: Singular Thomson Learning.

Johns, D. F. (Ed.). (1985). *Clinical management of neurogenic communicative disorders*. Boston: Little, Brown

Yorkston, K. M., Beukelman, D. R., & Bell, K. R. (1988). *Clinical management of dysarthric speakers*. Austin, TX: Pro-Ed.

Dysarthria: Specific Types. Variations in etiologic factors and symptoms of dysarthria that allow for a typological classification; consider the general symptoms, etiology, and assessment procedures described under Dysarthrias along with features unique to specific types described under this entry:

Ataxic Dysarthria. A type of motor speech disorder involving damage to the cerebellar system; characterized by slow, inaccurate movement and Hypotonia; distinguished from other types by its dominant articulatory and prosodic problems; basic cause is bilateral or generalized cerebellar lesions, degenerative ataxia including Friedreich's ataxia and olivopontocerebellar atrophy, cerebellar vascular lesions, tumors, traumatic brain injury, toxic conditions including alcohol abuse, drug toxicity, and such inflammatory conditions as meningitis and encephalitis; use the assessment procedures described under Dysarthrias and focus on the following that apply especially to ataxic dysarthria:

Major Symptoms

- Abnormal stance and gait; instability of the trunk and head, involving tremors and rocking motions; rotated or tilted head posture; hypotonia
- Ocular motor abnormalities
- Movement disorders: Over- or undershooting of targets; discoordinated movements; jerky, inaccurate, slow, imprecise, and halting movements
  - articulation disorders: imprecise production of consonants; irregular breakdowns in articulation; and distortion of vowels
  - prosodic disorders: excessive and even stress; prolonged phonemes and intervals between words or syllables; slow rate of speech
  - phonatory disorders: monopitch, monoloudness, and harshness
  - drunken speech quality

Diagnostic Criteria

- Clear evidence of cerebellar damage and a supportive neurologic diagnosis
- Listed speech characteristics

Differential Diagnosis

- Possible confusion between ataxic dysarthria and hyperkinetic dysarthria
  - the two are distinguished by involuntary movements of the jaw, face, and tongue (present in hyperkinetic dysarthria, absent in ataxic dysarthria)
  - strained-strangled voice quality, audible inspiration, voice tremor, and voice stoppages of hyperkinetic dysarthria are not prominent in ataxic dysarthria
- Possible confusion between ataxic dysarthria and unilateral upper motor neuron (UMN) dysarthria
  - the two are distinguished by unilateral lower facial and lingual weakness (present in UMN dysarthria and absent in ataxic dysarthria)

- distorted vowels, prolonged phonemes, and prosodic problems of ataxic dysarthria are not prominent in UMN dysarthria

Recommendations

- Communication treatment with an emphasis on modifying rate and prosody

Flaccid Dysarthria. A type of motor speech disorder due to damage to the motor units of cranial or spinal nerves that supply speech muscles (lower motor neuron involvement); neurologists tend to describe this as bulbar palsy; various causes including degenerative, vascular, traumatic, infectious, neoplastic, metabolic, toxic, and other factors creating neuropathology; such diseases as myasthenia gravis and botulism; vascular diseases and brainstem strokes; infections including polio, secondary infections in AIDS patients, and herpes zoster (a viral infection that tends to affect the Vth and VIIth nerve ganglia); demyelinating diseases including Guillain-Barré syndrome; myotonic muscular dystrophy; degenerative diseases including motor neuron diseases, progressive bulbar palsy, and amyotrophic lateral sclerosis (ALS); surgical trauma during neurosurgery, laryngeal and facial surgery, and chest/cardiac surgery; injury to the laryngeal branches of the vagus nerve; use the assessment procedures described under Dysarthrias and focus on the following that apply especially to flaccid dysarthria:

Common Sites of Lesions

- Trigeminal (Vth) nerve; bilateral damage to the motor branch causes significant articulation disorders involving bilabial, linguadental, and lingual-alveolar sounds; vowels may be distorted
- Facial (VIIth) nerve; unilateral and bilateral damage can cause articulation disorders involving bilabial and labiodental sounds; patient may be unable to produce them; pressure consonants may be weak
- Glossopharyngeal (IXth) nerve; isolated damage uncommon; usually associated with a lesion in the Xth nerve; effects on speech not clear

- Vagus (Xth) nerve; lesions cause breathiness, diplophonia, reduced pitch, pitch breaks, reduced loudness, short phrases, and mild to moderate hypernasality
- Accessory (XIth) nerve; effects on speech unclear or minimal; any effect it has is intertwined with that of the Xth nerve
- Hypoglossal (XIIth) nerve; involvement produces imprecise articulation
- Spinal nerve lesions, although their role in flaccid dysarthria is not well understood; possible indirect effects on respiration
- Multiple cranial nerve damage (bulbar palsy); a combination of effects depending on the specific nerves involved

Major Symptoms

- Muscle weakness, hypotonia, muscle atrophy, and diminished reflexes
- Fasciculations (isolated twitches of resting muscles) and fibrillations (contractions of individual muscles)
- Rapid and progressive weakness with use and recovery with rest (especially with neuromuscular junction diseases)
- Respiratory disorders: respiratory weakness in combination with cranial nerve weakness
- Phonatory disorders: breathy voice; audible inspiration; short phrases
- Resonance disorders: hypernasality; imprecise consonants (mostly due to resonance problems); nasal emission; and short phrases
- Phonatory-prosodic disorders: harsh voice; monopitch, and monoloudness
- Articulation disorders: May be significant especially with lesions of Vth, VIIth, and XIIth cranial nerves

Diagnostic Criteria

- Clear evidence of lesion in one or more of the cranial nerves; an associated medical-neurological diagnosis when appropriate; and the listed dominant phonatory and resonatory speech problems

Differential Diagnosis

- Breathiness, audible inspiration, and short phrases that characterize flaccid dysarthria are less pronounced in other types of dysarthria
- Hypernasality that occurs in spastic and hypokinetic dysarthrias is much more prominent in flaccid dysarthria
- Short phrases that occur in spastic and hyperkinetic dysarthria are not associated with other kinds of evidence of vocal fold weakness that are present in flaccid dysarthria
- Audible nasal emission that characterizes flaccid dysarthria is rare in other types
- Rapid speech deterioration and recovery after rest found in flaccid dysarthria are rare in other types of dysarthria

Recommendations

- Treatment to improve communication

Hyperkinetic Dysarthria. A type of motor speech disorder caused by damage to basal ganglia (extrapyramidal system); resulting in involuntary movement and variable muscle tone; a dominant symptom is prosodic disturbance; varied causes including degenerative, vascular, traumatic, infectious, neoplastic, and metabolic factors; also caused by neuroleptic and antipsychotic drugs that cause dyskinesia and dystonia and such degenerative diseases as Huntington's Disease; causes unknown in a majority of cases (about 59%); affected structures include the muscles of the face, jaw, tongue, palate, larynx, and respiration; use the assessment procedures described under Dysarthrias and focus on the following that apply especially to hyperkinetic dysarthria:

Major Symptoms

- Predominance of a variety of movement disorders mostly because of damage to the basal ganglia control circuit

- Orofacial dyskinesia (abnormal and involuntary movements)
- Myoclonus (involuntary jerks of body parts; may be single or repetitive; rhythmic or nonrhythmic); tics of the face and shoulders; tremor (involuntary trembling or quivering); chorea (random, rapid, and apparently meaningless movements)
- Ballism (abrupt and severe contractions of the extremities) and athetosis (writhing, involuntary movements, often in hands)
- Dystonia, which results from contractions of antagonistic muscles resulting in abnormal postures; spasmodic torticollis (intermittent dystonia and spasm of the neck muscles)
- Blepharospasm (forceful and involuntary closure of the eyes due to spasm of the orbicularis oculi muscle)
- Spasm (a sudden and involuntary contraction of a muscle or group of muscles); may be tonic (prolonged or continuous) or clonic (repetitive, rapid, brief in duration)
- Varied communication disorders depending on whether the dominant neurological condition is chorea, dystonia, athetosis, spasmodic torticollis, and so forth
- Phonatory disorders: voice tremor; intermittently strained voice; voice stoppage; vocal noise; harsh voice
- Resonance disorders: intermittent hypernasality
- Prosodic disorders: slower rate; excess loudness variations; prolonged inter-word intervals; inappropriate silent intervals; equal stress
- Respiratory problems: audible inspiration; forced and sudden inspiration/expiration
- Articulation disorders: imprecise consonants; distortion of vowels; inconsistent articulatory errors

Diagnostic Criteria
- Clear evidence of lesion or disease resulting in chorea, dystonia, athetosis, spasmodic torticollis, and so forth; associated medical-neurological diagnosis when appropriate

- Listed communication disorders

Differential Diagnosis
- Involuntary movements of the face and mouth distinguish hyperkinetic dysarthria from other types
- Regularity of vocal tremor and stoppages in conjunction with movement disorders also help distinguish hyperkinetic dysarthria from other types

Recommendations
- Treatment to improve communication

Hypokinetic Dysarthria. A type of motor speech disorder caused by damage to basal ganglia (extrapyramidal system); caused by varied factors including such degenerative diseases as progressive supranuclear palsy, Parkinson's disease (much more commonly) and Alzheimer's disease, Pick's disease; vascular disorders resulting in multiple or bilateral strokes, repeated head trauma, inflammation, tumor, antipsychotic or neuroleptic drug toxicity, and normal pressure hydrocephalus; the most typical form produced by Parkinson's disease although dysarthria occurs only in about half of the patients with Parkinson's disease; use the assessment procedures described under Dysarthrias and focus on the following that apply especially to hypokinetic dysarthria:

Major Symptoms
- Tremor at rest (tremor in relaxed facial, mouth, and limb structures that diminish when moved voluntarily; *pill-rolling* movement between the thumb and the forefinger);
- Rigidity; bradykinesia; hypokinesia
- Lack of facial expression (mask-like face); infrequent blinking; lack of smiling; reduced hand and facial movements during speech
- Micrographic writing (small print)
- Walking disorders (slow to begin, then short, rapid, shuffling steps)
- Postural disturbances (involuntary flexion of the head, trunk, and arm; difficulty changing positions)

- Decreased swallowing resulting in accumulated saliva in the mouth, possibly drooling
- Phonatory disorders: monopitch; monoloudness; harsh voice; continuously breathy voice; low pitch
- Prosodic disorders: reduced stress; inappropriate silent intervals; short rushes of speech; variable and increased rate in segments; short phrases
- Articulation disorders: imprecise consonants; repeated phonemes; resonance disorders; mild hypernasality (in about 25% of the cases)
- Respiratory problems: reduced vital capacity, irregular breathing, and faster rate of respiration

Diagnostic Criteria
- Evidence of lesion in the basal ganglia and the listed neurologic symptoms
- An associated medical-neurological diagnosis when appropriate
- Listed dominant phonatory and prosodic problems

Differential Diagnosis
- Hypokinesia, bradykinesia, and other neuromotor symptoms of hypokinetic dysarthria are not prominent in other types of dysarthria
- Dominant phonatory and prosodic problems, including monopitch, monoloudness, reduced loudness, reduced stress, inappropriate silent intervals, variable rate, short rushes of speech, and in some cases, increased rate distinguish hypokinetic dysarthria

Prognosis
- Varies with the associated neurologic disease and other factors listed under Dysarthrias

Recommendations
- Treatment to improve communication

Mixed Dysarthria. A type of motor speech disorder that is a combination of two or more pure dysarthrias; the neuropathology is varied and often multiple; any and all combinations of pure dysarthrias are possible; two types are mixed in about 84% of cases; three types may be mixed in about 12%; the flaccid-spastic dysarthria is the most common (42% of the mixed cases), followed by ataxic-spastic (23%); frequent causes include multiple strokes and degenerative, demyelinating, and vascular diseases; also caused by trauma, tumor, toxicity, infection, and toxic-metabolic diseases (e.g., Wilson's disease); the patterns of speech disorders also are varied and dependent on the types of pure dysarthrias that are mixed; more common than other pure types of dysarthria because more than 34% of all dysarthria patients have it; use the assessment procedures described under Dysarthrias and focus on the following that apply especially to mixed dysarthria:

Major Symptoms

- Constellation of symptoms found in specific types of dysarthria depending on the specific types of dysarthria that are mixed in a given patient
- Constellation of symptoms of mixed flaccid-spastic dysarthria associated with amyotrophic lateral sclerosis; the order of listing suggests most to least severe, as described by Darley, Aronson, and Brown (1969a, 1969b): imprecise production of consonants; hypernasality; harsh voice; slow rate; monopitch; short phrases; distorted vowels; low pitch; monoloudness; excess and equal stress or reduced stress; prolonged intervals; prolonged phonemes; strained-strangled quality; breathiness; audible inspiration; inappropriate silences; nasal emission

Diagnostic Criteria

- Evidence of lesion, often in multiple sites and an associated medical-neurologic diagnosis when appropriate
- Constellation of communication disorders as listed

Differential Diagnosis

- Differentiate the types of dysarthria that are mixed; use the guidelines given under specific types of dysarthria

Recommendations

- Treatment to improve communication

D

Spastic Dysarthria. A type of motor speech disorder caused by bilateral damage to the upper motor neuron (direct and indirect motor pathways); varied causes of neuropathology including degenerative, vascular, traumatic, metabolic, toxic, and other factors; lesions in multiple areas including cortical areas, basal ganglia, internal capsule, pons, and medulla; use the assessment procedures described under <u>Dysarthrias</u> and focus on the following that apply especially to spastic dysarthria:

Major Symptoms

- Spasticity; weakness, especially bilateral facial weakness; however, normal jaw strength and less pronounced lower face weakness
- Reduced range of movements; slowness of movement; slow nonspeech alternating motion rates
- Hyperactive gag reflex
- Loss of fine, skilled movement; increased muscle tone
- Generally, impaired movement patterns, not weakness of individual muscles
- Hyperadduction of vocal folds and inadequate closure of the velopharyngeal port
- Prosodic disorders: excess and equal stress; slow rate; monopitch; monoloudness; reduced stress; short phrases
- Articulation disorders: imprecise production of consonants; distorted vowels
- Phonatory disorders: continuous breathy voice; harshness; low pitch; pitch breaks; strained-strangled voice quality; short phrases; slow rate
- Resonance disorders: hypernasality

Diagnostic Criteria

- Evidence of damage to the direct and indirect activation pathways of the upper motor neuron and the resulting physical symptoms listed previously
- An associated medical-neurologic diagnosis when appropriate

- Dominance of slow rate, strained-strangled voice quality, and slow alternating speech-related movements that support a diagnosis of spastic dysarthria

Differential Diagnosis

- Abnormal reflexes, dysphagia, drooling, and uncontrolled crying or laughter support the diagnosis of spastic dysarthria
- The strained-strangled voice quality of hyperkinetic dysarthria is distinguished with its less frequent association with slow alternating motion rates and decreased speech rate, which characterize spastic dysarthria
- Slow rate found in other dysarthrias is less frequently associated with strained-strangled voice quality except in spastic dysarthria
- Slow rate and excess and equal stress are found in both spastic dysarthria and ataxic dysarthria; however, ataxic dysarthria is not associated with strained-strangled voice

Recommendations

- Treatment to improve communication

Unilateral Upper Motor Neuron (UUMN) Dysarthria.
A type of motor speech disorder caused by damage to the upper motor neurons that supply cranial and spinal nerves involved in speech production; most frequent causes of neuropathology are vascular disorders; with left hemisphere lesion, may coexist with aphasia or apraxia; with right hemisphere lesion, may coexist with right hemisphere syndrome; use the assessment procedures described under Dysarthrias and focus on the following that apply especially to UUMN dysarthria as described by Duffy (1995):

Major Symptoms

- Unilateral lower face weakness; unilateral tongue weakness; unilateral palatal weakness; hemiplegia/hemiparesis
- Articulation disorders: imprecise production of consonants, irregular articulatory breakdowns

- Phonatory disorders: harsh voice; reduced loudness; strained-harshness
- Prosodic disorders: slow rate; increased rate in segments; excess and equal stress; monopitch, monoloudness, low pitch, and short phrases may be present in some cases
- Resonance disorders: hypernasality
- Often associated dysphagia, aphasia, apraxia, and right hemisphere syndrome

Diagnostic Criteria
- Evidence of upper motor neuron lesion
- An associated medical-neurologic diagnosis when appropriate
- Dominant communication disorders as listed

Differential Diagnosis
- The presence of central facial weakness on either the right or the left side helps distinguish UUMN dysarthria from other types, except for flaccid dysarthria
- Overall, mild and temporary communication problems of UUMN dysarthria help distinguish it from other types
- Most difficult to distinguish UUMN dysarthria from flaccid and ataxic varieties because all three share imprecise articulation; however, infrequent occurrence of voice and resonance problems in UUMN dysarthria help distinguish it from these two varieties
- More regular alternating movement rates of UUMN dysarthria may help distinguish it from ataxic dysarthria

Recommendations
- Treatment to improve communication
  For details on treating types of dysarthria:
- See the cited sources and *PGTSLP* for details

Brookshire, R. (1997). *An introduction to neurogenic communication disorders* (5th ed.). St. Louis, MO: Mosby Year Book.

Darley, F. L., Aronson, A. E., & Brown, J. R. (1975). *Motor speech disorders*. Philadelphia: W. B. Saunders.

Darley, F. L., Aronson, A. E., & Brown, J. R. (1969a). Differential diagnostic patterns of dysarthria. *Journal of Speech and Hearing Research, 12,* 246–269

Darley, F. L., Aronson, A. E., & Brown, J. R. (1969b). Cluster of deviant speech dimensions in the dysarthrias. *Journal of Speech and Hearing Research, 12,* 462–496.

Duffy, J. R. (1995). *Motor speech disorders.* St. Louis, MO: C. V. Mosby.

Freed, D. (2000). *Motor speech disorders: Diagnosis and treatment.* San Diego: Singular Thomson Learning.

Johns, D. F. (Ed.). (1985). *Clinical management of neurogenic communicative disorders.* Boston: Little, Brown

Yorkston, K. M., Beukelman, D. R., & Bell, K. R. (1988). *Clinical management of dysarthric speakers.* Austin, TX: Pro-Ed.

Dysfluencies.   Behaviors that interrupt fluency; see <u>Stuttering</u> for a description of different forms and their assessment.

Dysgraphia.   Writing problems; the same as <u>Agraphia</u>.

Dysostosis.   Abnormal ossification; anomalous ossification of fetal cartilages; see Treacher-Collins syndrome under <u>Syndromes Associated With Communicative Disorders</u>).

Dysphagia.   Disorders of swallowing; problems in the execution of the oral, pharyngeal, and esophageal stages of swallow; includes problems in chewing the food, preparing it for swallow, initiating the swallow, propelling the bolus through the pharynx, and in passing the food through the esophagus; speech-language pathologists assess and treat oropharyngeal disorders of swallowing; esophageal swallowing disorders handled medically; causes include a variety of physical diseases and disorders including several neuropathologies resulting in paralysis of the muscles involved and cancer and the consequent surgical treatment (laryngectomy); a majority of patients assessed and treated in medical settings because of the associated diseases; may occur at any age although more common in the elderly.

Etiology

• Strokes, especially brainstem and anterior cortical strokes resulting in poor motor control of structures involved in swallowing (including the tongue and cricopharyngeal structures)

- Various neurologic diseases (e.g., Parkinson's disease, amyotrophic lateral sclerosis, multiple sclerosis, myasthenia gravis, muscular dystrophy, and dystonia)
- Tumors in the oral cavity or the pharynx
- Surgical treatment of oral, pharyngeal, and laryngeal cancer
- Any form of head, neck, and gastrointestinal surgery
- Radiation therapy for oral, pharyngeal, and laryngeal cancer
- Neurosurgical procedures
- Traumatic brain injury
- Cervical spine disease
- Poliomyelitis (polio)
- Pulmonary diseases, especially chronic, obstructive, pulmonary disease
- Cerebral palsy
- Dysautonomia (an inherited disorder associated with autonomic imbalance, sensory deficits, and motor incoordination)
- Side effects of certain prescription drugs (e.g., drugs that reduce spasticity, antipsychotic drugs, and neuroleptic drugs)

At-Risk Signals
Patients with the following symptoms are at risk of experiencing or developing swallowing disorders:
- Dysarthria
- Drooling
- Frequent coughing
- Choking on food and sputum
- Difficulty in chewing, excessively slow eating, weight loss
- Reported pain during swallowing; sense of reported obstruction during swallowing
- Confusion associated with neurologic disease or damage

Description of Normal Swallow and Swallowing Disorders
- Mastication: Chewing solid or semisolid food; an activity that precedes swallowing (deglutition)

Dysphagia

- Disorders of mastication: Symptoms include problems in chewing food; causes include reduced range of lateral and vertical tongue movement, reduced range of lateral mandibular movement, reduced buccal tension, and poor alignment of mandible and maxilla
- Oral preparatory phase: Preparation of masticated food for swallow; bolus preparation (collecting the masticated food into a mass)
- Disorders of the oral preparatory phase: Symptoms include difficulty in forming and holding the bolus; abnormal holding of the bolus; food falling into anterior and lateral sulcus; and aspiration before swallow; causes include weak lip closure, reduced tongue movement, inadequate tongue and buccal tension; and tongue thrust
- Oral phase: Begins with the posterior tongue action; moves the bolus posteriorly; ends as the bolus passes through the anterior faucial arches (and the swallowing reflex is initiated)
- Disorders of the oral phase: Symptoms include searching tongue movements; anterior instead of posterior tongue movement; weak tongue movement; food residue in various places (anterior and lateral sulcus, floor of the mouth, tongue surface, hard palate); premature swallow; and aspiration before swallow; causes include apraxia of swallow, tongue thrust, reduced labial, buccal, and tongue tension and strength; and reduced range of tongue movement and elevation
- Pharyngeal phase: Reflex actions of swallow that are triggered by the contact the food makes with the anterior faucial pillars; includes such functions as the velopharyngeal closure, laryngeal closure by an elevated larynx that seals the airway and the consequent interruption in breathing; reflexive relaxation of the cricopharyngeal muscle for the bolus to enter; reflexive contractions of the pharyngeal contractors to move the bolus down and eventually into the esophagus

D

D

- Disorders of the pharyngeal phase: Problems in propelling the bolus through the pharynx and into the P-E segment; symptoms include delayed or absent swallowing reflex; nasal and airway penetration of food; food coating on the pharyngeal walls; food residue in valleculae (space between the base of the tongue and epiglottis), on top of airway, in pyriform sinuses, and throughout the pharynx; aspiration before and after swallow; and generally delayed pharyngeal transmit time; causes include inadequate velopharyngeal closure; mucosal fold at base of the tongue; cervical osteophytes; reduced pharyngeal contractions; pharyngeal paralysis; reduced movement of tongue base; reduced laryngeal movement; inadequate closure of airway; and cricopharyngeal dysfunctions
- Esophageal phase: A swallowing phase not under voluntary control; begins when the food arrives at the orifice of the esophagus; food is propelled through the esophagus by peristaltic action and gravity and into the stomach; bolus entry into the esophagus results in restored breathing and depressed larynx and soft palate
- Disorders of the esophageal phase: Problems in passing the bolus through the cricopharyngeus muscle and past the 7th cervical vertebra; the main symptom is backflow of food from esophagus to pharynx; causes include weak cricopharyngeus, reduced esophageal contractions due to surgery, neurologic damage, or radiation therapy; diverticulum (a pouch that collects food); tracheoesophageal fistula; and esophageal obstruction (e.g., by a tumor)

Assessment Objectives/General Guidelines

- To assess the functioning of the different stages of swallow
- To assess various swallowing disorders
- To assess potential causes of the disorders to the extent possible
- To make both clinical and instrumental assessment of the symptom complex
- To assess treatment potential
- To suggest treatment options

Dysphagia

Case History/Interview Focus
- See **Case History** and **Interview** under Standard/Common Assessment Procedures
- Concentrate on the patient's medical history with an emphasis on those that are related to dysphagia, weight loss, intubation, and current method of feeding

Ethnocultural Considerations
- See Ethnocultural Considerations in Assessment

Assessment
- Assess patients who are at-risk for swallowing disorders
  - observe the conditions listed previously
- Assess the patient's mental status
  - ask questions about:
    - → time, date, year, and place
    - → his or her name; names of family members
    - → what he or she ate for breakfast or lunch
    - → what he or she did (in the morning, afternoon, evening, yesterday)
    - → why he or she is in the hospital
  - administer, if preferred or necessary, a screening test of mental status
- Screen speech, voice, language, and writing skills
  - screen speech sound articulation as you interview the patient
    - → take note of any errors
    - → measure the diadochokinetic rate
    - → make a more detailed assessment if necessary; see Articulation and Phonological Disorders
  - screen voice
    - → judge the quality of voice as the patient talks to you (take note of hoarseness, harshness, and breathiness)
    - → ask the patient to sustain a vowel; measure the duration and take note of vocal quality
    - → take note of the pitch and loudness of voice
    - → take note of hyponasality and hypernasality
  - screen the patient's language comprehension; give a series of:

D

> → simple verbal commands to assess their comprehension
> → written commands to assess their comprehension

- screen naming responses; have the patient:
  > → name a few common objects and geometric forms
  > → name pictures of family members
- screen spelling and writing skills; ask the patient to:
  > → copy a few printed words
  > → write words and phrases as you dictate them
  > → write a paragraph about anything
- screen comprehension of abstract meaning; ask the patient to:
  > → tell the meaning of a few proverbs
  > → tell the meaning of a few common phrases (e.g., go overboard, come out of the closet, elbow room, lame duck, top brass)
  > → define a few abstract terms (e.g., honesty, truthfulness, good, bad)
- screen visual-perceptual skills; ask the patient to
  > → copy geometric forms (e.g., a square, triangle, circle, rectangle)

- Make a laryngeal examination
  - with indirect laryngoscopy and/or endoscopic examination:
    > → inspect the base of the tongue, vallecula, epiglottis, pyriform sinuses, vocal folds, and ventricular folds
    > → evaluate the vocal fold functioning during such tasks as quiet breathing, forced inhalation, and phonation
  - refer the patient to an otolaryngologist for a medical examination
- Administer test swallows
  - take note of the patient's posture, alertness, intubation, ability to follow direction, language comprehension, and readiness for examination
  - use case history, medical charts, initial indications of the type of swallowing problems, and results of your observation to plan test swallows

- collect the necessary materials: a laryngeal mirror, a tongue blade, a cup, a spoon, a straw, a syringe; and various foods of different consistency (described later)
- use an appropriate posture during the test swallows
  - → in the case of tongue weakness and bolus manipulation problems, ask the patient to tilt the head downward as food is placed in the mouth and tilt the head backward when the swallow is initiated
  - → in the case of hemilaryngectomy, delayed triggering of swallowing reflex, and inadequate laryngeal closure, ask the patient to tilt the head downward to hold the food in the valleculae until the reflex is triggered
  - → ask the patient with pharyngeal paralysis to turn the head toward the affected side during swallowing
  - → ask the patient to tilt the head toward the more normal side in case of unilateral oral or lingual weakness or paralysis; have the patient tilt the head before placing food in the mouth
- make appropriate placement of foods in the mouth
  - → place food in the more normal side of the mouth
  - → use a straw or a syringe to place liquids posteriorly
  - → use a tongue blade to place thicker foods on various places on the tongue
- use different kinds of foods in evaluating test swallows
  - → use liquid foods or foods of thin consistency when the patient has limited oral control
  - → use liquid foods when the patient has reduced pharyngeal peristalsis or impaired functioning of the cricopharyngeus muscle
  - → use foods of thicker consistency when the patient's swallowing reflex is delayed or laryngeal closure is inadequate
  - → modify food consistency to suit a patient who has a combination of problems
- give appropriate instructions
  - → give the patient any special instructions (e.g., head tilting)

D

- → place food appropriately
- → ask the patient to swallow the material
- manually examine the swallowing movements
  - → place your index finger just below the chin, middle finger on the hyoid and the third and fourth fingers at top and bottom of the thyroid; do not press the structures
  - → take note of the submandibular, hyoid, and laryngeal movements during swallowing
  - → take note of lack of laryngeal movement causing aspiration
  - → take note of abnormally low position of the larynx in some elderly patients
  - → ask the patient to phonate a vowel soon after swallowing; take note of gargling sounds indicative of food material on the vocal folds
  - → ask the patient to pant for several seconds to shake loose foods in the pharyngeal recesses; ask the patient to vocalize
  - → take note of coughing and expectoration that suggest aspiration
  - → be aware that lack of signs of aspiration does not mean no aspiration; videofluorography is more definitive
- Make still radiographic assessment
  - use still radiographic procedure if videofluorography is not available
    - → take lateral still radiographs 2 seconds after you instruct the patient to swallow
    - → take note of food residue in the valleculae, the pyri form sinuses, or food coating on the pharyngeal wall that indicate swallowing problems
    - → note that still radiographic assessment provides only limited information on the nature of the disorder
- Make videofluorographic assessment
  - note that videofluorographic assessment (modified barium swallow: MBS) of oropharyngeal swallow function is

essential for a more complete assessment and diagnosis of dysphagia

- complete both lateral and anterior-posterior (A-P) plane examinations; note that the lateral examination provides the most information and the A-P examination provides information on the symmetry of the swallow
- note that procedure uses radiation and may be contraindicated in some cases; do not use the procedure if
  → no new information is likely to emerge
  → the patient is not alert and mouth feeding is not practical
  → the patient has no swallowing response at all
- if the patient is severely ill and the procedure is still judged necessary, request the presence of a physician, a nurse, or a respiratory therapist during the test
- note that a regular barium procedure is necessary to diagnose esophageal disorders; it should follow MBS and should not be done simultaneously
- begin with the lateral plane examination and then switch over to (A-P) plane examination; give calibrated boluses:
  → begin with liquid barium: 1 ml, 3 ml, 5 ml, 10 ml, and drinking from a cup
  → pudding: 1 ml
  → cookie: one quarter of a butter cookie
  → thicker liquids or foods of thicker consistencies
  → place the food in the mouth with a spoon or a syringe
  → ask the patient to hold the food in the mouth until asked to swallow; use gestures; check the patient's understanding of your instructions
- let the patient try two swallows of each kind/quantity
  → examine the anatomy and physiology of swallowing structures
  → identify swallowing disorders; take note of food residues in various structures; coughing; and aspiration

- in completing the assessment and interpreting the results, use a standard and detailed set of instructions and follow the prescribed procedures carefully; see Logemann (1993)
- Make a manometric assessment
  - note that an esophageal manometer measures pressure in the upper and lower esophagus
  - have the patient swallow 3 small pressure-sensitive tubes, one positioned at the upper esophageal sphincter, the other within the esophagus, and the last at the lower esophageal sphincter
  - measure pressure changes associated with various swallows
  - take note of pressure deviations (disruptions in peristaltic waves) and esophageal disorders associated with them
  - note that manometry may be conducted simultaneously with videofluoroscopy
- Make an electromyographic assessment
  - note that electromyographic examination is done by attaching electrodes on structures of interest (e.g., oral, laryngeal, or pharyngeal muscles)
  - note that electrical activity of the muscles involved in swallow can be measured with this technique
  - note that muscle weakness or paralysis can be identified with this technique
  - use the procedure described in the manual of the electromyographic instrument used in assessment
- Make an endoscopic assessment
  - note that endoscopic examination can reveal the movement of bolus only until it triggers the pharyngeal swallow
  - note that endoscopic examination can reveal food residue after swallow
  - note that endoscopic examination is useful in evaluating the vocal folds and related structures before and after swallow

Dysphagia

- Make an ultrasound examination
  - note that ultrasound equipment helps measure oral tongue movement and hyoid movement
  - place the ultrasound sensor under the chin
  - give measured foods of different amount and thickness
  - record the reflected and converted sound waves on tape
  - note the movements of the tongue and the hyoid bone

Related/Medical Assessment Data
- Consider the medical conditions listed under **Etiology** in an earlier section
- Integrate results of all medical, surgical, and radiological examinations with the results of dysphagia assessment
- Consider current physical condition of the patient

Standard/Common Assessment Procedures
- Complete the <u>Standard/Common Assessment Procedures</u>; pay special attention to:
  - the muscles of facial expression
  - muscles of mastication
  - tongue mobility and strength
  - lip closure
  - movement of the soft palate
  - oral sensation (stimulate with hot and cold stimuli and with pressure; note that reduced oral sensation is rarely a cause of dysphagia)
  - dryness or the amount of moisture in the mouth

Analysis of Results
- Analyze the results of clinical and bedside examination to make a preliminary assessment of dysphagia and its potential sites and causes
- Integrate the results of clinical examination with those of instrumental assessment (e.g., videofluoroscopy, EMG, manometry, endoscopy)
- Describe the specific symptoms and causes of dysphagia

Diagnostic Criteria/Guidelines
- Relate symptoms to phases of swallow outlined earlier and their anatomic and physiologic loci and physiologic and anatomic deviations (if any)

Dysphagia

Differential Diagnosis
- Greater difficulty with liquids may suggest neurological involvement (general weakening of the muscle movements)
- No or little difficulty with liquids but greater difficulty with solids may suggest physical obstructions including tumor
- Difficulty with both liquids and solids may suggest a greater involvement of esophageal structures
- Differential effects of cold and hot food (e.g., esophageal spasms or reduction of esophageal peristalsis due to cold food)
- Pain associated with swallowing may help rule out dysphagia of neurologic origin
- Hyperactive gag reflex, tongue thrusting, and tonic bite may suggest neurologic impairment
- Nasal penetration of food suggests velopharyngeal closure problems
- Chest pain may suggest esophageal motor disorder
- Dysphagia caused by drugs may help rule out esophageal involvement (as esophagus is rarely affected by drugs)
- Normal speech and voice may suggest swallowing problems due to cricopharyngeal (late pharyngeal stage) or esophageal dysfunction
- Normal eating and swallowing when food is presented without verbal instructions but difficulty in swallowing when such instructions are given suggest the presence of swallowing apraxia

Prognosis
- Varies, depending on the underlying anatomic and physiologic causes, associated diseases and their natural course, physical and mental condition of the patient, and the past, present, and the future medical and surgical treatment planned for the patient
- Most patients with oropharyngeal dysphagia with good mental condition are candidates for dysphagia treatment

Recommendations

- Treatment for oropharyngeal dysphagia by speech-language pathologist trained in dysphagia management
- Medical management for esophageal dysphagia
- See the cited sources and *PGTSLP* for details

Groher, M. E. (Ed.). (1992). *Dysphagia: Diagnosis and management.* Newton, MA: Butterworth-Heinemann.

Logemann, J. A. (1988). *Evaluation and treatment of swallowing disorders.* Austin, TX: Pro-Ed.

Logemann, J. A. (1993). A *manual of videofluoroscopic evaluation of swallowing* (2nd ed.). Austin, TX: Pro-Ed.

Logemann, J., A., & Zingeser, L. (1995). *Dysphagia: Latest in instrumental diagnostic procedures and service delivery issues.* [ASHA Teleseminar]. Washington, DC: American Speech-Language Hearing Association.

Miller, R. M. (1992). Clinical examination for dysphagia. In M. E. Groher (Ed.), *Dysphagia: Diagnosis and management* (pp. 143–162). Newton, MA: Butterworth-Heinemann.

Dysphonia. A general term that means disordered voice; any voice disorder with the exception of Aphonia.

Dysplasia. Abnormal growth and development; unusual shape and size of body parts.

Dystonia. Movements that are repetitive, slow, twisting, writhing, and flexing. Uncontrolled adductor and abductor laryngeal spasms occur; voice is breathy, strained, and hoarse.

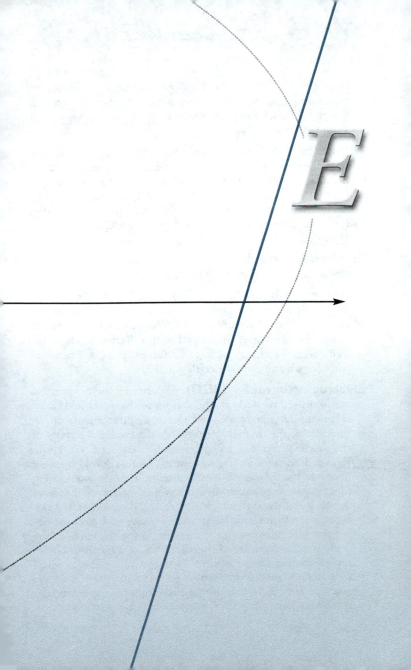

Ectrodactyly. Congenital absence of fingers or toes; part of some genetic syndromes including ectrodactyly-ectodermal dysplasia-clefting syndrome; see <u>Syndromes Associated With Communicative Disorders</u>.

Ectoderm. An embryo's outermost germ layer; gives rise to such organs as nails, hair, enamel of teeth, sweat glands, nervous system, and such sense organs as the ear and eye; ectodermal deformities are a part of certain genetic syndromes including ectrodactyly-ectodermal dysplasia-clefting syndrome; see <u>Syndromes Associated With Communicative Disorders</u>.

Ectodermal Dysplasia. Underdevelopment of organs or tissue that are derived from the <u>Ectoderm</u>.

Electroencephalogram (EEG). An established neuro-diagnostic method; a method to record the electrical impulses of the brain by surface electrodes; can show different kinds of brain waves associated with different kinds of activity (e.g., listening, talking, thinking); indicates cerebral pathology by abnormal electrical activity.

Electroglottography (EGG). A noninvasive, electrical method used to study the behaviors of the vocal folds; also called the <u>laryngograph</u>; uses electrode attachments on either side of the thyroid alae; records the electrical activity of the folds generated by their movement and vibration; recorded waveforms (Lx waveform) represent fold opening (increased resistance to electrical conductance) and closing (decreased resistance); also measures different phases of opening and closing and the degree and duration of fold closures; waveforms may be affected by several factors including the placement of the electrodes, tissue thickness in the neck area, and gender of the client (more difficult to obtain representative Lx waveforms in women); significant vocal fold lesions, mucus across the glottis, and paralysis of the folds reduce the reliability of assessment; a commercially available instrument is Kay Elemetrics Laryngograph.

Embolism. A sudden blocking of blood flow within an artery by clot or a mass of foreign material that had its origin elsewhere and traveled through the bloodstream to the site of lodgement and blocking; a common cause of stroke and the resulting aphasia.

Endoscopy. Use of a fiberoptic instrument to view internal bodily structures; naso- or oropharyngolaryngoscopes are of special interest to otorhinolaryngologists and speech-language pathologists because they permit viewing of the laryngeal or pharyngeal structures; may be inserted either through the nose (nasal endoscopy) or through the mouth (oral endoscopy) to view structures within the body; endoscopic examination of the laryngeal structures useful in diagnosing laryngeal pathologies, vocal fold vibrations, and associated voice disorders; endoscopic examination of the pharyngeal structures useful in observing the velopharyngeal structures and functions and thus useful in assessing these mechanisms in clients with clefts and velopharyngeal incompetence; invasive procedure, although trained speech-language pathologists working in medical settings may use it; may be connected to a stroboscope; a thin bundle of fibers carry light and illuminate the structures to be observed; another set of fibers brings the image back to a monitor; may be connected to a video recorder for recording images; should not be used as the sole data source for diagnosis as some distortions may be common.

Epicanthal Fold. A vertical layer of skin covering the inner canthus on either side of the nose; normal in individuals of certain races and a physical characteristic in certain syndromes, the prominent being Down syndrome (see <u>Syndromes Associated With Communicative Disorders</u>)

Ethnocultural Considerations in Assessment. Factors related to individual's cultural, ethnic, social, and personal variables that may affect assessment of communicative disorders; an important consideration in assessing

communicative disorders; often assumed to be of importance in assessing ethnic or cultural minority group members, but relevant to all individuals, including those belonging to majority ethnic or cultural groups; consider the
following in designing appropriate assessment procedures
for clients of all ethnocultural groups; note that the suggestions are only illustrative, not exhaustive:

- Understand the differences in prevalence rates of different disorders or related medical conditions in different
  ethnocultural groups
  - note that in African Americans:
    → high prevalence of hypertension and strokes
    → high prevalence of multi-infarct dementia, but possi-
      bly a low incidence of Alzheimer's disease
    → a high prevalence of head injury, especially due to
      gunshot wounds in youth
    → a high prevalence of laryngeal, lung, and esophageal
      cancers
    → a low incidence of cleft palate, especially cleft lip
    → generally low smoking rate
  - note that in Native Americans:
    → high prevalence of otitis media
    → high prevalence of cleft palate
    → generally high smoking rate
    → high prevalence of alcoholism and fetal alcohol
      syndrome
    → generally low prevalence of lung cancer
  - Note that in Asian Americans
    → a high prevalence rate of strokes
    → low prevalence of Alzheimer's disease, especially in
      Chinese Americans
    → high prevalence of cleft palate, especially in Chinese
      and Japanese
    → high prevalence of nasopharyngeal cancer in Chi-
      nese Americans
    → generally low smoking rate
    → generally low rate of alcoholism

- note that in Hispanics
  - → higher prevalence of strokes and diabetes than in whites
  - → high prevalence of cardiovascular diseases, especially correlated with low income
  - → low prevalence of esophageal cancer
  - → generally low smoking rate
- Take note of gender differences in the prevalence of various diseases or disorders
  - high prevalence of high blood pressure in older non-white women, especially the older African American women
  - high prevalence of laryngeal cancers in African American males
  - higher prevalence of laryngeal cancer in the African American females compared to white females
  - higher prevalence of high blood pressure and arteriosclerosis in Hispanic women than in Hispanic men
  - higher prevalence of multiple strokes in Hispanic men than in Hispanic women
  - generally higher incidence of laryngeal pathologies in the male than in the female
  - high prevalence of vocal nodules in white male children and in African American female children
  - higher prevalence of stuttering in the male than in the female
  - higher prevalence of articulation and phonologic disorders in the male than in the female
- Understand and explore during the interview different views and dispositions regarding diseases and disorders
  - understand how the client's culture views the etiology, effects, and social significance of diseases and disorders of interest
- Understand and explore during the interview different views and dispositions regarding communication and communication disorders

E

- understand how the client's cultural milieu views communication, its importance, and its need for social survival
- understand how language is used in different cultural groups and how the use of language varies depending on the communication partners
- understand how the parents of children being evaluated view communication problems for which they seek help
- note that in some minority cultures early cognitive changes associated with dementing diseases may be attributed to normal aging process or folk illnesses
- understand any social stigma attached to all or certain disorders of communication

- Understand and explore during the interview different views and dispositions regarding assessment and treatment of communicative disorders
  - understand how the family views assessment and treatment and what expectations they have of clinical services
  - explore the level of support the family members seem to offer for assessment and treatment of the client
- Understand and explore during the interview different geographic and socioeconomic barriers to access to, and underutilization of, clinical services
  - note the possibility of misclassification of minority children as being learning disabled
  - note that, probably due to healthcare access problems, dementia is underdiagnosed in nonwhite populations
  - note that undiagnosed depression in some elderly may be mistaken for dementia
  - note that many diseases and associated disorders may be in more advanced stage in minority groups because of lack of early diagnosis
- Study and understand dialectal differences including Black English
  - understand the semantic, morphologic, syntactic, and pragmatic differences of Black English
  - understand variations in English dialects as influenced by the client's primary language

Ethnocultural Considerations in Assessment

- Avoid cultural stereotypes; consider individual uniqueness
  - understand cultural patterns, but always treat a client as a unique individual
  - explore to what extent a member of a cultural group is different from the majority of that group (e.g., an African American who does not speak the Black English dialect or a southern rural white person who does)
  - understand that foreign-born individuals of minority groups who live in the United States will have changed to varying degrees
  - select standardized tests that have, in their standardization process, sampled the ethnocultural group to which the client belongs
  - avoid testing information about practices or events that are not culturally maintained or reinforced (e.g., do not celebrate anniversaries or birthdays)
  - consider the client's home environment and past experiences before formulating interview or assessment questions
  - consider the client's home environment and past experiences before selecting stimulus items to be used during assessment (e.g., exposure to certain kinds of toys, television shows, books)
  - if culturally appropriate standardized tests are not available, design Client-Specific Assessment Procedures
  - consider the bilingual/multilingual status of the client; select assessment tools that are appropriate for the bilingual/multilingual status
  - use trained interpreters in assessing bilingual/multilingual clients
  - determine whether a communication disorder exists in the primary language, the second language (which may be English), or both
  - be aware of differences in the same primary language (e.g., Spanish spoken by Mexican Americans or Cuban Americans)

E

- do not diagnose an articulation disorder based solely on a dialect influenced by primary language
- seek appropriate services to clients and families
- During assessment observe the client carefully and take note of the client's and accompanying persons':
  - general behavioral disposition
  - the level of ease and comfort in interacting with you
  - use of language with you and among themselves
  - expressed opinions about communication disorders, etiology, assessment, treatment, and clinical expectations

Battle, D. E., (1998). *Communication disorders in multicultural populations* (2nd ed.). Boston: Andover Medical Publishers.

Cheng, L. L. (1995). *Integrating language and learning for inclusion.* San Diego, CA: Singular Publishing Group.

Kayser, H. (1995). *Bilingual speech-language pathology: An Hispanic focus.* San Diego: Singular Publishing Group.

Roseberry-Mckibbin, C. (1995). *Multicultural students with special language needs.* Oceanside, CA: Academic Communication Associates.

Stockman, I. (1996). Phonological development and disorders in African American children. In A. G. Kamhi, K. E. Pollack, & J. L. Harris (Eds.), *Communication development and disorders in African American children* (pp. 117–153). Baltimore: Paul H. Brookes.

Expressive Aphasia. The same as Broca's aphasia; see Aphasia: Specific Types.

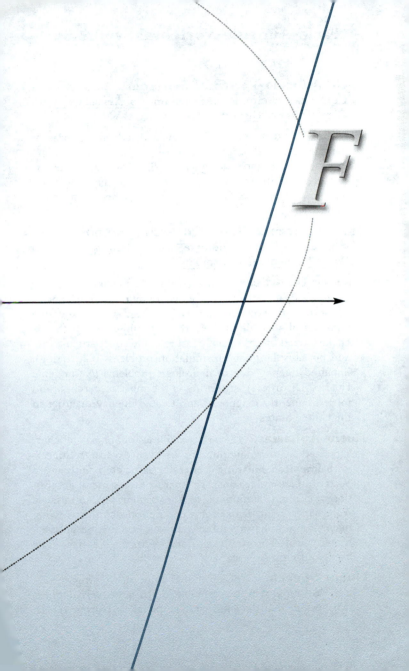

F

Facio-Auriculo-Vertebral Syndrome.   The same as Goldenhar syndrome; see <u>Syndromes Associated With Communicative Disorders</u>.

Familial Incidence.   Frequency with which a disease or disorder is found among blood relatives; many disorders (e.g., stuttering) show a higher familial incidence (if there is one person with the disorder, there are likely to be other persons among his or her blood relatives who also have the same disorder).

First and Second Branchial Arch Syndrome.   The same as Goldenhar syndrome; see <u>Syndromes Associated With Communicative Disorders</u>.

Fluency Disorders.   Speech disorders characterized by excessive dysfluencies or excessive duration of dysfluencies or both, and speech that is produced with excessive amounts of struggle and effort (<u>Stuttering</u>); speech that is characterized by excessively fast rate, indistinct articulation, and possibly language formulation problems (<u>Cluttering</u>); impaired fluency due to neurologic problems (<u>Neurogenic Fluency Disorders</u>); stuttering is the most researched and more frequently diagnosed and treated fluency disorder in the United States.

Fluent Aphasias.   Several syndromes of aphasia all characterized by normal-sounding or even excessive fluency with impaired meaning; generally associated with more posterior cerebral lesions; see <u>Aphasia</u> for a general description of etiology, symptoms, and assessment procedures; see <u>Aphasia: Specific Types</u> for a description of the following major fluent aphasias: anomic aphasia, conduction aphasia, transcortical sensory aphasia, and Wernicke's aphasia; see also <u>Nonfluent Aphasia</u>.

Fluent Speech.   Speech that is smooth, flowing, effortless, and rapid within acceptable limits; negatively defined, it is speech that does not contain excessive pauses, repetitions, sound and silent prolongations, interjections, and other forms of dysfluencies; speech that is not produced with excessive effort and struggle.

Functional Assessment.   Assessment of functional communication skills in naturalistic, socially meaningful contexts; whether a person achieves certain effects through any means (verbal, nonverbal, instrument-assisted, written) is the main focus of assessment; some assessment devices, and perhaps an increasing number, include functional components; several procedures within the traditional assessment can help target functional communication:

- Observe the client's communication with family members during assessment
- Always arrange a mother-child interaction that approximates their usual play-oriented interaction to observe more naturalistic communication than would be possible under typical testing conditions
- Whenever possible, with children and adolescents, arrange for a peer interaction situation and observe communication patterns; interview a peer on how the client communicates in social contexts
- Obtain one or more home speech and language samples; instruct the family to record natural and everyday communication interaction
- In educational (school) settings, observe the child in the classroom, in the playground, in the cafeteria, and so forth; obtain information from teachers about the child's communication skills; focus on target communication skills (e.g., fluency, language structures, voice quality, articulation)
- In medical settings, observe the patient's interaction with family members and health caregivers; interview them and obtain information on how the patient communicates with them (e.g., How does the patient communicate with the nurse? With the physician? With the physical therapist?)
- With adults, always interview at least one person with whom the client regularly interacts (spouse, friend, colleague)

Functional Communication

- Place emphasis on conversational speech; never make judgments based solely on purely imitative tasks or picture naming tasks; note, however, that such tasks are diagnostic and necessary in many cases (e.g., in assessing clients with dysarthria, apraxia, aphasia)
- Record a conversational speech (at least observe speech) outside the clinic room and in more naturalistic situations
- To the extent possible, structure assessment tasks that are meaningful (e.g., instead of having the client repeat sentences that have no bearing to his or her life, select sentences that include activities the client enjoys, names of the family members, and so forth)
- Document variations in the disorder in natural settings (e.g., in assessing a person who stutters, document the degree of fluency in such naturalistic contexts as ordering in a restaurant, purchasing at counters, talking on the telephone)
- Emphasize the effects communicative attempts produce rather than the language structure that the traditional assessment is often concerned with (e.g., whether a brain injured or stroke patient can successfully communicate his or her basic needs may be, at a certain stage in assessment, more important than how it is done); note, however, that this does not suggest that assessment of language structures is unimportant
- In essence, note that functional assessment requires the clinician to make targets, procedures, and settings of assessment as naturalistic as possible
- Select standardized methods or tests that are functionally oriented
- See ASHA FACS for adults as an example and develop similar procedures for your clients (American Speech-Language-Hearing Association: *Functional Assessment of Communication Skills for Adults* by C. M. Frattali, C. K. Thompson, A. L. Holland, C. B. Wohl, & M. M. Ferketic)

Functional Communication.   Effective, natural, meaningful communication in natural (social) environments; in assessment, often contrasted with noncommunicative responses given to special stimuli the clinician presents; for example, such responses as "red," "circle," "cup," "juice," "boy is walking," and so forth evoked by presenting pictures or objects in the clinic are not naturally communicative; however, similar responses in natural settings in the context of everyday communication are functional; not limited to verbal responses; any mode of response that achieves an effect or modifies the environment is functional communication.

F

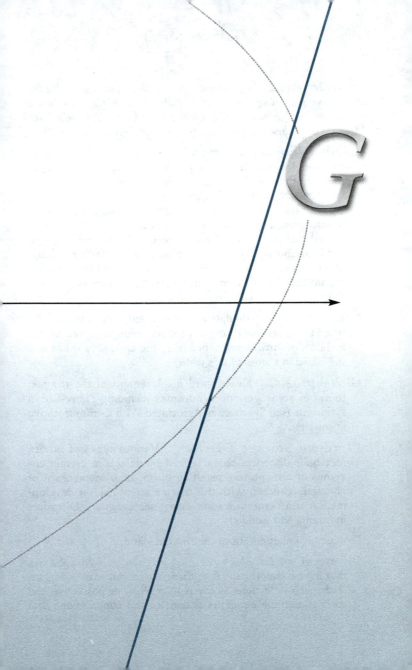

Galactosemia.   A group of genetic disorders caused by defective galactose metabolism; children with these disorders are at risk for developmental and communication delay; see Language Disorders in Infants and Toddlers.

Gestural Communication.   Method of communication that supplements oral communication with smiles and a variety of other facial expressions, body movements including shoulder shrugging, hand movements, pantomime, pointing, and head nodding or shaking; part of normal oral communication; in gestural communication, they play a more crucial role of communicating the speaker's messages; gestural communication may be unaided as in smiling or hand movements, or aided, as in gestures combined with a communication board; procedures described under Augmentative and Alternative Communication (AAC).

Glossing.   In articulation assessment, interpreting the word the child was trying to produce; adult interpretation of a child's misarticulated word (e.g., the child says *wawa* and the clinician's gloss of it is *water*).

Glossoptosis.   Downward displacement of the tongue; found in some genetic syndromes including Pierre-Robin syndrome (see Syndromes Associated With Communicative Disorders).

Glycogen Storage Disease.   Various types of inborn metabolic disorders characterized by defects in certain enzymes or transporters resulting in impaired metabolism of glycogen; children with this disease are at risk for developmental and communication delay; see Language Disorders in Infants and Toddlers.

Goiter.   Enlargement of the thyroid gland.

Grammatic Morphemes of Language.   Morphemes that have a grammatic value; change or modulate meaning; include such inflections as the regular plural or possessive and such grammatic elements as articles and conjunctions that modulate meaning; a significant aspect of language acquisition; an element that is usually omitted or misused by children who exhibit language disorders; an important element of language assessment in all clients, especially in children with language disorders; in all language assessment, consider the following:

Morpheme	Example
Present progressive *ing*	walk*ing*, runn*ing*, eat*ing*, work*ing*
Prepositions: *in* *on* *under* *behind*	 the ball is *in* the box the book is *on* the table the doll is *under* the blanket the car is *behind* the house
Regular plurals plural *s* plural *z* plural *vz* plural *ez*	 cat*s*, bat*s*, book*s* bag*s*, bear*s*, bed*s*, web*s* wol*ves*, dish*es*, match*es*, watch*es*
Irregular plurals	men, women, children, feet
Zero morpheme (the same plural and singular forms)	sheep, fish, deer
Past tense irregular verbs	went, came, ate, fell, meant, knew, sat, swam, sank, threw, wrote
Past tense regular verbs past *d* past *t* past *ed*	 kill*ed*, turn*ed*, burn*ed* chas*ed*, walk*ed*, bak*ed*, melt*ed*, board*ed*, hoard*ed*
Possessive nouns possessive *s* possessive *z* possessive *əz*	 bat*'s*, cat*'s*, Matt*'s*, goat*'s* boy*'s*, dad*'s*, dog*'s*, Joan*'s* mouse*'s*
	(continued)

G

(continued)

Morpheme	Example
Pronouns	he, she, it, we, they

Conjunctions
  coordinating
  correlative (used in pairs)
 	
  subordinating
	and, but, or, nor, so, and yet
	either . . . or; neither . . . nor;
	not only . . . but also;
	whether . . . or
	although, because, since, if,
	until, when, where, while

Uncontractible copula	here I *am*; *is* she coming?; she *was* here
Contractible copula	she's nice, she *is* nice; boy's good, boy *is* good
Articles	the, a
Regular third person singular	he *works*, she *smiles*, Tom *hits*
Irregular third person singular	he *does*, she *has*
Uncontractible auxiliary	she *is* (in response to a question like *who is coming?*); he *was*, she *was*, it *was*
Contractible auxiliary	she's running, she *is* running; mommy's coming, mommy *is* coming, it's eating, it *is* eating
Negation	*no* and *not*; *un*happy, *un*likely
Reflexive pronouns	them*selves*, my*self*
Comparatives/Superlatives	bet*ter*, big*gest* best (irregular)

Granulovacuolar Degeneration. A build-up of fluid-filled vacuoles and granular remains within nerve cells; a basic neuropathology of <u>Alzheimer's Disease</u> and found in some normal elderly people.

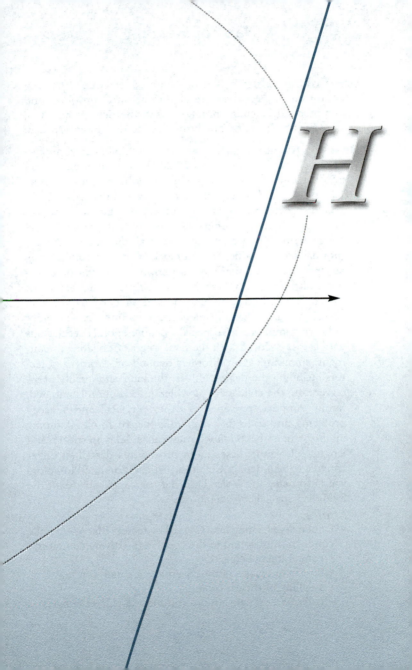

Hard of Hearing. Persons who have reduced hearing acuity but nonetheless are able to acquire, produce, and comprehend language primarily with the help of audition; may use amplification and visual cues to understand speech.

Hearing Impairment. Reduced hearing acuity; a hearing level that is greater than 25 dB HL in case of adults and 15 dB HL in case of young children who still are learning language; includes the Hard of Hearing and the Deaf; classified as shown under Hearing Loss; may be organic or nonorganic; nonorganic hearing loss may be malingering or psychogenic; may be peripheral or central; may be conductive (normal bone conduction and much worse air conduction), sensory (cochlear pathology), peripheral neural (involvement of the auditory branch of the VIIIth cranial nerve), or mixed (better bone conduction than air conduction); oral speech and language disorders are a common concomitant of hearing impairment, especially deafness; oral speech skills vary across children with the same degree of hearing impairment; communication disorders depend on a variety of factors including the degree of loss, the kind and quality of intervention, the child's age at which intervention is initiated, family support, presence of other physical and sensory problems, and so forth; even a mild loss of 15 dB HL during infancy and early childhood may cause delay in speech and language learning; assessment procedures described under Language Disorders in Children, Articulation and Phonological Disorders, and Voice Disorders are applicable with the following special considerations:

Etiology
- Conductive hearing loss: Caused by factors that prevent the conduction of sound to the cochlea (relatively common)
  - congenital or acquired
  - atresia or aplasia of the external ear canal
  - swelling of the ear canal
  - collapsed ear canal (more common in elderly females)

- osteomas (benign bony tumors of the ear canal)
- impacted cerumen (more common)
- foreign objects in the ear canal
- disarticulation of the auditory ossicular chain
- middle ear effusion (more common, especially in children)
- ossicular fixation
- Sensory hearing loss: Caused by interference with the normal functioning of the hair cells of the cochlea (relatively common)
  - congenital (genetic or acquired in utero) or acquired after birth
  - fetal alcohol syndrome
  - maternal drug addiction
  - low birth weight
  - mechanical injury to the cochlea
  - ototoxins, especially related to kidney malfunctioning
  - viral and bacterial infections
  - vascular accidents that restrict cochlear blood supply
  - noise exposure
  - normal aging process
- Peripheral neural hearing loss: Caused by the involvement of the auditory branch of the VIIIth cranial nerve (relatively rare)
  - VIIIth nerve tumor (the most common of the cranial tumors)
  - demyelinating diseases of the VIIIth nerve
- Mixed hearing loss: Caused by several factors that affect normal conduction of sound to the cochlea and the neural transmission of sound
  - factors that cause conductive loss
  - factors that cause neural loss
  - otosclerosis
  - noise-induced
- Nonorganic peripheral hearing loss: Caused by psychological/behavioral factors

H

- malingering to gain advantages by knowingly faking a hearing impairment
- psychogenic factors which suggest lack of awareness of motivating factors on the part of the individual; possibly due to difficult life situations
- Central auditory problems: Caused by abnormal central auditory processing of auditory stimuli; no discernible organic cause in some cases; pure tone thresholds may be normal; difficulty manifested mostly in speech discrimination and understanding (filtered or altered speech stimuli)
  - neoplasmas and tumors
  - demyelinating diseases (e.g., multiple sclerosis)
  - cerebrovascular diseases
  - central degenerative diseases (e.g., Alzheimer's disease)
  - various genetic disorders
  - asphyxia during birth
  - infections (e.g., HIV)
  - traumatic brain injury

Communication Disorders

Pattern and sequence of language acquisition in the hearing impaired follow the normal pattern and sequence

- Speech problems
  - omission of final consonants and in blends
  - omission of /s/ in almost all positions
  - omission of initial consonants
  - substitution of voiced consonants for voiceless consonants
  - substitution of nasal consonants for oral consonants
  - vowel substitutions
  - distortion of sounds, especially of stops and fricatives
  - imprecise production of vowels
  - increased duration of vowels
  - addition of sounds (sʌ top for *stop*)
  - breathiness before the production of vowels

- inappropriate release of final stops (cap^h)
- Language problems
  - generally limited vocabulary
  - poor comprehension of word meanings
  - lack of understanding of multiple meanings of words
  - difficulty understanding abstract, metaphoric, and proverbial phrases
  - Slower acquisition of grammatic morphemes; omission of many morphemes (omission or inconsistent production of articles, prepositions, conjunctions, past tense inflections, plural inflections, the present progressive *ing,* indefinite pronouns, quantifiers, and the third person singular)
  - Slower acquisition of verb forms
  - difficulty understanding and producing complex, compound, and embedded sentences
  - Shorter sentences
  - fewer varieties of sentences
  - pragmatic language problems including reluctance to speak
  - limited oral communication (saying very little)
  - lack of elaborated speech
  - insufficient background information
  - occasional irrelevance of speech
  - improper stress patterns
- Fluency problems
  - generally limited fluency
  - increased rate of dysfluencies
  - Slow rate of speech
  - inappropriate pauses
  - abnormal flow of speech
  - abnormal rhythm of speech
- Voice and resonance problems
  - voice quality deviations, especially in the deaf (high pitched voice, lack of normal intonation, harshness, and hoarseness

H

- hyponasal resonance on nasal sounds
- hypernasal resonance on non-nasal sounds
- Reading and writing problems
  - poor reading comprehension
  - writing that reflects the language problems listed (poor syntax; omission of grammatic morphemes; limited variety of sentences; minimal information offered)

Assessment Objectives/General Guidelines

- To assess all aspects of communication, including speech, language, voice, and fluency characteristics

Case History/Interview Focus

- See **Case History** and **Interview** under Standard/Common Assessment Procedures
- Concentrate on hearing loss, its onset, and effects on communication

Ethnocultural Considerations

- See Ethnocultural Considerations in Assessment

Assessment

An audiologist makes an evaluation of the type and the degree of hearing loss; speech-language pathologist makes an assessment of communication disorders

- Assess speech
  - take a comprehensive Speech and Language Sample (see Standard/Common Assessment Procedures)
  - pay special attention to the kinds of speech problems a hearing-impaired person is likely to exhibit
  - use the procedures described under Articulation and Phonological Disorders
  - list the kinds of *articulation problems the client exhibits*
  - if useful, make a phonological pattern analysis
- Assess language
  - use the recorded speech and language sample
  - pay special attention to the kinds of language problems a hearing-impaired person is likely to exhibit

- use the procedures described under Language Disorders in Children
- List the kinds of semantic, morphologic, syntactic, and pragmatic problems the client exhibits
- Assess fluency
  - use the recorded speech and language sample
  - use the assessment procedures described under Stuttering
  - count the number of individual dysfluencies and the number of words in the speech sample
  - calculate the percent dysfluency rate
  - describe the overall rhythm of speech
- Assess voice
  - use the recorded speech and language sample
  - use the procedures described under Voice Disorders to make an assessment of voice and resonance problems
  - observe and take note of voice deviations during the interview and speech and language sample
  - take note of resonance problems
  - list the voice and resonance problems of the client
- Assess nonverbal communication
  - Observe and take note of the nonverbal means of communication the client uses

Standardized Tests
- Administer selected tests listed under Articulation and Phonological Disorders and Language Disorders in Children

Related/Medical Assessment Data
- Obtain otological report from the client's otologist
- Obtain audiological assessment report from the child's audiologist
- Obtain reports from the child's regular teacher or special education specialist including the educator of the deaf
- Obtain psychological assessment reports
- Obtain any general medical reports that shed light on the child's health and hearing

Standard/Common Assessment Procedures
- Complete the Standard/Common Assessment Procedures

H

Analysis of Results
- Analyze and summarize the results of communication assessment; highlight the significant problems in speech and language production
- Relate communication assessment results with those of audiological, otological, general medical, educational, and psychological reports
- Take note of the client's strengths (including the use of a nonverbal system of communication) and limitations

Diagnostic Criteria/Guidelines
- An independent diagnosis of hearing impairment (including its type and severity level) based on otological and audiological examinations
- Pattern of oral communication disorders that support the diagnosis

Differential Diagnosis
- Differentiate hearing impairment with mental retardation; make the distinction based on specific speech, language, voice, and resonance problems of the former along with an independent diagnosis of hearing impairment

Prognosis
- Prognosis for oral communication depends on the individual client's or family members' philosophy of communication and emphasis on oral modes of communication
- Prognosis for oral communication also depends on the degree of hearing loss; the less severe the loss, the better the prognosis for sustained oral communication skills
- Prognosis for oral communication generally good for children who are hard of hearing (not deaf)
- Prognosis for sustained nonverbal means of communication generally good for persons who are deaf

Recommendations
- Early speech and language intervention for children who are hard of hearing

- Speech and language intervention for individuals with more severe hearing impairment depending on the client's and family's preference and acceptance
- See the cited sources and *PGTSLP* for details

Bernthal, J. E., & Bankson, N. W. (1998). *Articulation and phonological disorders* (2nd ed). Englewood Cliffs, NJ: Prentice-Hall.

Hegde, M. N. (1996). *A coursebook on language disorders in children.* San Diego, CA: Singular Publishing Group.

Kelly, B. R., Davis, D., & Hegde, M. N. (1994). *Clinical methods and practicum in audiology.* San Diego, CA: Singular Publishing Group.

Paul, R. (2001). *Language disorders from infancy through adolescence* (2nd ed.). St. Louis, MO: Mosby.

Hearing Loss.   Roughly the same as Hearing Impairment; classified as follows:
- Mild hearing loss: 16–40 dB HL
- Moderate hearing loss: 41–70 dB HL
- Severe hearing loss: 71–90 dB HL
- Profound hearing loss: 90 dB and higher

Hearing Screening.   See Standard/Common Assessment Procedures

Hemifacial Microsomia.   Underdevelopment of one side of the face.

Heterochromia.   Pigmentary disorder in which a part that should have the same color has multiple colors; in heterochromia iridis, for example, the two irides are of different color; a part of some genetic syndromes including Waardenburg syndrome; see Syndromes Associated With Communicative Disorders.

Hunter Syndrome.   A variety of mucopolysaccharidosis syndrome; see Syndromes Associated With Communicative Disorders.

Huntington's Disease (HD).   A degenerative neurological disease; also called *Huntington's chorea*; results in a variety of subcortical dementia; transmitted by an autosomal dominant gene on the short arm of chromosome 4; a 50% transmission rate to the offspring; typical onset in early 30s to early 40s; affects men and women equally; has a juvenile form with an onset as early as age 4; late onset in the 80s; caused by neuronal loss in the caudate nucleus and putamen along with diffuse neuronal loss in the cortex; symptoms include chorea and Dementia; associated with motor speech disorders and language impairment; see Dementia for general assessment procedures; also see hyperkinetic dysarthria under Dysarthria: Specific Types for assessment of motor speech disorders; use the following information specific to HD.

Etiology
• Autosomal dominant inheritance in Huntington's disease
• Other factors including drug toxicity, postencephalopathy, and arteriosclerotic diseases that produce chorea, the major neurologic symptom of Huntington's disease

Early Symptoms
• Gradual changes in behavior and personality
• Depression, irritability, and anxiety
• Suspicious, complaining, and nagging personality
• A false sense of superiority
• Emotional outbursts
• Abnormalities of movement (resembling fidgeting)
• Beginning problems of memory, judgment, and executive functions
• Disorganized speech in some cases
• Early signs of chorea
• Seizure, motor problems, confusion, or disorientation in some cases

Advanced Symptoms
• Aggravation of memory, judgment, and executive disturbances
• Generalized chorea (irregular, spasmodic, jerky, complex, rapid, and involuntary movements of the limb and facial muscles)

Huntington's Disease (HD)

- Intellectual deterioration
- Attention deficits
- Dysarthria, more often the hyperkinetic type
- Language impairment associated with dementia
- Confusion and disorientation
- Hostility and physical and verbal abuse
- Profound dementia
- Death within 10 to 20 years of onset

Case History/Interview Focus
- See **Case History** and **Interview** under Standard/Common Assessment Procedures
- Document the changes in cognition, general behavior, emotional responding, and communication skills

Ethnocultural Considerations
- See **Case History** and **Interview** under Standard/Common Assessment Procedures

Assessment
- Assess speech, language, memory, cognition (including orientation and confusion)
- Follow the procedures described under Dementia
- Follow the procedures described under hyperkinetic dysarthria (see Dysarthria: Specific Types)

Standardized Tests
- Consider using standardized tests described under *Dementia* and *Dysarthrias*

Related/Medical Assessment Data
- Integrate available medical, neurological, psychological, behavioral, and diagnostic medical laboratory findings with the results of communication assessment

Standard/Common Assessment Procedures
- Complete the Standard/Common Assessment Procedures

Diagnostic Criteria
- Basic diagnosis of Huntington's disease with chorea as the dominant symptom
- Dementia and dysarthria

Differential Diagnosis
- Distinguish Huntington's disease from related diseases that produce subcortical dementia (Parkinson's disease, progressive supranuclear palsy, and Wilson's disease)
- See <u>Dementia</u> to make a differential diagnosis of diseases associated with subcortical dementias

Prognosis
- Disease is progressive and irreversible

Recommendations
- Communication treatment in the initial stages; management of problems later
- Family counseling and management strategies
- See the cited sources and *PGTSLP* for details

Bayles, K. A., & Kaszniak, A. W. (1987). *Communication and cognition in normal aging and dementia.* Austin, TX: Pro-Ed.

Brookshire R. H. (1997). *An introduction to neurogenic communication disorders* (5th ed.). St. Louis, MO: Mosby Year Book.

Cummings, J. L., & Benson, D. F. (1983). *Dementia: A clinical approach.* Boston: Butterworth.

Lubinski, R. (1991). *Dementia and communication.* Philadelphia: B. C. Decker.

Ripich, D. N. (1991). *Geriatric communication disorders.* Austin, TX: Pro-Ed.

Hurler Syndrome.   A variety of mucopolysaccharidosis syndrome; see <u>Syndromes Associated With Communicative Disorders</u>.

Hydrophthalmos.   A variety of glaucoma in which the fibrous coats of the eye are enlarged and distended; part of some genetic syndromes; see Waardenburg syndrome under <u>Syndromes Associated With Communicative Disorders</u>.

Hypernasality.   Excessive nasal resonance on non-nasal sounds; see <u>Voice Disorders</u> for assessment procedures.

Hypertelorism.   Abnormally increased distance between two organs (e.g., the eyes); part of some genetic syndromes.

Hypodontia.   Absence of one or more teeth; part of some genetic syndromes.

Hyponasality.   Reduced or absent nasal resonance in the production of nasal sounds; the same as denasality; see Voice Disorders for assessment procedures.

Hypoplasia.   Underdevelopment or incomplete development of an organ; typically due to genetic or congenital reasons; associated with certain genetic syndromes.

Hypoplastic Philtrum.   Underdevelopment of the vertical groove of the middle part of the upper lip.

Hypotonia.   Reduced tone or tension.

H

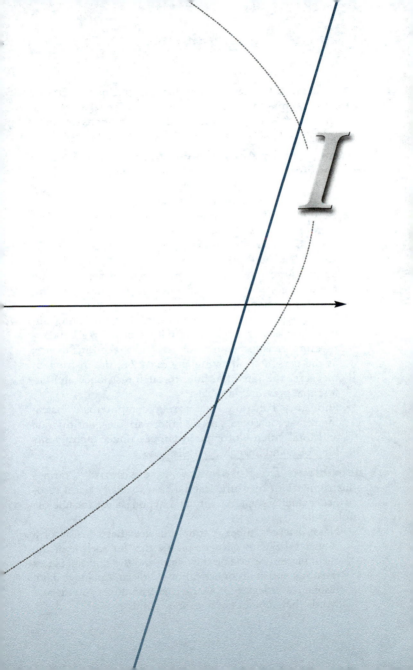

I

Incontinence.   Loss of voluntary control over excretory functions; may be urinary incontinence or fecal incontinence; associated with various medical conditions including Dementia.

Instruments for Aerodynamic Measures of Phonatory Functions.   Various instruments to measure aspects of respiratory functions that are relevant for voice and speech production; include the following:

• Aerophone II Voice Function Analyzer (Kay Elemetrics Corporation): A special hardware and software system used in a microcomputer to analyze various voice and speech characteristics and functions including airflow, air pressure, and sound pressure; includes face mask for measuring aerodynamic variables; gives computer printouts for permanent record.

• Pneumotachograph: An instrument for measuring airflow; consists of a face mask with acoustic resistance, a pressure transducer, an amplifier, and a recording device; as the person speaks with the mask on, the instrument measures the rate of airflow through resistance and differential pressure variables.

• Phonatory Function Analyzer: A computerized instrument that measures, among other variables, airflow rate and total volume of expired air; see under Instruments for Voice and Speech Analysis.

Instruments for Resonance Assessment.   Various instruments to measure resonance, especially nasal resonance including hypernasality and hyponasality; include the following:

• Nasal listening tube: A simple device that consists of a rubber tube with glass or plastic tips on each end; the client places one end on the nostril and the clinician places the other end in his or her ear; the clinician can judge nasal resonance or lack of it as the client produces sounds and words that contain nasal or oral sounds.

- Nasometer (Kay Elemetrics Corporation): A computerized instrument to measure nasal resonance; as the client speaks into two microphones that are separated by a nasaloral separator, the instrument measures relative nasal resonance; gives instantaneous feedback to the client.

Instruments for Voice and Speech Analysis.   A variety of electronic and increasingly computerized instruments to assess various aspects of voice and speech; include the following:

- Visi-Pitch (Kay Elemetrics Corporation): A special hardware and software system used in a microcomputer to analyze various aspects of voice and speech including speaking fundamental frequency, the lowest and the highest frequencies, average loudness of a speech sample (relative intensity), minimum and maximum loudness, voice onset time, glottal attacks, and intonation and stress patterns; gives digital and oscilloscopic displays.
- Phonatory Functional Analyzer: A computerized instrument to measure aspects of phonation and airflow; measures phonation time, frequency, intensity, airflow rate, and total volume of expired air; with a face mask, can measure pitch in continuous speech; because it takes simultaneous measures of these variables, the interaction among them may be documented; the effects of changes induced in one variable may be documented; provides computer print-out of data for permanent record.
- Fundamental Frequency Indicator: An instrument to measure pitch; patient holds a microphone to the larynx or under the nose and produces various vowels and syllables; gives read-outs of habitual pitch, the best pitch, and the pitch range.

Intention Tremor.   Tremor that is absent during periods of rest, but manifests itself during voluntary movements.

Interview.   See <u>Standard/Common Assessment Procedures</u>.

Intubation Granuloma.   A lesion of the larynx that occurs at or near the vocal process of the arytenoid because of trauma caused by the insertion, positioning, or removal of an endotracheal tube; treatment is surgical; no voice therapy except for vocal rest.

I

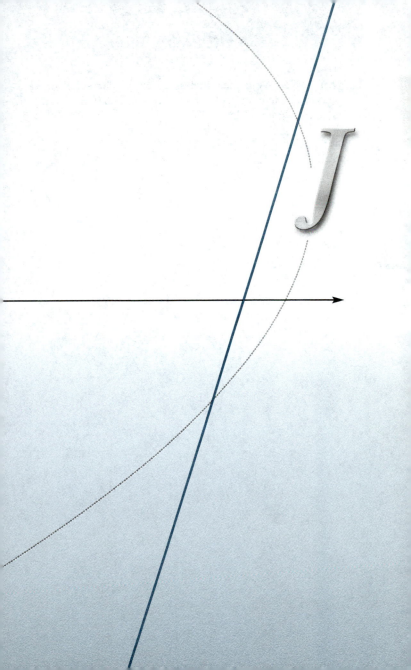

Jargon. Fluent but meaningless speech; a characteristic of aphasia; also may mean the technical vocabulary of sciences and professions.

J

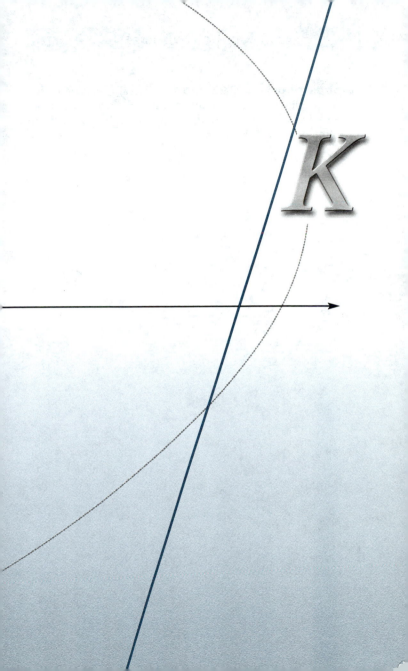

Kyphoscoliosis.   Backward and lateral curvature of the spinal column; eventually affects lung and hearing function; see Refsum syndrome under <u>Syndromes Associated With Communicative Disorders</u>.

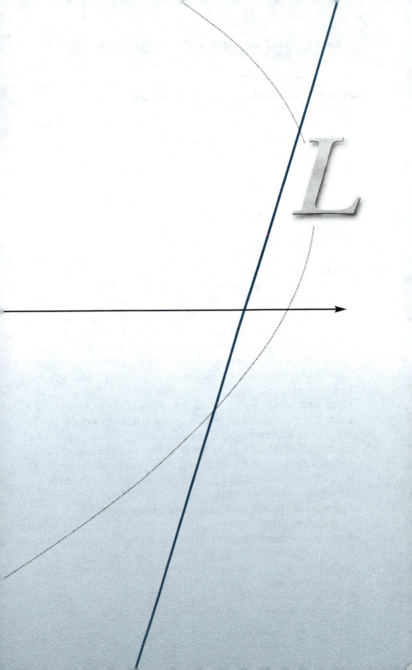

L

Language Disorders in Adolescents

Language Disorders in Adolescents. Semantic, morphologic, syntactic, and pragmatic language problems of adolescents; include problems that persist from early childhood and those that are due to a failure to acquire more advanced skills of language and literacy; problems in reading, writing, advanced discourse, and critical, logical, and scientific reasoning; relatively less research on adolescents' language compared to the language of preschool children; research suggests that language learning continues during the adolescent years and even beyond; changes are more subtle and gradual (hence more difficult to identify); phonologic and morphologic changes are not significant during the adolescent years; normative data are extremely limited; research shows gradual but noticeable increase in sentence length during adolescent years; changes may be measured in C-units (communication units) or T-units (terminable units); both contain an independent clause and subordinate clauses but the C-units also may be incomplete sentences produced in response to questions; the two units show regular increase from 6th through 12th grades; increases in language structures that occur at low frequency are significant; learning scientific, technical, literate, academic, logical, and discipline-specific terms and terms used in advanced reasoning and scholarly analysis also is a part of adolescent language acquisition; skills in word retrieval, word definitions, word relations, and skills in the use of figurative language continue to improve; learning advanced syntactic structures and pragmatic features also is evident during the adolescent years.

Factors Related to Language Disorders in Adolescents

- Language disorders in early childhood; hence most all factors listed under Language Disorders in Children
- Persistence of language problems from the early childhood years
- Difficulty in learning more advanced features of language that are learned in adolescent years

Language Disorders in Adolescents

Description of Language Disorders in Adolescents
- Semantic problems
  - difficulty in understanding and correctly using literate lexicon necessary for thinking, logical reasoning, verbal analysis, and scholarly and scientific discourse (e.g., such terms as interpret, presume, assume, hypothesize, infer, summarize, define, compare, contrast, criticize, evaluate, support, reject, discriminate, explain, conclude, assert, predict)
  - difficulty in understanding and correctly using figurative language (e.g., proverbs, metaphors, and idioms) with or without verbal contexts
  - difficulty in learning peer group slang
  - difficulty in understanding and correctly using words with abstract and multiple meanings
  - word-retrieval problems in conversational speech resulting in false starts, pauses, revisions, repetitions, and other kinds of dysfluencies
  - deficient word-definition skills; difficulty may be especially evident in defining literate, technical, and scientific words
  - word-relation problems; difficulty in understanding and correctly using words that are related by similar or contrastive meanings (synonyms and antonyms)
  - difficulty in using precise terms with clear referents (e.g., excessive use of such terms as "this," "that," "you know what I mean," "this thing," "that stuff," etc.)
- Syntactic problems
  - limited sentence lengths (often measured in C-units or T-units and expressed in number of words per unit)
  - limited use of low-frequency structures (e.g., passive sentences, such noun phrase postmodifications as "a tree *called the oak*" or "Mr. Thomas *the history teacher*")
  - difficulty using complex sentences containing subordinate clauses (e.g., such nominal subordinate clauses as "Jane did not know that she was the winner"; such adverbial clauses as *"When you get your pilot's license,* you can start

281

flying on your own"; and such adjectival clauses as "The man, who was *sleeping on the sidewalk*, had a sign that said *residentially challenged*")

- difficulty using concise and precise grammatical constructions that suggest greater syntactic sophistication (e.g., "once licensed, you can start flying on your own" instead of the lengthier adverbial clause); note that sentence length does not always suggest greater syntactic skill
- difficulty using cohesion devices or connectives (e.g., the use of such expressions as *therefore, for example, similarly, moreover, consequently, furthermore, because, while, as well as, rather than, neither, either*, etc.)
- lack of agreement (e.g., noun-verb agreement)
- use of ambiguous pronouns
- persistence of syntactic errors from earlier language problems
- Pragmatic problems
  - difficulty using the correct register (e.g., the use of slang register with peers, but a more formal register with teachers)
  - inappropriate use of gestures
  - difficulty maintaining topic of conversation
  - difficulty distinguishing facts from opinions
  - tactless expressions
  - difficulty modifying statements or adding new information (restatement of the same information)
  - difficulty sequencing events correctly
  - maze behavior (false starts and repeated attempts to express the same ideas)
  - difficulty asking relevant questions and making relevant comments during conversation
  - deficient listening skills
- Reading and writing problems
  - reading errors and revisions
  - difficulty comprehending read material
  - spelling errors in writing

- poor formation of letters
- lack of punctuation skills
- poor organization of essays
- sparse information, lack of detail
- deficient grammar
- use of nontechnical language instead of technical language
- lack of cohesion
- infrequent use of low-frequency structures

Assessment Objectives/General Guidelines
- To evaluate semantic, syntactic, morphologic, and pragmatic aspects of language
- To evaluate reading and writing skills
- To relate communication skills to academic demands and performance
- To suggest treatment targets
- Note that adolescent language assessment may be more protracted than assessment of language in a younger child because of the need to obtain writing samples, extended narratives, use of such abstract statements as proverbs, definition of terms, and so forth

Case History/Interview Focus
- See **Case History** and **Interview** under Standard/Common Assessment Procedures
- Obtain information from parents, teachers, and peers about the adolescent's communication patterns

Ethnocultural Considerations
- See Ethnocultural Considerations in Assessment; pay special attention to Bilingual/Multilingual Status described under this entry

Screening
- When a language disorder is not obvious, screen language to determine if a more detailed assessment is needed
  - evoke a brief conversation from the adolescent and take note of language disorders; note that some language

problems of the adolescent may be too subtle to be detected by brief conversational samples
- administer one of the following standardized screening tests or measures; note that only a few adolescent screening tests are available:

Test	Purpose
Adolescent Language Screening Test (D. L. Morgan & A. M. Guilford)	To assess vocabulary, sentence construction, morphologic features, and pragmatic aspects (11 to 17 yrs)
Clinical Evaluation of Language Fundamentals—Revised Screening (E. Semel, E. Wiig, & W. Secord)	To assess morphologic, syntactic, and semantic features and auditory comprehension (5 to 16 yrs)
Screening Test of Adolescent Language (E. M. Prather, S. V. Breecher, M. L. Stafford, & E. M. Wallace)	To assess vocabulary, auditory memory span, language processing, and verbal expression (6 to 12 yrs)

- Refer the adolescent who fails a screening test according to the test protocol for a language assessment

Assessment
- Obtain an extended speech and language sample (see Standard/Common Assessment Procedures) for a typical analysis of language functions; note that you need especially structured tasks to assess many problems of the adolescent speaker
- Obtain a sample of conversation between the client and a peer; between the teacher and the client; and between the client and a family member or members
- Assess semantic skills
  - assess difficulty in understanding and correctly using literate (academic, scholarly, learned) lexicon; make a list of such words as the following:

assume	suppose	infer	interpret	hypothesize	define
compare	contrast	criticize	evaluate	summarize	predict
explain	describe	conclude	confirm	support (a statement)	discriminate
imply	concede	presume	guess	reject (a statement)	allude
fact	opinion	evidence	belief	contradictory	logical

- ask the client to define the terms on the list
- ask the client to contrast the meaning of terms:
  - → fact and opinion
  - → description and explanation
  - → inference and assumption
  - → suggestion and hypothesis
  - → belief and theory
  - → illusion and allusion
  - → since and because
  - → further and farther
  - → affect and effect
  - → alternate and alternative
  - → latter and later
- assess difficulty in understanding and correctly using figurative language; make a list of common proverbs, metaphors, and idioms and then ask the client what they mean; for example:
  - → a stitch in time saves nine
  - → a penny saved is a penny earned
  - → put the cart before the horse
  - → put all your eggs in one basket
  - → don't kill the goose that lays golden eggs
  - → he is cold as ice
  - → she is fit as a fiddle
  - → time is money
  - → they wanted to bury the hatchet
  - → off the wall
  - → off the record
  - → she looks like a million bucks

L

→ skeleton in the closet

- assess word-retrieval problems in conversational speech; take note of false starts, pauses, revisions, repetitions, and other kinds of dysfluencies; take note of words that are retrieved with difficulty
- assess deficient word-definition skills; in addition to having the client define literate words, obtain a list of words from the teacher or from the client's textbooks; ask the client to define them
- assess word-relation problems by having the client define and contrast synonyms and antonyms; analyze a writing sample to see if the same words are overused (instead of words with similar meanings)
- assess difficulty in using precise terms during conversation and narrative tasks; take note of the frequency with which such expressions as "this," "that," "you know what I mean," "this thing," "that stuff," etc., are used; infer the precise words that were not produced

- Assess syntactic skills
  - use the speech and language sample, narratives, writing samples, and several behavior-specific tasks to make a syntactic skills analysis
  - assess sentence lengths in C-units or T-units; count the number of words per unit and calculate both the mean and the mode (the most frequently observed length)
  - assess the use of low-frequency structures; take note of low-frequency structures that the client used and those that he or she did not use
  - assess the use of complex sentences containing subordinate clauses; use the C- and T-units; take note of the clause structures the client used and those the client did not use; calculate the number of clauses used in utterances (e.g., "I only saw lions and snakes" contains 1 T-unit (one main clause); however, "that was a person who knew everything but did not know anything" has 3 T-units (the main clause *that was a person* and two subordinate clauses *who knew everything* and *but did not know anything*)

- assess the use of more precise (hence shorter) expressions instead of wordy, vague, and roundabout expressions
- assess the use of cohesion devices or connectives; take note of the contexts in which such devices should have been used but the client did not
- assess agreement (e.g., noun-verb agreement) in both connected speech and writing samples
- assess the use of ambiguous pronouns; take note of the pronouns that the client did not use or used infrequently
- take note of all other syntactic and morphologic errors, some of which may have persisted from early childhood
- Assess pragmatic skills
  - use the speech and language sample and narratives
  - assess the use of correct register depending on the situation; use role play (e.g., you play the role of a peer and then that of a teacher); if practical, obtain speech samples from home and classroom; observe the speech as the client interacts with a peer; obtain a teacher's report
  - note inappropriate use of gestures in conversation
  - Systematically introduce several topics and judge the acceptability of topic maintenance
  - ask the client to clarify certain statements; ask for more information; judge whether the client modifies statements or just repeats; judge the amount of new information the client adds
  - ask the client to narrate a story or retell a story he or she reads; judge event sequencing skills
  - count the frequency of maze behavior (false starts and repeated attempts to express the same ideas)
  - take note of irrelevant comments
  - make vague and nonspecific statements and take note of requests for clarification
  - assess the frequency with which the client asks you to repeat information suggesting poor listening skills
- Assess reading and writing skills
  - ask the client to read printed material that is at his or her grade level and analyze the reading errors

- ask questions about the material read to assess reading comprehension
- analyze multiple writing samples for spelling errors, poor formation of letters, general organization, and handwriting problems
- analyze punctuation skills
- analyze the writing sample for its content; judge the adequacy of information offered and details given
- analyze errors of syntax in the written samples
- judge the appropriateness of the language used; take note of technical word usage
- analyze the written passage for cohesion and correct use of words that indicate cohesion
- count the use of low-frequency syntactic structures (e.g., such noun phrase postmodifications as "an aircraft *called the airbus*," "Mr. Johnson *the teacher*," or "the woman *who does not work here*"; such passive sentences as *"the man was hit by the train"*)

Medical, Psychological, and Educational Assessment Data

- Obtain any available medical data of importance in evaluating language disorders
- Obtain results of audiological evaluation
- Obtain psychological data including the results of intelligence testing and cognitive functioning
- Obtain data on the adolescent's educational achievement and assessment that might suggest learning disabilities
- Obtain writing samples from the adolescent's teachers
- Examine the adolescent's textbooks to select words and phrases that might be included in assessment

Standard/Common Assessment Procedures

- Complete the Standard/Common Assessment Procedures

Standardized Tests of Adolescent Language Skills

- Administer one or more of the following standardized tests or measures:

Test	Purpose
Adapted Sequenced Inventory of Communication Development for Adolescents and Adults with Severe Handicap (S. E. McClennen)	To assess communication skills in severely handicapped individuals with sensory and neuromotor involvement (adolescent to adulthood)
Bilingual Syntax Measure II (M. K. Burt & H. C. Dulay)	To assess expressive syntactic skills in English and Spanish (3rd to 12th grade)
Clinical Evaluation of Language Fundamentals—Third Edition (E. Semel, E. Wiig, & W. Secord)	To assess semantic and syntactic skills (5 to 16 yrs)
Evaluating Communicative Competence (C. S. Simon)	To assess language processing, metalinguistic skills, and pragmatic aspects (9 to 17 years)
Fullerton Language Test for Adolescents (A. R. Thorum)	To assess morphologic skills, oral commands, syntactic skills, and idoms (11 yrs to adult)
Rhode Island Test of Language Structure (E. Engen & T. Engen)	To assess receptive syntax, especially in hearing-impaired children and adolescents (3 to 20 yrs)
Test of Adolescent Language—3 (D. D. Hammill, V. L. Brown, S. C. Larsen, & J. L. Weiderholt)	To assess language, reading, writing, and auditory comprehension skills (12 to 24;11 yrs)
Test of Adolescent/Adult Word Finding (D. J. German)	To assess naming, nouns, verbs, sentence completion, description, and categories (12–80 yrs)
Test of Word Knowledge: Two levels (E. Wiig & W. Secord)	To assess definitions of words, antonyms, synonyms, and multiple meanings (5 to 8 & 8 to 17;11 yrs)

L

Language Disorders in Adolescents

Analysis of Results
- Analyze the speech and language sample for semantic, syntactic, morphologic, and pragmatic problems
- List the deficiencies and strengths of the client
- Relate your assessment data to educational demands and curricular materials

Diagnostic Criteria/Guidelines
- Significant deficiencies in advanced language skills as listed

Differential Diagnosis
- Distinguish between persistence of early childhood problems and additional language problems due to a failure to acquire more advanced features of language

Prognosis
- Variable depending on the adolescent, the family support, time of intervention, and the intensity of intervention
- Most adolescents with language disorders benefit from treatment

Recommendations
- Language intervention to strengthen the advanced features of language
- Working with the adolescent's teachers to coordinate treatment activities with academic activities
- Home intervention programs implemented by family members or other primary caretakers
- See the cited sources and *PGTSLP* for details; use methods described under <u>Language Disorders in Children</u>

Larson, V. L., & McKinley, N. (1995). Language disorders in older students: Preadolescents and adolescents. Eau Claire, WI: Thinking Publications.

Nippold, M. A. (1993). Developmental markers in adolescent language: Syntax, semantics, and pragmatics. *Language, Speech, and Hearing Services in Schools, 24,* 21–28.

Paul, R. (2001). *Language disorders from infancy through adolescence* (2nd ed.). St. Louis, MO: C. V. Mosby.

Reed, V. (1994). *An introduction to children with language disorders* (2nd ed.). New York: Macmillan.

Ripich, D. N., & Creaghead, N. A. (1994). *School discourse problems* (2nd ed.). San Diego, CA: Singular Publishing Group.

Language Disorders in Adults. Difficulty in comprehending, formulating, and producing language; often refer to loss of language functions due to physical diseases, especially neurologic diseases; includes Aphasia, Dementia, and language disorders associated with Right-Hemisphere Injury and Traumatic Brain Injury; see these alphabetical entries for assessment procedures.

Language Disorders in Children. Difficulty in learning to comprehend and/or produce semantic, phonologic, syntactic, morphologic, and pragmatic aspects of language; deficient and/or inappropriate verbal behavior in children; found in a varied group of children, some of whom have associated clinical conditions (e.g., autism or mental retardation) and others who present no other conditions; 10 to 15% of 2-year-olds and 4 to 7.5% of 3-year-olds may have language disorders; may be subtle in some children; some residual problems in most treated children; some school-age children with language disorders may be classified as learning disabled; associated with significant effects on social and academic behavior of children; Specific Language Impairment refers to language problems with no other problems, also controversial; found in many genetic syndromes in children that affect communication; see Syndromes Associated With Communicative Disorders; see Mental Retardation, Autism, and Hearing Impairment for assessment of language disorders associated with these conditions; see also Language Disorders in Infants and Toddlers and Language Disorders in Adolescents; for phonological problems, see Articulation and Phonological Disorders; this section describes language disorders and their assessment in children with no other significant mental, behavioral, or psychiatric conditions; most of the assessment procedures described also may be used, with suitable modifications, to assess language disorders associated with such other clinical conditions as mental retardation, autism, hearing impairment, and various genetic syndromes.

L

Language Disorders in Children

Factors Related to Language Disorders in Children
- No specific associated clinical conditions that could satis-factorily account for language disorders (in children des-cribed in this section)
- Higher familial incidence of language disorders suggesting the influence of genetic factors whose precise role is not clearly understood

Description of Language Disorders in Children
- Slower or delayed onset of language
  - possibly, delayed babbling
  - delayed acquisition of vocabulary
  - slower vocabulary growth rate
  - slower acquisition of language milestones
- Limited amount of language
  - generally limited verbal repertoire
  - limited number of words produced
  - limited range of vocabulary learned and produced
  - limited variety of vocabulary comprehended
  - lack of complex or longer word productions
  - lack of abstract words in the repertoire
- Deficient learning and inappropriate use of <u>Grammatic Morphemes of Language</u>
  - omission of various grammatic morphemes of language, including the present progressive *ing*, the regular and irregular plural morphemes, regular and irregular past tense inflections, articles, third person singular *s*, auxil-iary and copula, prepositions, and pronouns
  - incorrect use of learned grammatic morphemes, includ-ing overgeneralizations (e.g., *womans* for *women*, *goed* for *went*)
  - difficulty with comparatives and superlatives (e.g., big, bigger, biggest)
- Deficient syntactic skills
  - generally limited syntactic structures
  - single words or phrases instead of sentences
  - shorter sentences instead of longer sentences
  - simpler sentences instead of more complex sentences

- limited variety of syntactic structures (use of only a few types of sentences)
- Deficient or inappropriate use of language
  - difficulty in using acquired language in social situations
  - difficulty in initiating conversation
  - difficulty in maintaining a topic of conversation
  - difficulty in conversational turn-taking
  - difficulty in using conversational repair strategies
  - difficulty in maintaining eye contact during conversation
  - deficient narrative skills including confused chronological sequence, misidentified characters, missing details, lack of logical progression from the beginning to the end, and limited word output
  - language that may be irrelevant to time, space, and person with whom the child interacts (less common)
- Difficulty in comprehending spoken language
  - difficulty in comprehending meaning of complex words, phrases, and sentences
  - difficulty in comprehending abstract terms
  - difficulty in comprehending syntactically longer productions

Assessment Objectives/General Guidelines

- To assess the extent and nature of language delay or disorder
- To measure various aspects of language skills
- To assess language comprehension
- To assess or rule out the presence of associated clinical conditions (e.g., mental retardation, hearing impairment, or autism)
- To assess the family constellation and communication patterns
- To diagnose a language disorder
- To assess the educational demands made on the child
- To suggest potential treatment targets

Case History/Interview Focus

- See **Case History** and **Interview** under Standard/Common Assessment Procedures
- Concentrate on language, speech, gestures, and developmental sequence of communication

Language Disorders in Children

Ethnocultural Considerations
- See <u>Ethnocultural Considerations in Assessment</u>
- See <u>Language Disorders in African American Children</u> following this main entry
- See <u>Language Disorders in Bilingual Children</u> following this main entry

Screening
- When a language disorder is not obvious, screen language to determine if a more detailed assessment is needed
  - evoke a brief conversation from the child and take note of deficiencies, if any, in semantic, morphologic, syntactic, and pragmatic aspects of language
- Administer one of the following standardized screening tests or measures:

Test	Purpose
Bankson Language Screening Test (N. W. Bankson)	To screen semantic, morphologic, and syntactic skills and auditory and visual perception (4 to 7 yrs)
The Communication Screen (N. Striffler & S. Willig)	To assess vocabulary and auditory comprehension skills (2;10 to 5;9 yrs)
Denver Developmental Screening Test II (W. K. Frankenburg and associates)	To assess language, personal social, and motor development (2 wks to 6 yrs)
Fluharty Preschool Speech and Language Screening Test-R (N. B. Fluharty) (continued)	To screen basic language skills (2 to 6 yrs)
Northwestern Syntax Screening Test (L. Lee)	To screen syntactic, morphologic, and semantic skills (3 to 8 yrs)
Preschool Language Screening Test (E. Hannah & J. Gardner)	To assess visual, motor, and auditory perceptual concepts (3 to 5;6 yrs)

Language Disorders in Children

- Refer the child for a language assessment if the skills fall below expectations (either based on the conversational speech sample or the screening test)

Assessment

- **Assess word production and usage (semantic skills)**
  - obtain parental reports on the types and number of words the child uses at home
  - obtain parental reports on the use of single words as the primary mode of communication
  - ask the parents to list words the child produces, especially if the child produces only a limited number of words
  - observe interactions between the child and the mother, father, another caregiver, or another family member and note the types and frequency of single-word productions
  - record a speech sample; engage the child in play-oriented interaction
  - have the child name pictures (not point to them) as you show them
  - have the child name objects and toys as you show them
  - have the child talk about pictures, objects, and toys
  - have the child describe pictures and other stimuli presented
  - have the child name actions depicted in pictures
  - have the child tell a story depicted pictorially
  - have the child retell a short story you tell
  - take note of any unusual word usage
  - take note of overextension of words (e.g., use of the word *mother* to refer to all adult women or the use of the word *ball* to refer to all things round)
  - take note of underextensions (e.g., only the family Ford is a car and all other cars are not cars)
  - take note of signs of misunderstanding or misinterpretation of words
  - take note of the use of general terms for more specific terms (*this, this thing, that, that thing*)

L

- classify words according to <u>Semantic Relations</u>; note that there is no conclusive evidence to suggest that theoretical and abstract semantic relations are empirically real for children
- **Assess production of grammatic morphemes**
  - record an extended Speech and Language Sample (see <u>Standard/Common Assessment Procedures</u>)
  - use all connected speech-language evoking procedures including picture descriptions, description of activities you and the child engage in, interaction between the child and family member, storytelling with the help of pictures, story retelling, narrating personal experiences (e.g., favorite vacation, movie, TV shows, friends, sports, other activities), and so forth; see Speech and Language Sample under Standard/Common Assessment <u>Procedures</u> for details
  - design behavior-specific tasks to evoke production of particular grammatic morphemes; for example:
    → ask the child to name pictures of one or more objects to assess the production of plural morphemes (e.g., ask "what is this?" and "what are these?" as you show the picture of a book and that of two or more books; show multiple exemplars)
    → ask the child to name pictures that depict irregular plural nouns (e.g., show pictures of children, men, or women, and ask the child "who are these?")
    → ask the child to describe actions depicted in pictures to assess production of present progressive *ing* and the auxiliary verbs (e.g., ask "what is the boy doing?" or "what is the girl doing?" as you show pictures of a *boy running* and a *girl smiling*)
    → ask the child to say where an object is as you manipulate its location to assess the production of prepositions (e.g., ask the child "where is the ball?" as you place it in a box, on the box, behind the box, beside the box, under the box, etc.)

→ ask the child to tell "which is bigger?" "which is smaller?" "which is the smoothest?" and so forth to assess the production of comparatives and superlatives; to evoke verbal responses, show appropriate paired objects without naming them or without pointing to them

→ ask the child such questions as "whose hat is this?" "whose shoes are these?" and "whose shirt is this?" to evoke the possessive morpheme in such responses as *man's hat, woman's shoes*, and *boy's shirt*; show appropriate pictures and point to the relevant portion of the picture

→ ask such questions as "what moves?" and "who walks?" after demonstrating movement of a car and walking by a puppet to evoke the production of third person singular in such responses as *car moves* and *puppet walks*

→ ask the child to complete such sentences as *this boy is . . . ("big"); this girl is . . . ("tall"); this ball is . . . ("red")* and so forth to assess the production of adjectives; show appropriate pictures to evoke responses

→ show various pictures and tell the child a brief story and ask relevant questions to evoke the production of irregular past inflections (e.g., tell the child that *the man is now yawning; he did the same yesterday; what did he do yesterday? Or, the man is now painting; he did the same yesterday; what did he do yesterday?*)

• **Assess syntactic skills**
  • use the recorded speech and language sample to assess production of syntactic structures
  • administer one of the standardized tests of syntactic skills
  • use the elicited imitation technique to assess imitative production of sentences that the child did not produce in spontaneous speech
    → write four to six sentences of a particular type (e.g., active declarative, passive, questions, requests, negations)

Language Disorders in Children

→ model each of the sentences for the child to imitate
→ record the child's response for a precise analysis of missing or mismanaged elements
→ if time permits, administer each sentence on three trials to improve reliability; if time does not permit, make sure to repeat the procedure with three trials in establishing baselines before starting treatment
→ calculate the percent correct imitation for each of the sentence types presented
→ be aware that correct imitation of a structure is not always an indication of correct spontaneous production

- assess syntactic productions; calculate the percent correct use of major syntactic structures, elements of syntactic structures (such as adjectives), or those that are of special relevance to the child being evaluated; consider the following:
    → noun phrases: a noun with one or more modifier preceding it, often an adjective (e.g., *my shoes, big hat, that pencil*)
    → verb phrase: words or phrases that describe action or state of being; consider the auxiliary and copular verbs as well (e.g., *he is running, that is nice*)
    → prepositional phrase: a construction with a preposition, a noun or pronoun, and a modifier (e.g., *the toys in the box are mixed up*)
    → independent or main clause: a grammatically complete and correct sentence that can stand alone (e.g., *the lion growled*)
    → subordinate clause: a construction that includes a subject and a predicate but cannot stand alone as grammatically correct (e.g., *because you are nice; though I like to play*); these can become complete sentences only when combined with independent clauses (*because you are nice, I like you; though I like to play, I have no time*)

→ simple sentence: an independent clause with no subordinate clause (e.g., *I tried; she went*)

→ declarative sentences: a construction that makes a statement (e.g., *this is a ball; the sun is shining*)

→ compound sentence: a sentence with minimally two independent clauses joined by a comma and a conjunction or with a semicolon; containing no subordinate clauses (e.g., *John is not as nice as Toni, but he can be nice on occasions;* or, *I went to see Jane; I only found her dog*)

→ complex sentences: a sentence with one independent clause and one or more subordinate clauses (e.g., *I tried some small talk while we were in the elevator*)

→ active sentences: sentences in which the subject performs the actions of the verb (e.g., *Jenny hit the car*)

→ passive sentences: sentences in which the subject receives the action of the verb (e.g., *the car was hit by Jenny*)

→ questions: sentences that require more information or require a yes/no answer

→ negatives: sentences that reject or deny an affirmation (e.g., *that is a boy, not a girl; I don't like it; not for me, for him; not the car, but the puppet*)

→ requests: sentences that ask others to perform certain actions (e.g., *please give me that car; please say yes; please hand me that*)

→ imperatives: sentences that require others to perform certain actions; they are like commands (*look at me; stop that*)

• use one of the computerized language sample analysis programs to evaluate the production of syntactic structures

• **Assess language use (pragmatic skills)**
  • assess conversational repair. Assess skills of handling breakdown in communication; these include such skills as asking questions when messages are not clear and responding effectively to requests for clarification

L

Language Disorders in Children

- *Assess the frequency with which the child makes requests for clariflcations from a speaker*
- during conversational speech sampling, make several ambiguous or unclear statements (e.g., say "Give me the car" when you have displayed several toy cars; "Pick up the toy" when the child faces several toys)
- wait for the child to request clarification
- count the frequency of such ambiguous statements you made and the number of acceptable requests for clarification the child made during the assessment session
- to assess stimulability, model a request for clarification ("ask me what do you mean?"; "ask me which car?")
- count the frequency of modeled requests for clarification and the frequency with which the child imitated your request
- do not give positive or corrective feedback for the presence or absence of requests for clarification
- calculate the percent correct requests for clarification (the total number of ambiguous statements made divided by the number of correct requests for clarification the child made multiplied by 100)
- repeat the procedures in a later session (such as at the beginning of reassessment when the child returns for treatment; during treatment when other language skills are being taught)
- *Assess the frequency with which the child responds appropriately to requests for clariflcation*
- during conversational speech sampling, play the role of a listener who does not fully understand the expressions of the child
- ask the child to repeat
- ask the child "What do you mean?"
- tell the child "I do not understand"
- negate a child's utterance so the child will clarify by assertion ("You did not go on the roller coaster 20 times, did you?"; the child might say "No, I went on it two times")

- wait for a few seconds for the child to respond to your indication of lack of understanding
- take note of adequate, inadequate, and lack of response
- do not give differential feedback for inadequate clarifications, lack of clarifications, or acceptable clarifications
- count the number of times you made requests for clarification and the number of times the child made a satisfactory clarification of his or her statements
- to assess stimulability, model clarified statements ("You mean you went on the roller coaster two times, right?")
- rephrase the child's utterance into a question and say it with a rising intonation ("You went on the roller coaster 20 times?")
- ask the child to say it differently
- count the number of times the child imitated the modeled requests for clarification
- calculate the percent correct compliance for requests for clarification and the percent correct imitation of modeled compliance for requests for clarification
- **Assess topic initiation.** A pragmatic, conversational skill; the skill in introducing new topics for conversation; a language assessment target; children with language disorders either fail to initiate topics or introduce inappropriate topics
  - during conversational speech sampling, arrange a variety of stimuli that could trigger new topics of conversation: objects, pictures, storybooks, topic cards (for children who can read), toys, structured play situations such as a kitchen, a doll house, and so forth
  - introduce one of the stimulus items or situations and draw the child's attention to it (e.g., a picture of a family setting up a tent in a park)
  - wait for the child to initiate conversation about the picture and the story
  - count the number of times the child initiated a topic upon stimulus presentation
  - if the child does not initiate a topic, instruct the child to say something about the picture

- count the number of times the child initiated a topic when asked to say something
- if the child still does not initiate a topic, prompt it by beginning the story ("they are setting up a . . . .)
- count the number of times the child initiated topics upon specific verbal prompting
- accept statements that are remotely connected to the topic at hand; discount those that in your judgment are irrelevant or inappropriate
- do not give differential feedback for correct or incorrect responses and for no responses
- count the total number of stimulus presentations under each category (e.g., stimulus presentation and verbal prompting) and the total number of appropriate topic initiations; calculate the percent correct topic initiations
- repeat the measures on reassessment or at the beginning of treatment
- **Assess topic maintenance.** A pragmatic language skill of talking about a single general topic for extended duration; children with language disorders tend to abruptly and frequently switch conversational topics; a language assessment target
  - during conversational speech sampling, let the child select topics of interest for talking; prompt and suggest topics if necessary, but let the child lead you
  - measure the duration (seconds or minutes) for which the child maintained the same topic of conversation; start a stop watch as the child introduces a new topic, stop the clock as the child stops talking on that topic, or shifts to another topic
  - to assess stimulability of topic maintenance skills, use such devices as *Tell me more, What about that?, What happened next?, Who said what?, Where was it?, When did that happen?*; measure the duration for which the child maintained a topic with such prompts
  - do not give differential feedback to the child for topic maintenance or lack of it

- summarize the range of durations (the briefest and the longest) for which the child maintained topics
- calculate the typical duration (statistical mode, not the mean) for which the child maintained topics; for example, if the child talked on four topics, what was the most frequently observed duration for which the child maintained the topic?
- repeat the measures upon reassessment or before initiating treatment
- **Assess conversational turn taking**. Appropriate exchange of speaker and listener roles during conversation; a pragmatic language skill and a language assessment target; interrupting a speaker and not responding to cues to talk are characteristic of children with language disorders
  - during conversational speech sampling, observe the turn-taking behavior; if necessary, devote a few minutes of assessment time to measure turn-taking behaviors
  - count the number of times the child interrupted your speech and thus took inappropriate turns
  - count the number of times the child appropriately took conversational turns without special signals
  - to assess stimulability, count the number of times the child took turns when you signaled (e.g., when you give such verbal cues as "Your turn" or give non-verbal cues as a hand gesture to suggest *you speak*)
  - do not give differential feedback for correct or incorrect turn-taking behaviors
  - repeat the measures during reassessment or just before starting treatment on turn taking
- **Assess eye contact.** A potential pragmatic communication target behavior for certain children who do not look at the listener while speaking or at the speaker while talking
  - potentially culturally determined; find out if avoiding direct eye contact during conversation, especially with an authority figure (such as a clinician, teacher, or parents), is a cultural practice in the community to which the child belongs

- during conversational speech sampling, take note of lack of eye contact; if it is a significant problem sure the durations for which the child maintained eye contact and the durations for which the child did not
- to assess stimulability, instruct the child (e.g., "look at me as you talk to me") to maintain eye contact and measure the duration for which the child maintains eye contact
- use clinical judgment in evaluating the measures as there are no specific guidelines on appropriate durations of eye contact in conversational exchanges
- repeat the measures during reassessment or just before starting treatment

- **Assess narrative skills.** A conversational skill illustrated by a speaker's description of events (stories, episodes) and experiences in a logically consistent, cohesive, temporally sequenced manner; an advanced language skill targeted for assessment

  - during conversational speech sampling, observe and take note of narrative skills
  - note that overall narrative styles, amount of detail and elaboration offered, use of emotional expression, organization and sequencing of events may be influenced by the child's cultural background
  - ask the child to describe such events as grocery shopping, eating in a restaurant, birthday parties, camping trips, vacations, playing certain games, and so forth to assess narrative skills
  - read aloud or tell a story to the child and ask him or her to retell it
  - retell the same story to the child and pause before important phrases or critical descriptions to assess whether the child will supply them
  - to assess stimulability, prompt phrases and descriptions as the child hesitates; observe if the child picks up details and sequences
  - tell a story with the help of pictures, and ask the child to retell it while looking at the pictures

L

- Analyze the narratives for proper temporal sequence of events, inadequate character descriptions, misplaced story settings, missing details, sparse descriptions, abrupt ending, confused characters, and so forth
- **Assess language comprehension**
  - observe the child's responses while taking a conversational speech sample to assess comprehension of your speech
  - note irrelevant or inappropriate responses that suggest lack of comprehension
  - note the response complexity level at which comprehension breaks down (e.g., correct comprehension of phrases but not sentences)
  - give specific commands to assess comprehension; use or modify such strategies as the following:
    → ask the child to point to a set of common pictures as you name them (e.g., "point to the *car*" or "point to the *dog*"); score the correct and incorrect responses
    → ask the child to manipulate objects or toys (e.g., "put the block on the book" or "make the car go"); score the correct and incorrect responses
    → ask the child to follow simple to progressively more complex commands (e.g., "please stand up"; "please shut that door"; and, "please shut the door and open the drapes"); score the correct and incorrect responses
    → ask the child to point to correct pictures that help assess comprehension of grammatic morphemes and syntactic structures (e.g., "show me *the boy* is *running*"; "show me *the girl is riding*"; "show me *two cups*"; "show me *the ball is in the box*"; "show me *the car is on the table*"; "show me *he is smiling*"; "show me she *is walking*"); score the correct and incorrect responses
  - assess comprehension of abstract statements by asking the child to explain the meaning of proverbs you expect the child to have heard; note that proverbs and typical expressions are extremely culture-bound

L

Language Disorders in Children

Administer Selected Standardized Tests of Children's Language Skills

- Use the Speech, Language, and Motor Development guidelines in assessing children
- Administer one or more of the following standardized tests or measures; use the following matrix to make initial selection of tests to be administered to a child; please see their respective alphabetical entries for more information:

Test	Purpose
Assessment of Children's Language Comprehension (R. Foster, J. J. Giddan, & J. Stark)	To assess comprehension of words and phrases (3 to 6;11 yrs)
Test of Auditory Comprehension of Language-Revised (E. Carrow-Woolfolk)	To assess comprehension of word categories, grammatic features, and syntactic con structions (3 to 9;11 yrs)
Expressive One-Word Picture Vocabulary Test—Revised (M. Gardner)	To assess production of single words (2 to 11;11 yrs)
Peabody Picture Vocabulary Test—Revised (L. M. Dunn & L. A Dunn)	To assess comprehension of single words (2;3 to 40;11 yrs)
Bankson Language Test (N. W. Bankson)	To assess production of semantic, syntactic, and morphologic skills (4 to 8 yrs)
Boehm Test of Basic Concepts (A. E. Boehm)	To assess comprehension of basic semantic concepts (K through 2nd grade)
Basic Language Concepts Test (S. Englemann, D. Ross, & V. Bingham)	To assess basic language skills necessary to succeed in initial grades (4 to 6;6 yrs)
Carrow Elicited Language Inventory (E. Carrow-Woolfolk)	To assess imitative production of syntactic skills (3 to 7;11 yrs)
	(continued)

306

(continued)

Test	Purpose
Clinical Evaluation of Language Fundamentals—3rd Edition (E. Semel, E. Wiig & W. Secord)	To assess production of semantic, syntactic, phonologic, and memory skills (6 to 21;11 yrs)
Evaluating Communicative Competence (C. S. Simon)	To assess comprehension and production of pragmatic skills (9 to 17 yrs)
Sequenced Inventory of Communication Development—Revised (D. L. Hedrick, E. M. Prather, & A. R. Tobin)	To assess comprehension and production of communication skills (4 months to 4 yrs)
Wiig Criterion-referenced Inventory of Language (Wiig, 1990)	A criterion-referenced assessment tool for semantic, syntactic, morphologic, and pragmatic skills (4 to 13 yrs)
Test for Examining Expressive Morphology (K. G. Shipley, T. Stone, & M. Sue)	To assess production of morphological skills (3 to 8;11 yrs)
Test of Early Language Development—2nd Edition (W. P. Hiresko, D. K. Reid, & D. D. Hammill)	To assess comprehension and production of semantic and syntactic structures (2;7 to 7;11 yrs)
Test of Language Development—2 Primary (P. L. Newcomer & D. D. Hammill)	To assess comprehension and production of words; articulation; and some grammatic features (4 to 8;11 yrs)
Test of Language Development—2 Intermediate (P. L. Newcomer & D. D. Hammill)	To test comprehension and production of words; articulation; and grammatic features 8;6 to 12;11 yrs)
Preschool Language Scale—3 (I. R. Zimmerman, V. G. Steiner, & R. E. Pond)	To assess comprehension and production of language skills (birth to 6;11 yrs) *(continued)*

L

(continued)

Test	Purpose
Utah Test of Language Development—3 (M. J. Mecham)	To assess language production and comprehension (3 to 9;11 yrs)
Test of Word Finding (D. J. German)	To assess single-word retrieval skills (6;6 to 12;11 yrs)
Test of Word Finding in Discourse (D. J. German)	To assess word retrieval deficits in conversation (6;6 to 12;11 yrs)
Test of Pragmatic Skills—Revised (B. B. Schulman)	To assess verbal and nonverbal pragmatic skills (3 to 8;11 yrs)
Wiig Criterion-referenced Inventory of Language (E. H. Wiig)	To make a criterion referenced assessment of semantic, syntactic, morphologic, and pragmatic skills (4 to 13 yrs)

L

Medical, Psychological, and Educational Assessment Data

- Obtain any available medical data of importance in evaluating language disorders
- Obtain results of audiological evaluation
- Obtain psychological data including the results of intelligence testing and cognitive functioning
- Obtain data on the child's educational achievement and assessment that might suggest learning disabilities and educational demands made on the child

Standard/Common Assessment Procedures

- Complete the <u>Standard/Common Assessment Procedures</u>

Analysis of Results

- Analyze the results of comprehension assessment; identify the levels at which comprehension is adequate (e.g., correct comprehension of words or phrases)
- Identify the levels at which comprehension breaks down (e.g., poor comprehension of sentences; questions; two-element commands; requests; etc.)

- Estimate the level of comprehension of connected, spoken speech (e.g., 80% of words, phrases, or sentences comprehended)
- Analyze the kinds of words the child uses (e.g., nouns only; nouns and a few verbs; few or no adjectives); if possible, estimate the size of the child's vocabulary, especially if the child is producing mostly single words
- Calculate the <u>Mean Length of Utterance (MLU)</u>
- Calculate the length of most frequently produced utterances (statistical mode, not the mean)
- Identify the shortest and the longest utterance
- List the grammatic morphemes the child produced with 100% accuracy in conversational speech and standardized tests
- List the grammatic morphemes the child failed to produce or produced at some inadequate level in either conversational speech or during standardized testing; quantify these observations (e.g., 0% production of past tense *ed* inflection; 10% accurate production of the present progressive *ing*)
- List the sentence types the child produced in conversational speech (e.g., simple, active declarative; questions; negation; passive; requests; complex sentences; compound sentences; embedded sentences, etc.)
- List the sentence types the child did not produce in either conversational speech or during standardized testing
- Summarize the pragmatic features the child correctly used or managed (e.g., appropriate eye contact, acceptable turn taking, adequate topic initiation skills, etc.); to the extent possible, quantify these observations (e.g. appropriate topic initiation 80% of the opportunities)
- Summarize the pragmatic features the child did not use or used inappropriately (e.g., lack of topic maintenance; poor narrative skills, inadequate response to request for clarification, lack of request for clarification, etc.); to the extent possible, quantify these observations (e.g., 100% failure in responding to requests for clarification)

L

- Summarize the child's phonological skills; make a thorough analysis as described under <u>Articulation and Phonological Disorders</u> if the data warrant
- Make a clinical judgment of voice; take note of voice problems, if any; conduct a voice assessment if data warrant it
- Make a clinical judgment of fluency; conduct a fluency assessment if data warrant it
- Use such computer software programs as Lingquest 1, Systematic Analysis of Language Transcripts, and Computerized Profiling

Diagnostic Criteria/Guidelines
- Significantly limited or deficient language skills affecting all aspects of language (semantic, syntactic, morphologic, and pragmatic skills)
- Absence of sensory deficits, intellectual deficiency, neuromotor problems, and psychiatric problems

Differential Diagnosis
- Rule out the presence of associated clinical conditions
  - differentiate language disorders associated with autism by its basic characteristics: a pervasive developmental disorder characterized by a lack of responsiveness to people and their feelings; no or abnormal seeking of comfort when ill; no or impaired imitation (echolalia), no or abnormal play; lack of interest in play; abnormal, idiosyncratic, irrelevant, and stereotypic speech; stereotypic body movements; preoccupation with objects; insistence on routines; reluctance to be hugged, held, or touched; and preference to be left alone
  - differentiate language disorders associated with hearing impairment by these specific characteristics: an audiological assessment that documents the type and degree of hearing impairment; reluctance to speak; significant phonological problems including omission of final consonants, simplification of blends, and substitution of voiced consonants for voiceless consonants and vice versa; greater difficulty in producing fricatives; distor-

tions of various sounds; hyper- and hyponasality; significant voice problems especially with deafness; abnormal flow of speech; and slower rate of speech

- differentiate language disorders associated with mental retardation on the basis of the following: an independent diagnosis of mental retardation by a psychologist; a medical diagnosis of a genetic syndrome or associated medical conditions that cause mental retardation (e.g., Down syndrome, prenatal lead poisoning, fetal alcohol syndrome, postimmunization encephalitis, etc.); note that generally simplified language associated with mental retardation is similar to language disorders found in otherwise normal children who show language problems
- differentiate language disorders associated with various kinds of brain injury on the basis of the following: an independent diagnosis of brain injury and its cause (e.g., vehicular accident, falls, assault and gunshot, physical abuse); initial symptoms of coma (in some cases), confusion and posttraumatic amnesia; retrograde amnesia; irritability, aggression, lethargy, anxiety, withdrawal and other behavioral problems; motor dysfunctions including rigidity, tremors, spasticity, ataxia, or apraxia; mutism; and significant word retrieval problems

Prognosis

- Variable depending on the child, family support, time of intervention, and the intensity of intervention
- Most children with language disorders benefit from treatment
- Some deficits may continue into adolescent and adult years

Recommendations

- Language intervention
- Parent training in language stimulation and maintenance activities at home
- Working with the child's teacher to coordinate treatment objectives and activities with academic goals and activities

- See the cited sources and *PGTSLP* for details

Hegde, M. N. (1995). *A coursebook on language disorders in children.* San Diego, CA: Singular Publishing Group.

Lund, N. J., & Duchan, J. F. (1993). *Assessing children's language in naturalistic settings* (3rd ed.). Boston, MA: Allyn & Bacon.

Nelson, N. W. (1993). *Childhood language disorders in context.* New York: Merrill.

Paul, R. (2001). *Language disorders from infancy through adolescence* (2nd ed.). St. Louis, MO: C. V. Mosby.

Reed, V. (1994). *An introduction to children with language disorders* (2nd ed.). New York: Macmillan.

Ripich, D. N., & Creaghead, N. A. (1994). *School discourse problems* (2nd ed.). San Diego, CA: Singular Publishing Group.

Language Disorders in African American Children. Limited language skills in, or a failure to acquire language normally by, African American children; see Language Disorders in Children for a description of language disorders that applies to most children; the disorder may be evident in African American English (AAE), Standard American English (SAE), or both; children who speak AAE are more likely to use both AAE and a variety of SAE; not all African American children speak AAE and, therefore, clinicians should not stereotypically assume that all African American children need to be assessed for AAE; assessment presents challenges to clinicians who do not know the syntactic, semantic, and pragmatic properties of AAE; inappropriate assessment practices include: (1) a mistaken diagnosis of a language disorder in SAE when an African American child's patterns of communication simply reflect the influence of AAE and (2) overdiagnosis or underdiagnosis of a language disorder in AAE; both can be avoided with (1) a good knowledge of AAE, (2) a general understanding that AAE is a product of unique historical and cultural forces; that it is a recognized form of English with its own phonologic, syntactic, semantic, and pragmatic rules and conventions; see Ethnocultural Considerations in Assessment for general guidelines

Factors Related to Language Disorders in African American Children

- No unique factors that cause language disorder in African American children have been convincingly demonstrated
- Specific language impairment as described in this section, by definition, is free from such other associated clinical conditions as developmental disabilities and hearing impairment

Description of Language Disorders in African American Children

- Note that for the most part, African American children with language disorders exhibit the same kinds of language deficiencies as other children: limited vocabulary, limited syntactic structures, errors in morphologic use, and inappropriate or deficient use of language
- Note also that the issue is not whether African American children exhibit unique patterns of language deficiencies; it is whether a given pattern of language usage should or should not be diagnosed as a language disorder in light of the language, culture, and family communication systems of African Americans
- See under Language Disorders in Children for a summary of common language deficiencies found in children who have language disorders

Assessment Objectives/General Guidelines

- To analyze language disorders in AAE and in SAE if a child speaks both the forms; note that this requires knowledge of AAE and the unique communication styles and needs of the individual child and his or her family members
- To analyze language problems in SAE the child speaks that are *not* due to the influence of AAE; note that such problems do constitute a true language disorder; note, too, that this task requires knowledge of the AAE and the unique communication pattern of the child and his or her family

L

- To analyze an African American child's language patterns of SAE usage that vary from those of SAE but are a function of AAE patterns; note that such variations are not a basis to diagnose a language disorder; this analysis is done to achieve a comprehensive understanding of the child's communication styles and patterns; however, treatment may be offered if the child, the family, or both wish to minimize variations in SAE usage
- To identify potential language treatment targets that are ethnoculturally appropriate for the child and are consistent with the wishes, needs, and the cultural background of the child and his or her family

Case History/Interview Focus

- See **Case History** and **Interview** under Standard/Common Assessment Procedures
- Ask questions designed to obtain information on the family communication patterns; for instance:
  - do the family members speak only AAE at home?
  - do the family members also speak SAE at home?
  - how is the talking time roughly distributed across the two forms of English?
  - what is the level of SAE proficiency of family members?
  - what is the level of AAE proficiency of family members?
  - do they all effectively code-switch depending on communicative situations?
  - what are the parents' expectation regarding clinical services? Are they concerned about proficiency in SAE?
  - what kinds of educational demands are made on the child?
  - does the child's classroom teacher accept AAE?
  - how is the child doing in the classroom?
  - is there an indication of poor performance due to limited SAE proficiency, AAE proficiency, or both?
  - are there any associated clinical conditions that might affect prognosis (e.g., developmental disabilities, hearing loss, neurological impairment, genetic syndromes)?
  - what are the recommendations of the child's teachers?

- what are the educational and career goals of the client or as envisioned by the parents?

Assessment of Language Disorders in African American Children

- Note that few satisfactorily standardized tests are available to evaluate language proficiency in African American children; currently, using nonstandardized, systematic, client-specific procedures with a good background in AAE is the best diagnostic approach
- Note that most standardized tests of language skills may not have adequately sampled African American children in their standardization process
- Note that SAE patterns need to be assessed even if no diagnosis of a disorder is made solely on this basis; because the parents and the child may opt for language treatment geared toward standard English usage, it is essential to make a thorough analysis of deficiencies in both the forms of English
- Take extended, representative samples of connected speech and language productions in both English and the primary language of a bilingual child; use the general procedures for obtaining a speech and language sample described under Standard/Common Assessment Procedures; note that when one form of English is more dominant than the other, the samples will differ in their extent or complexity
- Use the assessment procedures described under Language Disorders in Children to assess aspects of language production including word production and usage, production of grammatic morphemes, syntactic skills, language use, and language comprehension; however, in selecting stimulus materials to evoke speech and language structures, consider the child's family and cultural background; let the parents guide the selection of materials that are familiar to their child
- Let the patents interact with the child as you tape record the conversational interaction; assist the parents in manip-

ulating the stimulus materials to evoke a variety of language productions to sample all aspects of language

Medical, Psychological, and Educational Assessment Data

- Obtain results of intellectual and behavioral assessment in cases of children with mental retardation and behavioral disorders
- Obtain information on academic and language performance and academic demands made on the child
- Obtain information on physical, medical, or neurological disabilities
- Obtain information on audiological assessment
- Obtain information on other sensory impairments if relevant

Standard/Common Assessment Procedures

- Complete the Standard/Common Assessment Procedures

Analysis of Results

- Use the procedures described under Language Disorders in Children
- Obtain the help of an African American SLP or one with a good knowledge of AAE
- Analyze language variations or deviations in AAE in light of the AAE language patterns; only productions that are inconsistent with AAE language patterns are a basis to diagnose a language disorder in AAE
- Analyze variations in SAE productions that may be a function of the AAE patterns; these variations are *not* a basis to diagnose a language disorder
- Analyze language deviations in SAE that are independent of AAE patterns; these errors are a basis to diagnose a language disorder in SAE

Diagnostic Criteria for African American Children

- Note that many aspects of AAE language usage are similar to SAE usage; only certain syntactic structures and communication styles of AAE vary from those in SAE

- Assess aspects of AAE language usages that differ from those of SAE but are indeed characteristics of AAE; in making this assessment, consider the following language patterns of AAE as summarized by Roseberry-McKibbin (1995); note that the following table contrasts the mainstream American expressions and AAE expressions; the described AAE characteristics and expressions are accepted in AAE, and hence, are *not* a basis to diagnose a language disorder:

AAE Characteristic	Mainstream American English	Sample AAE Utterance
Noun possessives may be omitted.	That's the woman's car. It's John's pencil.	That the *woman* car. It *John* pencil.
Noun plurals may be omitted.	He has 2 boxes of apples. She gives me 5 cents.	He got 2 box of *apple*. She give me 5 *cent*.
Third person singular may be omitted	She walks to school. The man works in his yard.	She *walk* to school. The man *work* in his yard.
Forms of to be (*is, are*) may be omitted.	She is a nice lady. They are going to a movie.	*She a* nice lady. *They going* to a movie.
Present tense is may be used regardless of person or number.	They are having fun. You are a smart man.	*They is* having fun. *You is* a smart man.
Person or number may not agree with past and present forms.	You are playing ball. They are having a picnic.	You *is* playing ball. They *is* having a picnic.
Present tense forms of auxiliary *have* may be omitted.	I have been here for 2 hours.	I been here for 2 hours. He done it again.
Past tense endings may be omitted.	He lived in California. She cracked the nut.	He *live* in California. She *crack* the nut.
Past tense was may be used regardless of number and person.	They were shopping. You were helping me.	They *was* shopping. You *was* helping me.

(continued)

(continued)

AAE Characteristic	Mainstream American English	Sample AAE Utterance
Multiple negatives may be used to add emphasis to the negative meaning.	We don't have any more. I don't want any cake. I don't like Broccoli.	We don't have no more. I don't never want no cake. I don't never like Broccoli.
None may be substituted for *any*.	She doesn't want any.	She don't want *none*.
In perfective constructions, *been* may be used to indicate that an action took place in the past.	I had the mumps when I was 5.	I *been had* the mumps when I was 5. I *been known* her.
Done may be combined with a past tense form to indicate that an action was started and completed	He fixed the stove. She tried to paint it.	He *done fixed* the stove. She *done tried* to paint it.
The form *be* may be used as the main verb.	Today she is working. We are singing.	Today *she be* working. *We be* singing.
Distributive *be* may be used to indicate actions and events over time.	He is often cheerful. She's kind sometimes.	*He be* cheerful. *She be* kind.
A pronoun may be used to restate the subject.	My brother surprised me. My dog has fleas.	My brother, *he* surprise me. My dog, *he* got fleas.
Them may be substituted for *those*.	Those cars are antiques. Where'd you get those books?	*Them* cars, they be antique. Where you get *them* books?
Future tense is and *are* may be replaced by *gonna*.	She is going to help us. They are going to be there.	She *gonna* help us. They *gonna* be there.
At may be used at the end of *where* questions.	Where is the house? Where is the store?	Where is the house *at*? Where is the store *at*?
Additional auxiliaries may be used.	I might have done it.	I *might could have* done it.
Does may replace *do*.	She does funny things. It does make sense.	*She do* funny things. *It do* make sense.

- Note that a diagnosable language disorder for a child who speaks AAE is a disorder in the context of AAE (and SAE), not in the sole context of SAE

Differential Diagnosis

- Differentiate language disorder from language difference in light of the listed AAE characteristics
- Use all of the guidelines for differential diagnosis summarized under <u>Language Disorders in Children</u>
- Note that the most critical task of differential diagnosis is to separate language errors in AAE and those in SAE that are not a function of AAE patterns; take note of all variations in SAE; however, diagnose a disorder in SAE only if the errors are not due to the language patterns of SAE
- Diagnose language problems in AAE only when they are inconsistent with AAE patterns

Prognosis

- No systematic evidence suggests that prognosis for improved language skills in African American children is any different from that in other children
- Most if not all children may be expected to improve with systematic treatment
- The presence of such additional variables as developmental disabilities, genetic syndromes, and sensory disabilities (e.g., hearing loss) may affect the rate of improvement

Recommendations for African American Children

- Recommend treatment for language disorders in AAE; recommend treatment targets that are consistent with AAE
- Recommend treatment for language variations in SAE only if the client or the family members request such treatment because of the advantage standard English offers in educational, social, and occupational settings
- Recommend treatment on a priority basis for errors that are common to AAE and SAE

- See the cited sources and the *PGTSLP* for treatment details

Hegde, M. N. (1996). *A coursebook on language disorders in children*. San Diego: Singular Publishing Group.

Massey, A. (1996). Cultural influences on language: Implications for assessing African American children. In A. G. Kamhi, K. E. Pollock, & J. L. Harris (Eds.), *Communication development and disorders in African American children* (pp. 285–306). Baltimore: Paul H. Brookes.

Roseberry-McKibbin, C. (1995). *Multicultural students with special needs*. Oceanside, CA: Academic Communication Associates.

Washington, J. A. (1996). Issues in assessing the language abilities of African American children. In A. G. Kamhi, K. E. Pollock, & J. L. Harris (Eds.), *Communication development and disorders in African American children* (pp. 35–54). Baltimore: Paul H. Brookes.

Language Disorders in Bilingual Children. Limited language skills in, or failure to develop language normally by, bilingual children whose primary language is other than English; see <u>Language Disorders in Children</u> for a description of language disorders that applies to most children; the disorder may be evident in one or both the languages spoken by a large and varied group of children in the United States; for the most part, these children include those whose primary language is Spanish, an Asian language, or a Native American language; may include children of European background who speak a language other than English; present assessment challenges because of the variety of primary languages that influence the secondary English spoken in the United States; see <u>Ethnocultural Considerations in Assessment</u> for general guidelines.

Factors Related to Language Disorders in Bilingual Children

- No unique factors that cause language disorders in bilingual children have been convincingly demonstrated
- Factors that are associated with language disorders in monolingual children also may be associated with such

disorders in bilingual children; see under <u>Language Disorders in Children</u> for a summary of these factors

Description of Language Disorders in Bilingual Children

- Note that, for the most part, bilingual children exhibit the same language deficiencies as monolingual children: limited vocabulary, limited syntactic structures, errors in morphologic use, and inappropriate or deficient use of language
- Note also that the issue is not whether bilingual children exhibit unique language disorders; it is whether a given pattern of language production should or should not be diagnosed as a language disorder in light of bilingual children's first language
- See under <u>Language Disorders in Children</u> for a summary of common error patterns found in children with language disorders

Assessment Objectives/General Guidelines

- To analyze deficiencies in language production and comprehension that are evident in the primary language of the child; note that this requires knowledge of the primary language's semantic, grammatic, and pragmatic aspects along with an understanding of the cultural communication patterns of the child and his or her family; in the absence of such knowledge, refer the child to a speech-language pathologist (SLP) who speaks the child's primary language or who has acquired the necessary knowledge or use a qualified interpreter
- To analyze errors of language production in English that are *not* due to the influence of the primary language; note that this task, too, requires knowledge of a bilingual child's primary language
- To analyze the child's patterns of English usage that vary from those in Standard or a regional American English that *are* due to the influence of the child's primary lan-

guage; such an analysis need not result in a diagnosis of a language disorder; this analysis is done to achieve a comprehensive understanding of child's language skills; however, treatment may be recommended if the child, the family, or both wish to minimize the educational, social, and occupational effects of variations in standard English usage

• To identify potential treatment targets that are ethno-culturally appropriate for the child and are consistent with the wishes and needs of the child and his or her family

Case History/Interview Focus

• See **Case History** and **Interview** under <u>Standard/Common Assessment Procedures</u>

• Ask questions designed to obtain information on the family communication patterns; for instance:

  • what percentage of the time do the family members speak the primary language, such as Spanish or Hmong, at home?

  • what is the level of English proficiency of family members?

  • what is the level of primary language proficiency of family members?

  • what is the specific variety of primary language spoken at home (e.g., Mexican Spanish or Puerto Rican Spanish)?

  • do they speak English, and if so, what percentage of the time or in what kinds of communicative situations?

  • is one or the other language dominant in certain speaking situations?

  • what are the parents' expectation regarding clinical services? Are they concerned about proficiency in Standard English?

  • what kinds of educational demands are made on the child? Is the child in a regular classroom or in a special bilingual program?

Language Disorders in Bilingual Children

- how is the child doing in the classroom? Is there an indication of poor performance due to English language deficiency, primary language deficiency, or deficiency in both the languages?
- are there any associated clinical conditions that might affect prognosis (e.g., developmental disabilities, hearing loss, neurological impairment, genetic syndromes)?
- what are the recommendations of the child's teachers?
- what are the educational and career goals of the client or as envisioned by the parents?

Assessment of Language Disorders in Bilingual Children

- Note that very few satisfactorily standardized tests are available to evaluate language proficiency in bilingual children; a few tests of Spanish language may be available, but for bilingual children who speak an Asian language, a Native American language, or one of several other secondary languages spoken in the United States, standardized tests are more limited or nonexistent
- Make sure that an available test of Spanish language skills samples the specific variety of Spanish (e.g., Mexican Spanish or Cuban Spanish) the child and the family members speak
- Note that English usage needs to be assessed even if no diagnosis of a disorder is made solely on this basis; because the parents and the child may opt for language treatment geared toward standard English, it is essential to make a thorough analysis of errors in both the languages
- Take extended, representative samples of connected speech and language in both English and the primary language of a bilingual child; use the general procedures for obtaining a speech and language sample described under Standard/Common Assessment Procedures; note that when one language is more dominant than the other, the samples will differ in their extent

- Use the procedures described under <u>Language Disorders in Children</u> to assess aspects of language production including word production and usage, production of grammatic morphemes, syntactic skills, language use, and language comprehension; however, in selecting stimulus materials to evoke speech and language structures, consider the child's family and cultural background; let the parents guide the selection of materials that are familiar to their child
- Let the patents interact with the child as you tape record the conversational interaction; assist the parents in manipulating the stimulus materials to evoke a variety of language productions to sample all speech language

Medical, Psychological, and Educational Assessment Data

- Obtain results of intellectual and behavioral assessment in cases of children with mental retardation and behavioral disorders
- Obtain information on academic and language performance and academic demands made on the child
- Obtain information on physical, medical, or neurological disabilities
- Obtain information on audiological assessment
- Obtain information on other sensory impairments if relevant

Standard/Common Assessment Procedures

- Complete the <u>Standard/Common Assessment</u> Procedures

Analysis of Results

- Use the procedures described under <u>Language Disorders in Children</u>
- Obtain the help of a bilingual speech-language pathologist who knows the child's primary language
- Analyze separately the child's errors in the primary language and the secondary English
- Analyze language problems in English that may be a function of the primary language; in this case, the prob-

lems are variations and not a basis to diagnose a language disorder
- Analyze language problems in English that may be independent of the characteristics of the child's primary language; these are a basis to diagnose a language disorder in English
- Analyze language problems in the primary language in light of the characteristics of that language; these are a basis to diagnose a language disorder in that language

Diagnostic Criteria for Selected Bilingual Children

- In diagnosing language disorders in **Hispanic Children**:
  - first ascertain the variety of Spanish the child and the family members speak, as the Spanish spoken in the United States may be of different origin (e.g., Mexican, Puerto Rican, Cuban)
  - find out the language and communication characteristics of the variety of Spanish the child speaks; also use the general characteristics of Spanish-influenced English summarized next
  - determine first if a Hispanic child is a bilingual speaker; then follow the guidelines offered in this section
  - develop a database of varieties of Spanish spoken in your service area and prepare lists of their language and communication patterns
  - make a diagnosis of language disorders based on such patterns
  - use all the guidelines specified in this section to evaluate the language difference or disorder in light of those characteristics
- Use the following characteristics of **Spanish-influenced English**, as summarized by Roseberry-McKibbin (1995), in diagnosing a language disorders in a child whose primary language is Spanish; see also Assessment of Articulation Disorders in Bilingual Children to understand the phonological properties of Spanish; note that these lan-

Language Disorders in Bilingual Children

guage and phonological characteristics, when they influence the production of English as a second language, are
not the bases to diagnose a language disorder in English:

Spanish-Influenced Language Characteristics	Sample English Utterances
1. Adjective comes after the noun.	The house green.
2. s is often omitted in plurals and possessives.	The girl book is . . . .
3. Past tense –ed is often omitted.	We walk yesterday.
4. Double negatives are required.	I don't have no more.
5. Superiority is demonstrated by using mas.	This cake is more big.
6. The adverb often follows the verb.	He drives very fast his motorcycle.

Roseberry-McKibbin, C. (1995). *Multicultural students with special needs.* Oceanside, CA: Academic Communication Associates.

- In diagnosing language disorders in **Asian American Children**:
  - first ascertain the Asian language the child and the family members speak, as the Asian American families are a diverse group that speaks literally hundreds of major Asian languages (e.g., languages of China, the Indian subcontinent, South East Asia)
  - find out the language and communication characteristics of the variety of Asian language the child speaks; also use the general characteristics of Asian languages as summarized next; however, note that because of the diversity of Asian languages—they belong to different language families with diverse language properties—a general description of language characteristics or communication patterns may be of limited practical use

- determine first if an Asian American child is a bilingual speaker; then follow the guidelines offered in this section
- use all of the guidelines specified in this section to evaluate the language difference or disorder in light of those characteristics
- develop a database of Asian languages spoken in your service area and prepare lists of their language and communication patterns
- make a diagnosis of language disorders based on such patterns
- Use the following characteristics of Asian communication patterns, as summarized by Roseberry-McKibbin (1995), in diagnosing a language disorder in a child who speaks an **Asian language**:

Asian Language Characteristics	Sample English Utterance
Omission of plurals	Here are two piece of toast. I got 5 finger on each hand.
Omission of copula	He going home now. They eating.
Omission of possessive	I have Phuong pencil. Mom food is cold.
Omission of past tense morpheme	We cook dinner yesterday. Last night she walk home.
Past tense double marking	He didn't went by himself.
Double negative	They don't have no books.
Subject-verb-object relationship differences/omissions	I messed up it. He like.
Singular present tense omission or addition	You goes inside. He go to the store.
Wrong ordering of interrogatives	You are going now?

(continued)

(continued)

Asian Language Characteristics	Sample English Utterance
Misuse or omission of prepositions	She is in home. He goes to school 8:00.
Misuse of pronouns	She husband is coming. She said her wife is here.
Omission and/or overgeneralization of articles	Boy is sick. He went the home.
Incorrect use of comparatives	This book is gooder than that book.
Omission of conjunctions	You _____I going to the beach.
Omission, lack of inflection on auxiliary "do"	She _____not take it. He do not have enough.
Omission, lack of inflection on forms of "have"	She have no money. We _____been the store.
Omission of articles	I see little cat.

Roseberry-McKibbin, C. (1995). *Multicultural students with special needs.* Oceanside, CA: Academic Communication Associates.

- In diagnosing language disorders in **Native American Children**
  - first ascertain the Native American language the child and the family members speak, as the Native American families are a diverse group that speaks literally hundreds of major languages in North America alone
  - note that many children of Native Americans do not speak their parents' language or have only extremely limited proficiency in it
  - note that there are useful websites on American Indian or Native American culture and languages that offer information on certain languages and their properties; use these resources in understanding aspects of Native American languages

Language Disorders in Bilingual Children

- determine first if a Native American child is a bilingual speaker; then follow the guidelines offered in this section
- find out the language and communication characteristics of the Native American language the child speaks; also use the general characteristics of Native American communication patterns as summarized next; however, note that because of the diversity of Native American languages—they belong to different language families with diverse language properties—a general description of language characteristics or communication patterns may be of limited practical use
- use all of the guidelines specified in this section to evaluate the language difference or disorder in light of those characteristics
- develop a database of Native American languages spoken in your service area and prepare lists of their language and communication patterns
- make a diagnosis of language disorders based on such patterns
- Use the following characteristics of **Native American** cultural and communication patterns, as summarized by Roseberry-McKibbin (1995), in diagnosing a language disorder in a Native American child:
  - mutual respect is a high cultural value; avoiding eye contact and looking down is a standard method of showing respect
  - children are especially taught not to maintain eye contact while talking to adults; maintaining eye contact during conversation with an adult is a sign of rudeness and defiance
  - Native American mothers, especially those in the Navajo population, may not talk much while caring for their infants
  - children are taught to listen, observe, and learn thereby
  - in the judgment of parents, their children may have better auditory comprehension skills than their expressive language skills

- some parents may not encourage their children to speak their native language until their articulation is acceptable; therefore, children in the early years may be deprived of language learning opportunities
- a long period of nonverbal communication (pointing and gesturing) may pass before children begin to use words
- talking too much or talking English may be viewed as imitating the White Man
- Native American etiquette requires that a speaker pause before answering a question; quick answers imply that the question did not require much thought
- if unsure of an answer, children may not respond to a question
- children may be reluctant to express their opinions until the adults indicate that they have earned their right express their own opinions
- public expression of strong feelings is generally discouraged
- expression of grief in the presence of outsiders may be acceptable only during official mourning ceremonies

Roseberry-McKibbin, C. (1995). *Multicultural students with special needs.* Oceanside, CA: Academic Communication Associates.

Differential Diagnosis

- Differentiate a language disorder from language difference in light of the characteristics of the child's primary language
- Use all the guidelines for differential diagnosis summarized under Language Disorders in Children
- Note that the most critical task of differential diagnosis in bilingual children is to separate language errors in the child's secondary English that are not a function of the child's primary language; take note of all variations in the secondary English; however, diagnose a disorder in English only if the errors are not due to the patterns of the primary language
- Diagnose language problems in the primary language only when they are inconsistent with patterns of that language

Prognosis

- No systematic evidence suggests that prognosis for improved language skills in bilingual children is any different from that in other children
- Most if not all bilingual children may be expected to improve with systematic treatment
- The presence of such additional variables as developmental disabilities, genetic syndromes, and sensory disabilities (e.g., hearing loss) may affect the rate of improvement

Recommendations for Bilingual Children

- Recommend treatment for language disorders in the first language in accordance with the patterns of that language
- Recommend treatment for disorders in English that are not just variations due to the influence of the primary language
- Recommend treatment for language variations in standard English only if the client or the family members request such treatment because of the advantage standard English offers in educational, social, and occupational settings
- Recommend treatment for language errors that are common to the child's primary language and the secondary English on a priority basis
- Refer the child to a bilingual clinician who knows the child's primary language
- See the cited sources and *PGTSLP* for treatment details

Hegde, M. N. (1996). *A coursebook on language disorders in children.* San Diego: Singular Publishing Group.

Kayser, H. (1995). *Bilingual speech-language pathology: An Hispanic focus.* San Diego: Singular Publishing Group.

Roseberry-McKibbin, C. (1995). *Multicultural students with special needs.* Oceanside, CA: Academic Communication Associates.

Language Disorders in Infants and Toddlers. Problems in the acquisition of language in infants and toddlers; various kinds of communication deficits become apparent as the infant grows older; not only oral language, but all aspects of communication, including nonverbal communication, may be deficient; communication delay may be associated with developmental disabilities; the prevalence rate may be as high as 10% of children under age 3; generally seen in two groups of children: those with established risk and those who are at risk for developing communication problems (often along with other developmental delays or disabilities) children with established risk have conditions known to be associated with overall developmental delay including language delay or disorders (e.g., children with genetic syndromes, neurological diseases, hearing loss, etc.); children who are at risk experience variables that are likely to produce language problems, especially if early and effective intervention is not provided; both biological and environmental variables place children in a risk category; any variable that interrupts or impedes the normal interaction between the child and his or her verbal environment is a risk factor; depending on the age of the children in this group there may be no language disorder yet, only some initial signs of impending delay or disorder, delayed onset of preverbal behaviors, or delayed onset of early communicative behaviors; assessment concerns all aspects of communication, especially family communication and emergence of preverbal and early verbal behaviors.

Etiology of Established Risk

Most of the established risk factors are biological or disease-related (Rossetti, 1996):

- Various genetic syndromes including Down syndrome, Fragile X syndrome, Waardenburg syndrome, and cri-du-chat syndrome; see Syndromes Associated With Communicative Disorders
- Various neurologic disorders including cerebral palsy, progressive muscular dystrophy, Wilson's disease, intracranial hemorrhage, intercranial tumors, neurofibromatosis, seizure disorders, and head and spinal cord injury

- Various congenital malformations including cleft palate, hypoplastic mandible, Treacher Collins syndrome, microcephaly, spina bifida, and Noonan syndrome
- Various metabolic disorders including mucopolysaccharidoses syndromes (including Hunter, Hurler, and Sanfilippo syndromes), galactosemia, pituitary diseases, glycogen storage disease, phenylketonuria (PKU), and Tay-Sachs disease
- Various sensory disorders including hearing loss, visual impairment and blindness, and congenital cataract
- Various atypical developmental disorders including autism and failure to thrive
- Severe toxic exposure including maternal PKU, cocaine and other drugs, fetal alcohol syndrome, lead poisoning and mercury poisoning
- Chronic illnesses including chronic hepatitis, diabetes, renal disorders, cancer, cystic fibrosis, and heart problems
- Severe infectious diseases including HIV, bacterial and viral meningitis, herpes, rubella, and encephalitis

Etiology of At-Risk Conditions

The etiological factors of at-risk condition include environmental factors, genetic background, and some disease-related conditions; however, many are environmental (Rossetti, 1996):

- Serious questions about parenting and child's development raised by the parent, a professional, or a caregiver
- Mental illness, mental retardation, chronic or severe physical illness, in one or both of the parents or in the primary caregiver
- Drug and alcohol abuse in a parent or the primary caregiver; maternal substance use or abuse; parental or caregiver history of abuse
- Family history of predisposing medical or genetic conditions
- Chronically impaired interaction among family members
- Adolescent mother or single parent
- Four or more siblings, all preschool age
- Parental unemployment and parental education below 9th grade

- Physical or social isolation of the child and separation of the child from the parent or primary caregiver
- Bad, dangerous, or unstable living conditions or homelessness
- Poor family health care; inadequate prenatal care; lack of health insurance
- Serious prenatal and natal complications
- Asphyxia, low birth weight (<1,500 g), and small for gestation age (<10th percentile)
- Early signs of behavior disorders including irritability and excessive crying
- Child's tendency for frequent and unusual accidents
- Chronic middle ear infections (otitis media)

Characteristics of At-Risk Children and Their Caregivers

- A group of parents or primary caregivers with varied genetic, medical, behavioral, family, and environmental conditions that may adversely affect interaction with their child
- A diverse group of children with varied genetic, medical, behavioral, family, and environmental conditions that may adversely affect interaction with their environment and parents/caregivers; early signs of the following suggest children at risk:
  - poor physical growth and health
  - poor motor skills including early feeding problems
  - behavioral disorders
  - emotional problems
  - deficient intellectual development
  - communication delay or disorder
  - poor interpersonal relations
  - not developing satisfying emotional attachment
  - poor academic performance

Assessment Objectives/General Guidelines

- To make a family-centered communication assessment of infants and toddlers in both the clinic and home settings

- To begin assessment as early as possible and to repeat assessment throughout the childhood period
- To assess the family constellation, family communication patterns, family resources, and family strengths and limitations
- To work with other professionals and make interdisciplinary decisions regarding assessment and how the outcome of assessment will be used
- To suggest an early intervention program that includes both treatment in a clinical facility and intervention activities at home by parents, other caregivers, and other family members (Individual Family Service Plans)
- Note that, in assessing prematurely born children, the duration of prematurity (weeks by which the child was born prematurely) is subtracted from the child's chronological age (CA) to derive the corrected gestational age (CGA) of the child; this correction is used throughout the first year
- Note that interdisciplinary assessment is the most useful

Case History/Interview Focus

- See **Case History** and **Interview** under Standard/Common Assessment Procedures
- Focus on family communication patterns, family strengths and weakness, maternal health during pregnancy, early development of the infant, and family resources

Ethnocultural Considerations

- See Ethnocultural Considerations in Assessment
- Focus on cultural practices in child rearing; mother-child interactions; family communication patterns; culturally accepted roles for children in adult-child interactions

Assessment

Note that an infant or toddler needs a comprehensive interdisciplinary assessment and that some of the assessment areas described may be handled by other professionals (e.g., audiologists, medical professionals, child psychologists); the speech-language pathologist takes greater responsibility for communication assessment and per-

haps feeding and oral motor development but contributes to assessing other areas as well.

- Assess feeding and oral motor development
  - assess suckling action (primitive form of sucking involving approximate lip closure, jaw movement, and extension and retraction of the tongue in the newborn, often in the newborn intensive care unit [NICU])
  - assess sucking (negative intraoral air pressure, elevated tongue tip, firm lip closure, and more precise jaw movements)
  - assess rooting (a reflexive turning toward tactile stimulation)
  - assess phasic bite reflex (bite and release movements when a nipple is placed in the mouth)
- Assess hearing and need for aural rehabilitation
  - advocate an early assessment of hearing of an infant in NICU
  - refer the infant to an audiologist
  - counsel the family members about hearing conservation and aural rehabilitation
- Assess general behavior and alertness
  - assess the infant's physiological and attentional state in NICU (including deep or light sleep states, drowsiness, alertness, eye opening, infant's level of toleration of handling, amount of stimulation the infant can take, crying, etc.); administer *Assessment of Preterm Infant Behavior* for this purpose (see Standardized Tests, Developmental Scales, or Screening Devices described later)
- Assess infant readiness for communication
  - assess the infant's readiness for communication; observe whether the child is too sick to respond; the *in-tuned* or *physiological state* in the Gorski, Davidson, and Brazelton (1979) terms
  - observe if the baby has recovered from illness and is beginning to respond to environmental stimuli; the *coming out* state in the Gorski, Davidson, and Brazelton (1979) terms

- observe whether the baby begins to show reciprocal interaction with the environment; *reciprocity state* in the Gorski, Davidson, and Brazelton (1979) terms
- Assess language comprehension and response to social stimuli
  - during the first 6 months, assess:
    → the baby's response to sound (alertness, diminished activity)
    → response to familiar face (watching the face)
    → response to familiar faces and mother's voice (becomes quiet, smiles)
    → response to emotional tones (e.g., fear at hearing loud or angry voice)
    → response to sight of food (anticipatory reaction)
    → response to his or her name
    → response to soft, affectionate, and pleasant speech directed to the baby (e.g., adult's smile, approach)
    → ask parents about the child's comprehension of language and response to social stimuli
  - During 6 to 12 months of age, assess:
    → response to names of family members (e.g., looking in certain directions, looking at the person whose name is called)
    → response to strangers (e.g., signs of apprehension, moving away from the stranger)
    → response to object names when the object is present (e.g., looking at it, reaching for the object)
    → response to sounds made by toys (e.g., looks at the object when sound is heard)
    → response to "No" (e.g., cessation of activity; hesitancy; unpleasant facial expression)
    → response to scolding (e.g., frowning, crying, unpleasant facial expression)
    → response to action words (understands a few action words)

L

→ response to gestures (e.g., claps when clapping is modeled; touches body parts when this is modeled)
→ ask parents to list words the baby understands and to describe social reactions

- during 12 to 18 months of age, assess:
  → response to names of people and objects that are present (correct recognition of familiar names and objects)
  → response to some names of objects and persons when the objects and persons are not present
  → comprehension of possessor + possession (e.g., *Mommy's shoes*)
  → response to simple commands
  → response to more gestures
  → ask parents about further comprehension of language and social stimuli; note that parents tend to think that the baby understands everything although the research has not substantiated this

- during 18 to 24 months of age, assess:
  → response to absent objects more precise and varied response to absent persons more precise and varied
  → response to two-word combinations
  → response to simple requests (e.g., can locate a missing object when requested) response to simple commands ask parents about the baby's comprehension of language structures

- during 24 to 36 months of age, assess:
  → response to three-word sentences (correct comprehension of simple three-word sentences)
  → response to commands (give two-, three-, and four-element commands to determine the level at which the child's comprehension breaks down)
  → response to requests (give progressively more complex requests to determine the level at which the child's comprehension breaks down)

L

→ ask questions involving *what, who,* and *where* and judge the appropriateness of responses to evaluate comprehension

→ ask parents and other caregivers about the child's response to language stimuli and social interactions

- Assess verbal communication
  - during the first 6 months, assess:
    → normal crying
    → vegetative sounds associated with feeding
    → grunting and sighing
    → vowel-like sounds
    → sound vocalizations
    → increased range of vocalizations
    → differentiated facial expressions
    → emergence of pleasure sounds (e.g., *mmmm*)
    → ask parents or caregivers to list the kinds of sounds the baby makes
    → possible emergence of marginal babbling (consonant-like sounds in babbling)
  - during 6 to 12 months of age, assess:
    → more frequent babbling (consonant-vowel syllable productions like *babababa* or *mamama*) emerging around 6 months of age
    → soon, addition of other sounds produced in the front of the mouth (e.g., /p/, /t/, /d/)
    → nonreduplicated babbling
    → turn taking in vocalization
    → increased production of consonant-like sounds
    → imitation of adult vocalizations or gestures
    → begins to point to things
    → emergence of social interaction and joint attention
    → emergence of phonetically consistent forms (specific sounds in specific situations; (e.g., one vowel sound to suggest a desire for an object and another sound to suggest disapproval)

L

→ intonation in babbling; emergence of prosodic features around 6 months of age
→ emergence of intentional communication between 9 and 10 months of age (e.g., specific gesturing or pointing; vocalizing while making eye contact)
→ have parents describe the speech sounds, babbling, and other communicative behaviors of the child

- during 12 to 18 months of age, assess:
  → expanded repertoire of sounds produced
  → increased use of gestures and vocalizations to obtain objects, draw attention, and regulate the behavior of caregivers
  → production of first words
  → have parents or caregivers describe the speech sounds, meaningful vocalizations, and other communicative behaviors of the child

- during 18 to 24 months of age, assess:
  → expansion and differentiation of single word classes (nominals, action words, modifiers or adjectives)
  → more meaningful and consistent use of 10–15 words
  → production of two-word phrases
  → speech intelligibility at least 50% to caregivers
  → unintelligible strings of syllables produced with a sentence-like intonation
  → combination of intelligible and unintelligible syllables with a sentence intonation
  → have parents or caregivers describe words, phrases, gestures, and other communicative behaviors of the child

- during 24 to 36 months of age, assess:
  → emergence of simple sentences
  → three- and four-word sentences; five-word sentences toward the end of this period
  → questions
  → increased intelligibility of speech (up to 75%) increased expressive vocabulary (at 24 months, just under 300 words; at 36 months, 900 to 1000 words)

→ take a Speech and Language Sample (see Standard/ Common Assessment Procedures), especially with the child at the end of this period; use informal play to evoke language productions

→ have parents or caregivers describe words, phrases, sentences, gestures, and other communicative behaviors of the child

- Assess infant-caregiver interaction
  - use the Observation of Communication Interaction by Klein a Briggs (1986) and the Mother-Infant Play Interaction Scale by Walker and Thompson (1982); these instruments offer suggestions of the following kind; observe:

    → the baby and the mother or another caregiver, preferably in the home setting; if in the clinical setting, arrange a natural interactive situation for the child and the mother; note the following:

    → how the mother handles and stimulates the baby; holding, cuddling, stroking, rocking, and so forth

    → how the mother expresses her affection for the baby; smiling and laughing in general and contingent smiling and laughing in particular

    → how the mother plays with the child; quiet play or play with speech and vocalizations; the tone of speech and vocalization; presence or absence of contingent response to child's reactions

    → how the mother visually concentrates on the baby; note whether the mother places or holds the infant at her eye level

    → the infant's mood and affect: note responsiveness and alertness or nonresponsiveness and disinterested disposition

    → how the mother responds contingently to infant's behavior

    → how the mother modifies her interaction when the infant gives negative cues

L

- Assess play activities
  - observe the child engaged in play with another child; make unobtrusive observations; take note of the child's pattern of interaction during play; observe whether the child
    → plays cooperatively with the other child or children
    → engages in parallel play or isolated play
    → indulges in constructive activities alongside or with other children
    → engages in role playing and pretend play
    → exhibits uncooperative or aggressive behaviors
    → does not share toys
    → does not talk much during play
    → simply watches others play

Standardized Tests, Developmental Scales, or Screening Devices

- Note that, in assessing children under 3, few standardized instruments are available; most are developmental scales that help structure observations of the child to take note of the presence or absence of behaviors of interest
- Use the Speech, Language, and Motor Development guidelines in assessing infants and toddlers
- Consider using the following instruments:

Instrument	Purpose
Assessment of Preterm Infant Behavior (H. Als, B. Lester, E. Tronick, & T. Brazelton)	To assess the infant's physiological and attentional state in NICU
Birth to Three Developmental Scale (T. Bangs & S. Dodson)	To assess developmental delays
Communication and Symbolic Behavior Scales (A. M. Wetherby & B. Prizant)	To assess nonverbal and verbal communication in infants and children up to 6 yrs
The Language Development Survey (L. Rescorla)	To screen language in toddlers
Rossetti Infant-Toddler Language Scale (L. Rossetti)	To assess communication and interaction in infants and toddlers

(continued)

(continued)

Instrument	Purpose
Sequenced Inventory of Communication Development—Revised (D. Hedrick, E. Prather, & A. Tobin)	To assess verbal and nonverbal communication in infants and children up to 4 yrs
Preschool Language Scale (I. Zimmerman, V. Steiner, & R. Pond)	To assess receptive and expressive language in infants and children up to 6;11 yrs

Related/Medical Assessment Data

- Obtain medical information about the baby's illness, treatment plans, and prognosis
- Obtain psychological or behavioral assessment data describing the child's behavioral development
- Integrate communication and related assessment information with related/medical data

Standard/Common Assessment Procedures

- Complete the Standard/Common Assessment Procedures

Analysis of Results

- Analyze the results of assessment along with parent interview information
- List the infant's or toddler's strengths and limitations
- Describe the child's communication deficits
- Describe the family communication patterns, mother-child interactions, and problems in this area

Diagnostic Criteria/Guidelines

- Note that in making an infant-toddler assessment, the examiner is more concerned with assessing the child in his or her family context than rendering a clinical diagnosis
- Deficiencies in preverbal, verbal, and nonverbal communication skills

Prognosis

- Generally good with early intervention and parent training

Recommendations

- Early intervention within the framework of a family service plan

- Parent training in language stimulation
- Both home-based and center-based intervention when warranted
- Periodic assessment
- More intensive center-based treatment if repeated assessment results suggest it
- See the cited sources and *PGTSLP* for details; in the *PGTSLP*, use procedures described under <u>Language Disorders in Children</u>

Gorski, P., Davidson, M., & Brazelton, T. (1979). Stages of behavioral organization in the high risk neonate: Theoretical and clinical considerations. *Seminars in Perinatology, 3,* 61.

Klein, D., & Briggs, M. (1986). Observation of Communicative Interaction. DHS Publication No. MCJ 0635 1 -0 1 -0. Washington, DC: U.S. Government Printing Office.

Rossetti, L. M. (1996). *Communication intervention birth to three.* San Diego, CA: Singular Publishing Group.

Nelson, N. W. (1993). *Childhood language disorders in context.* New York: Merrill.

Paul, R. (2001). *Language disorders front infancy through adolescence* (2nd ed.). St. Louis, MO: C. V. Mosby.

Reed, V. (1994). *An introduction to children with language disorders* (2nd ed.). New York: Macmillan.

Walker, L., & Thompson, E. (1982). Mother-infant play interaction scale. In S. Humenick-Smith (Ed.), *Analysis of current assessment strategies in the health care of voting children and childbearing families* (p. 56). Norwich, CT: Williams & Wilkins.

Language Sampling.   See Speech and Language Sampling under <u>Standard/Common Assessment Procedures</u>.

Laryngectomee or Laryngectomized Person.   A person who has had a partial or total <u>Laryngectomy</u>.

Laryngectomy.   Surgical removal of all or part of the larynx because of disease or trauma; results in a loss of the natural source of sound to produce speech; results in significant changes in the anatomy of the laryngeal area; creates a need to breathe through a surgically created stoma (hole) in the neck; creates a need to learn alternative modes of sound generation and then to produce speech with it.

Laryngectomy

Major Types of Laryngectomy

Note that most basic procedures have variations.

- Total laryngectomy: Surgical removal of the entire larynx
- Near total laryngectomy: Removal of most of the structures except for a small, healthy portion of one fold
- Pharyngo-laryngectomy: Total laryngectomy with portions of the pharynx also removed
- Partial laryngectomy: Removal of certain parts of the larynx:
  - Hemilaryngectomy: Removal of one half of the larynx; one fold is removed along with some related structures and the other fold is saved
  - Supraglottic laryngectomy: Removal of structures above the vocal folds
- Removal of other structures: Depending on the spread of cancer, removal of parts of esophagus, tongue, and lymphatic system in the neck (radical neck dissection)

Reasons for Laryngectomy

- Cancer of the larynx and related structures; 11,000 to 13,000 cases a year in the United States; higher prevalence in older males than in females although the gender ratio has been shrinking; the greatest prevalence rate for African American males.
  - supraglottal tumors (laryngeal cancer above the folds); (24% to 42% of all cases of laryngeal cancer)
  - glottal tumors (cancer of the vocal folds); the most frequent type (55% to 75%)
  - subglottal tumors (laryngeal cancer below the vocal folds); rare (1% to 6%)
- Laryngeal trauma resulting in severely damaged larynx that cannot be repaired; laryngectomy due to trauma and related factors less frequent than that due to laryngeal cancer
  - blow to the larynx
  - gunshot wounds
  - severe damage in automobile and other kinds of accidents
  - unsuccessful partial laryngectomy that necessitates a total laryngectomy

- total loss of control over the laryngeal structures due to brainstem strokes

Potential Etiology of Cancer of the Larynx
- Smoking (cigarettes, pipes, cigars)
- Alcohol intake (moderate to heavy drinking)
- Increased risk with combined smoking and moderate to heavy drinking
- Increased risk with combined smoking and occupational exposure to carcinogenic factors (e.g., exposure to asbestos)
- Possible link to diet (low consumption of vitamin A and C)
- Possible link to radiation exposure

Assessment Objectives/General Guidelines
- To counsel the patient about available options for communication after laryngectomy
- To help select the best methods of communication for the patient by getting the entire family involved in the process
- To make periodic assessments to evaluate need for change in the rehabilitation program
- Note that no form of alaryngeal speech can be rejected without careful consideration, assessment of candidacy with trial therapy

Case History/Interview Focus
- See **Case History** and **Interview** under Standard/Common Assessment Procedures
- Focus on the patient's surgical and medical treatment and rehabilitation and the family communication patterns and preferences

Ethnocultural Considerations
- See Ethnocultural Considerations in Assessment

Alaryngeal Speech Options
- Pneumatic devices: A unit that contains vibrating reed, a tube that carries the sound to the mouth, and a shallow cup that fits over the stoma from which the air passes through the reed
  - advantages include simplicity, ease of use, use of patient's own breath supply, normal phrasing, and suitability for early communication attempts after surgery

- disadvantages include the need to use the stoma which is normally kept covered, need to use one hand to hold the cup over the stoma, visual distraction, and low pitch, especially for the female speaker
- Electronic larynxes: Relatively small, battery-powered units that contain a vibrator when turned on; sound may be carried into the mouth by a tube or the unit may be held against the neck to transmit the sound via skin into the mouth; sound is articulated into speech; many varieties on the market
  - advantages include ease of use, volume and pitch controls, sufficient loudness of speech produced, and good speech intelligibility when well trained
  - disadvantages include electronic noise, problems in using on tender or scarred neck tissue, need for good articulation skills, and repair costs
- Esophageal speech: Speech produced by supplying air into the esophagus, creating vibration in the pharyngeal esophageal (P-E) segment, and articulating the sound into speech
  - advantages include more natural sound and lack of a hand-held mechanical device
  - disadvantages include difficulty in learning the method and low intensity of speech produced
- Tracheoesophageal speech: Speech produced with a voice prosthesis inserted into a small fistula or puncture made through the tracheal wall into the esophagus in a surgical procedure called tracheoesophageal fistulization or puncture (TEF/TEP); during exhalation, air from the lungs is directed into the prosthesis by occluding the stoma with a finger; air then passes through the prosthesis and into the esophagus; sound is produced as the air passes through the vibrating P-E segment; sound is then articulated
  - advantages include a more natural air supply into the esophagus (compared to the laryngectomy without TE/TEP), rapid learning of speech, and inexpensive prostheses

L

- disadvantages include the small risk involved in additional surgical procedure (TE/TEP), stenosis of the fistula or the stoma, and aspiration of the prosthesis

Assessment

- Note that a main assessment task is to familiarize the client with available options for alaryngeal communication; to determine candidacy for a particular type of alaryngeal speech by trying different methods; and then to select one for more intensive therapy
- Visit the patient prior to surgery and describe the effects of surgery on communication and options for alternative modes of communication
  - note that patients may or may not be in a favorable disposition to appreciate all you say
  - provide sufficient positive information on the possibilities of developing new forms of communication
  - let the client know that, with few exceptions, it is possible to resume work and lead a normal life
  - tell them to be patient with themselves after surgery
  - offer information about financial assistance
  - let them know about the support groups
  - have a rehabilitated laryngectomized person visit the client or the family only if they welcome this suggestion
  - have the client and the family meet other members of the professional team
  - get the family members involved in this preoperative counseling session
  - counsel the family about taking care of the patient immediately after he or she returns home
  - leave printed information about surgery, postoperative care, and methods of alaryngeal communication with the patient and the family
- After surgery, begin a more detailed discussion and demonstration of alaryngeal modes of communication and the options available to the patient and family members:
  - show, describe, and demonstrate the use of a pneumatic device

348

- show, describe, and demonstrate the use of an electronic larynx
- describe and demonstrate esophageal speech
- describe and demonstrate tracheoesophageal speech
- describe availability, cost, and maintenance of different devices
- briefly mention some of the advantages and disadvantages of different approaches; do not overemphasize limitations of a particular approach or device at this time so that the client does not prematurely rule out an option or options
- tell the client that initially he or she may use one method (e.g., a pneumatic device) and another method later (e.g., an electronic larynx or esophageal speech)
- let the client try the different options to the extent the physical condition permits (e.g., a pneumatic device may be easier to try at this initial phase; neck tenderness may prevent a trial of electrolarynx)
- give the patient and the family members as much printed information as available
- Assess the client's preference
  - during the demonstration of options, note the client's reactions
  - note the hand dexterity, skill in handling the device, and initial success
  - do not let the client become discouraged about initial failure in using a particular device or method; emphasize that practice is the key to success and what seems difficult initially may be easier later on, especially as the client recovers from surgery
  - ask about his or her preferences and reasons for preferences
  - ask family members about their preferences although the client's success with a method may be most important
- Assess candidacy for a pneumatic device
  - note that a Pneumatic device may be especially useful for early communication (soon after surgery)

- let the client try the unit as soon as possible and use it as found appropriate; observe:
  → how the client holds and handles the unit
  → the rate at which the client learns to use the unit
  → how well the client articulates speech sounds
- try devices from different manufacturers to find out a more suitable unit
- note any client reactions that might suggest acceptance or rejection of the device
- ask the client for his or her preferences and find out the reasons for selection or rejection
- let the client know that it is best to try all possibilities before selecting one for more permanent use; do not let the client rule out other possibilities without trying them
- reinforce and encourage the client for his or her willingness to consider all options and for showing signs of success
- Assess candidacy for an electronic larynx
  - show, describe, and demonstrate the use of a pneumatic device
  - assess how well and how efficiently the client: places the device on the neck articulates speech sounds note how well the patient handles the unit
  - note the presence or absence of manual dexterity in manipulating the switches of the unit
  - note the rate of learning (fast, slow, or little progress over several trials)
  - try units from different manufacturers to find out which one suits the client best
  - let the client express concerns and ask all questions
  - ask the client about preferences and reasons for preferences
  - discuss the problems noted and positively reinforce any sign of success
- Assess candidacy for esophageal speech

Laryngectomy

- note that assessing candidacy for esophageal speech takes time because persistent efforts often are needed to see initial success that helps select the method
- note that the following factors suggest success with esophageal speech, although individual differences may override some or all of them; in efficient learning of esophageal speech:
  → younger clients are more successful than older clients; after age 60, the success rate may be 50%
  → hearing loss is a negative factor
  → integrity of tongue strength and mobility is a necessary factor (for both air injection and articulation of sounds)
  → structural and functional integrity of the esophagus (no rupture or stricture) is essential
  → P-E segment should neither be too lax nor too tensed
  → oral and pharyngeal tissue damage due to radiation may make it a more difficult task
  → combination of total glossectomy and laryngectomy is detrimental, requiring surgical and prosthetic rehabilitation
- try the injection (positive pressure) and inhalation (negative pressure) methods; note that most clinicians prefer the injection method
  → describe, explain, and demonstrate each method
  → give sufficient practice before making a judgment about its suitability
  → ask the client to be patient and persistent
  → take note of problems and discuss them with the patient
  → encourage any sign of success
  → note that the injection method is inappropriate for patients with glossectomy
  → note that for patients with glossectomy, inhalation (not injection) is the only method of producing esophageal speech

Laryngectomy

- Assess candidacy for tracheoesophageal speech
  - note that tracheoesophageal speech requires additional surgery (tracheoesophageal fistulization or puncture [TEF/TEP] described earlier) and the use of a voice prosthesis
  - assess the presence of pharyngoesophageal spasm which will prevent success with TEP/TEP; administer an insufflation test; use such a standard procedure as the Blom-Singer insufflation test kit:
    → insert a catheter through the nose until the end rests below the P-E segment (as indicated by a 25 cm mark, which should be at the nostril)
    → place the other end with its stoma housing over the stoma
    → ask the patient to inhale and immediately close the stoma adapter with his or her thumb and then to exhale through the mouth while producing /a/
    → after a few practice trials, ask the patient to sustain the vowel as long as possible and in 5 trials; ask the patient to count from 1 to 15
    → pass criterion is 8 seconds of sustained vowel and counting from 1 to 15
    → note that a failed insufflation test indicates too much tension, constriction, or spasm in the P-E segment which indicates the segment to be a poor source of vibration
    → note that a radiological assessment is needed to confirm tension and spasm of the P-E segment
  - note that the surgeon may recommend either the pharyngeal constrictor myotomy or the pharyngeal plexus block (neurectomy) for those who fail the insufflation test
    → myotomy involves unilateral cutting of the laryngeal constrictors (inferior and middle pharyngeal constrictor muscles) to reduce constriction and spasm
    → pharyngeal plexus block involves sectioning the nerves that supply the pharyngeal constrictor mus-

cles, especially the middle constrictor, to reduce spasm and tension

→ note that, if an insufflation test is done prior to TEF/TEP, myotomy or neurectomy may be performed along with TEF/TEP

- visual acuity and manual dexterity in removing and inserting the voice prosthesis
- adequate depth and diameter of the stoma to use the voice prosthesis
- mental and emotional stability
- understanding of the care and use of the voice prosthesis
- Select a method of alaryngeal speech for systematic training
  - consider all initial selections tentative
  - be prepared to reassess, select another mode of alaryngeal communication, and retrain the patient

Related/Medical Assessment Data

- Integrate medical, surgical, and general health data into your assessment data in selecting the method of alaryngeal mode of communication

Standard/Common Assessment Procedures

- Complete the Standard/Common Assessment Procedures

Prognosis

- Prognosis for survival varies across patients; many variables including the general health of the patient, the extent of cancerous growth, recurrence of cancer, and the effectiveness of surgical treatment
- Significant hearing loss with no amplification negatively affects the learning and maintenance of alaryngeal speech
- Prolonged and intense radiation therapy may retard the progress of alaryngeal communication rehabilitation
- Prognosis for learning one or the other form of communication is good for most if not all patients

Recommendations

- Communication treatment with an optimal method of alaryngeal speech determined through assessment and trial therapy

- Periodic assessment preceding and following additional surgical or medical treatment
- See the cited sources and *PGTSLP* for details

Casper, J. K., & Colton, R. H. (1993). *Clinical manual for laryngectomy and head and neck cancer rehabilitation.* San Diego, CA: Singular Publishing Group.

Doyle, P. C. (1994). *Foundations of voice and speech rehabilitation following laryngeal cancer.* San Diego, CA: Singular Publishing Group.

Keith, R. L., & Darley, F. L. (Eds.). (1994). *Laryngectomy rehabilitation* (3rd ed.). Austin, TX: Pro-Ed.

Salmon, S. J., & Mount, K. H. (Eds.). (1991). *Alaryngeal speech rehabilitation: For clinicians by clinicians.* Austin, TX: Pro-Ed.

Laurence-Moon-Bardet-Biedl Syndrome. The same as Laurence-Moon syndrome (See <u>Syndromes Associated With Communicative Disorders</u>)

Laurence-Moon-Biedl Syndrome. The same as Laurence-Moon syndrome. (See <u>Syndromes Associated With Communicative Disorders</u>)

LeFort III Osteotomy. A surgical procedure designed to correct developmental deficiencies in the midface region.

Lobate. Containing lobes.

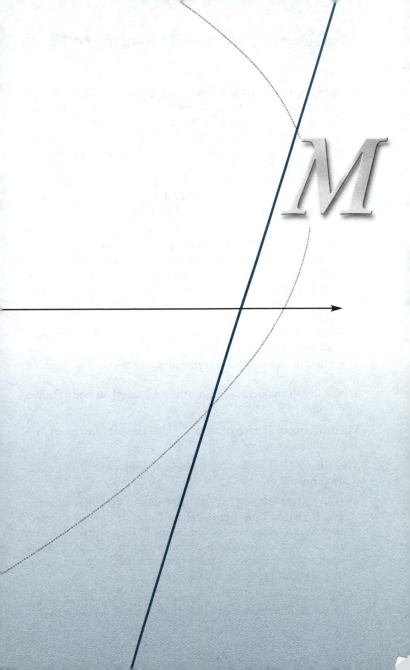

Magnetic Resonance Imaging (MRI). A neurodiagnostic method based on alignment and realignment of nuclei of atoms in the cell when a structure is placed in a strong magnetic field; variations introduced in the amount of magnetic radiation will cause alignment and realignment of nuclei; such changes produce electromagnetic signals that a computer analyzes to produce images of the structure; similar to CT scanning, but (MRI) produces clearer images; can detect lesions missed by CT scan.

Malocclusions. Deviations in the shape and dimensions of the upper and lower jaw bones and the positioning of individual teeth; misalignment of the upper and lower jaw and the upper and the lower row of teeth; the degree of deviation varies across cases and types of malocclusion; may affect articulation in extreme cases; include the following types:

- Class I malocclusion: normally aligned arches but misaligned individual teeth
- Class II malocclusion: protruded upper jaw and receded lower jaw
- Class III malocclusion: protruded lower jaw and receded upper jaw

Mandibular Hypoplasia. Underdevelopment of the mandible (lower jaw).

Maxillary Hypoplasia. Underdevelopment of the maxilla (upper jaw).

Maximum Phonation Duration. The duration for which a person can hold phonated sounds; typically, clients are asked to phonate /s/ and /z/ for as long as possible; the duration is measured in seconds; diagnostic of general phonatory efficiency; useful in voice diagnosis; see Voice Disorders for procedures and norms.

Mean Length of Utterance (MLU). The average length of utterances measured in morphemes; an index of language acquisition or performance of children; needs 50 utterances that are consecutive and intelligible; following guidelines have been suggested by Brown (1973) and Chapman (1981):

- Transcribe each intelligible utterance on a separate line; discard unintelligible segments
- Count each word as one
- Count a bound morpheme as one (e.g., the plural *s* morpheme)
- Count contracted morphemes as one (the result is two morphemes because the word and the contraction are both counted; e.g., *he's* is counted as two)
- Count all grammatic morphemes as one (e.g., *-ing, -ed*)
- Count all words repeated for emphasis
- Count compound words (e.g., *birthday*) as one
- Do not count fillers (e.g., such interjections as *mm*)
- Divide the total number of morphemes with the total number of utterances to obtain MLU

Brown, R. (1973). *A first language: The early stages.* Cambridge, MA: Harvard University Press.

Chapman, R. (1981). Exploring children's communicative intents. In J. Miller (Ed.), *Assessing language production in children* (pp. 111–138). Needleham Heights, MA: Allyn & Bacon.

Meningiomas.   Tumors within the meninges; one of the causes of cerebral infarct affecting language skills.

Meninges.   Membranes that cover the brain.

Mental Retardation.   Intellectual, social, and adaptive behaviors that are significantly below normal during the developmental period which extends up to age 18; communicative problems are a significant aspect of retardation; varied causes; varied degrees of retardation; profoundly retarded need institutional care; associated with physical problems in some cases; mildly retarded individuals may hold jobs and function in societies; in schools, often in need of special educational services; mostly, the assessment procedures described under <u>Language Disorders in Children</u> and <u>Articulation and Phonological Disorders</u> are applicable with the following special considerations:

Etiology

- Prenatal factors including maternal rubella, prenatal lead poisoning, mercury poisoning, prenatal immunization, maternal anoxia, prenatal trauma, X-ray and radiation, prematurity and low birth weight, fetal alcohol syndrome, and maternal drug abuse
- Natal factors including fetal anoxia and brain injury during birth due to such factors as birth canal compression and malpositioning of the baby
- Postnatal factors including postimmunization encephalitis, rabies vaccine, lead poisoning, or toxicity
- Head trauma due to vehicular and other kinds of accidents, child abuse, and gunshot wounds
- Metabolic disorders including phenylketonuria (PKU) and lipid metabolic errors (e.g., Tay-Sachs disease)
- Endocrine disorders including hypothyroidism
- Cranial abnormalities including anencephaly (absence of cranial bones), microcephaly (extremely small head), hydrocephaly (enlargement of the head due to excessive collection of spinal fluids within the cranial vault), and macrocephaly (enlargement of the head due to abnormal increase in the brain size)
- Hereditary and genetic factors resulting in such syndromes as Down syndrome, fragile X syndrome, Prader-Willi syndrome, and cri du chat syndrome (See <u>Syndromes Associated With Communicative Disorders</u>)

Theoretical Issue

- Some experts have suggested that language of the mentally retarded children is unique whereas others have suggested that their language is simpler and quantitatively, not qualitatively, different; the latter position generally supported by research data

Language of Children With Mental Retardation

- Phonologic problems
  - deletion of consonants in final positions (most frequent errors)
  - simplification of consonant clusters
  - distortions of consonants
  - substitution of consonants
  - errors similar to those of non-retarded children with articulation problems
  - phonologic processes similar to those of non-retarded children with articulation problems
  - see Articulation and Phonological Disorders for details
- Semantic problems
  - later and slower acquisition of first few words
  - relatively faster acquisition of single words than syntactic features
  - slower acquisition of new words
  - acquisition of fewer words at any given unit of time
  - smaller and limited vocabulary
  - less varied and more concrete vocabulary (e.g., mostly nouns)
  - fewer adjectives and adverbs
  - generally similar to the semantic problems described under Language Disorders in Children
- Morphologic problems
  - omission of many morphologic features including the regular plural, the possessive, the present progressive *ing*, the past tense inflections, prepositions, the auxiliary, and the copula
  - generally similar to the morphologic problems described under Language Disorders in Children
- Syntactic problems
  - generally simplified sentence structures
  - fewer sentence types; lack of transformational variety
  - lack of complex, compound, and passive sentence forms
  - fewer relative clause usages

M

- generally, less elaborate language
- generally similar to the syntactic problems described under <u>Language Disorders in Children</u>
- Pragmatic problems
  - reluctance to talk in social situations
  - difficulty in initiating conversation
  - abrupt and short answers to questions
  - responses that are inappropriate to time, place, person, and topic of conversation
  - difficulty in topic maintenance
  - difficulty in adding new information during conversation
  - problems in using conversational repair strategies (e.g., lack of appropriate responses to request for clarification and lack of requests for clarification when utterances are unclear)
  - limited generalization of learned language and other skills
  - deficient narrative skills
  - generally similar to the pragmatic problems described under <u>Language Disorders in Children</u>
- Fluency problems
  - generally limited fluency possibly due to limited language skills
  - repetitions, pauses, and other forms of dysfluencies
- Hearing problems
  - auditory disorders more frequent in children with retardation than in those without retardation
  - build-up of ear wax due to poor self-care skills
  - history of middle ear infections and conductive hearing loss
  - sensorineural hearing loss
- Language comprehension problems
  - difficulty in understanding syntactic constructions that are complex, long, or both
  - difficulty in comprehending the meaning of abstract words

M

Mental Retardation

- problems in understanding abstract statements (e.g., proverbs, metaphors, similes)

Assessment Objectives/General Guidelines

- To assess and describe articulation and phonological disorders
- To assess and describe language disorders
- To assess other communication problems including dysfluencies
- To screen hearing and request audiological assessment when the child fails the hearing screening

Case History/Interview Focus

- See **Case History** and **Interview** under Standard/ Common Assessment Procedures
- Concentrate on the prenatal, natal, and postnatal factors that are known to be associated with mental retardation and on speech, language, and motor development

Ethnocultural Considerations

- See Ethnocultural Considerations in Assessment

Assessment

- Assess phonologic problems
  - record a Speech and Language Sample (see Standard/ Common Assessment Procedures
  - list the sounds misarticulated; classify them according to omissions, distortions, and substitutions
  - identify the phonological processes
  - use the procedures described under Articulation and Phonological Disorders
- Assess semantic problems
  - assess word usage, vocabulary size, and variety of words used
  - use the procedures described under Language Disorders in Children
  - describe the classes of words that are especially difficult for the child
- Assess morphologic problems

M

- use the recorded speech and language sample in assessing production of morphologic features
- use the procedures described under Language Disorders <u>in Children</u>
- list the morphologic features the child produces and those the child does not produce; calculate the percent correct response rate for assessed morphologic features
- Assess syntactic problems
  - use the recorded speech and language sample in assessing production of syntactic features
  - use the procedures described under Language Disorders <u>in Children</u>
  - list the syntactic features the child produces and those the child does not
- Assess pragmatic problems
  - use the recorded speech and language sample in assessing pragmatic structures of language
  - use the procedures described under Language Disorders <u>Children</u>
  - list the pragmatic features the child produces and those the child does not

- Assess fluency problems
  - use the recorded speech and language sample in assessing
  - use the procedures described under <u>Stuttering</u>
  - list the types of dysfluencies the child produces
  - list the total frequency of each dysfluency in the speech sample
  - count the number of spoken words in the sample
  - calculate the percent dysfluency rate
- Screen hearing
  - use the standard screening procedure
  - refer the child who fails the hearing screening to an audiologist for an audiological diagnosis
- Assess language comprehension problems
  - observe the child for auditory language comprehension problems

- use the procedures described under <u>Language Disorders in Children</u>

Standardized Tests

- Use the selected standardized tests listed under <u>Articulation and Phonological Disorders</u> and <u>Language Disorders in Children</u>
- Be aware that children with mental retardation tend to perform less well on standardized tests than in conversational speech exhibited in natural settings

Related/Medical Assessment Data

- Obtain medical information of relevance
- Obtain audiological assessment data if hearing has been evaluated
- Obtain educational assessment data if available

Standard/Common Assessment Procedures

- Complete the <u>Standard/Common Assessment Procedures</u>

Diagnostic Criteria

- An independent diagnosis of mental retardation by a psychologist
- Significant intellectual and behavioral deficiencies
- Communication disorders as described

Differential Diagnosis

- Differentiate different syndromes of mental retardation; see <u>Syndromes Associated With Communicative Disorders</u>

Prognosis

- Varied across children; depends on the intellectual level of the child
- Generally good prognosis for improved communication skills

Recommendations

- Early communication treatment
- Parent training in early language stimulation
- Coordination of communication treatment with academic programs in the case of school-age children
- Coordination of communication treatment with psychological services being received

- See the cited sources and *PGTSLP* for details

Nelson, N. W. (1993). *Childhood language disorders in context.* New York: Merrill.

Paul, R. (2001). *Language disorders from infancy through adolescence* (2nd ed.). St. Louis, MO: C. V. Mosby.

Reed, V. (1994). *An introduction to children with language disorders* (2nd ed.). New York: Macmillan.

Microcephaly.   Abnormally small head associated with mental retardation.

Microdontia.   Abnormally small tooth or teeth due to a genetic or congenital developmental disorder; a symptom of certain genetic syndromes.

Micrognathia.   Underdeveloped lower jaw (mandible); associated with certain genetic syndromes, including the fetal alcohol syndrome (see Syndromes Associated With Communicative Disorders).

Microphthalmia.   Reduced eye size due to developmental disorders; part of several genetic syndromes including the fetal alcohol syndrome (see Syndromes Associated With Communicative Disorders).

Microtia.   Gross underdevelopment of the pinna and absent external auditory canal; part of some genetic syndromes; see Goldenhar syndrome and oro-facial-digital syndrome type 11 (see Syndromes Associated With Communicative Disorders).

Mohr Syndrome.   The same as oro-facial-digital syndrome type 11 (see Syndromes Associated With Communicative Disorders).

Motor Aphasia.   The same as Broca's aphasia (see Aphasia: Specific Types).

Motor Speech Disorders.   A group of speech disorders associated with neuropathology affecting the motor control of speech muscles or motor programming of speech movements; varied etiological factors creating a variety of symptoms and subtypes; include <u>Apraxia of Speech</u> and <u>Dysarthrias</u>; also see <u>Dysarthria: Specific Types</u> for ataxic dysarthria, flaccid dysarthria, hyperkinetic dysarthria, hypokinetic dysarthria, mixed dysarthria, spastic dysarthria, and unilateral upper motor neuron dysarthria.

Multi-Infarct Dementia (MID) or Vascular Dementia.

A form of <u>Dementia</u> due to multiple strokes; second highest in frequency, dementia of the Alzheimer's type (DAT) being the highest; a form of mixed dementia because of both cortical and subcortical involvement; named *vascular dementia* in the DSM-IV; due to repeated strokes associated with a history of hypertension and arteriosclerosis; no familial pattern; varied symptom complex; younger age of onset compared to DAT; more frequent in men than in women; the frequency may be just as high in non-White older women; may be more frequent in non-White populations because of their high frequency of vascular diseases.

Etiology

- History of hypertension
- History of arteriosclerosis
- Strokes due to large vessel occlusions in the major cerebral arteries (anterior, middle, posterior cerebral arteries) often producing focal damage
- Lacunar states (strokes resulting from ruptures of small arterial branches) causing damage to the basal ganglia, thalamus, midbrain, and brainstem
- Binswanger's disease associated with multiple infarcts causing damage to subcortical white matter

Symptoms

- Abrupt onset with step-wise deterioration
- Confusion in some patients
- Inconsistent memory impairment (total inability to recall an event to sudden, total recovery)
- Early signs of cognitive impairment
- Patchy distribution of impairment (some skills impaired while others remain intact)

Multi-Infarct Dementia or Vascular Dementia

- Focal neurological signs including pseudobulbar palsy, gait abnormalities, and weakness of an extremity
- Deterioration in memory and other cognitive skills as in other forms of dementia
- Impaired language (aphasia)
- Motor speech disorders
- Better preserved personality and behavior than in other forms of dementia

Case History/Interview Focus
- See **Case History** and **Interview** under Standard/Common Assessment Procedures
- Document changes in cognition, general behavior, emotional responding, and communication skills

Ethnocultural Considerations
- See Ethnocultural Considerations in Assessment
- Take note of the high frequency of vascular diseases in non-White populations

Assessment
- Assess speech, language, memory, cognition (including orientation and confusion)
- Follow the procedures described under Dementia
- Follow the procedures described under Dysarthrias

Standardized Tests
- Consider using standardized tests described under Dementia and Dysarthrias

Related/Medical Assessment Data
- Integrate available medical, neurological, psychological, behavioral, and diagnostic medical laboratory findings with the results of communication assessment

Standard/Common Assessment Procedures
- Complete the Standard/Common Assessment Procedures

Diagnostic Criteria
- Basic diagnosis of repeated strokes either due to large vessel pathology, lacunar state, or Binswanger's disease
- Dementia (and Dysarthrias)
- Step-wise course of deterioration and patchy deficits

Differential Diagnosis
• See **Differential Diagnosis** under Dementia

Prognosis
• Irreversible disease

Recommendations
• Communication treatment in the early stages
• Management and coping strategies in later stages
• Family counseling and management strategies
• See the cited sources and *PGTSLP* for details; use procedures described under Dementia

American Psychiatric Association. (1994). *Diagnostic and statistical manual of mental disorders* (4th ed.) (DSM-IV). Washington, DC: Author.

Bayles, K. A., & Kaszniak, A. W. (1987). *Communication and cognition in normal aging and dementia*. Austin, TX: Pro-Ed.

Cummings, J. L., & Benson, D. F. (1983). *Dementia: A clinical approach*. Boston: Butterworth.

Brookshire, R. H. (1997). *An introduction to neurogenic communication disorders* (5th ed.). St. Louis, MO: Mosby Year Book.

Lubinski, R. (199 1). *Dementia and communication*. Philadelphia: B. C. Decker.

Ripich, D. N. (1991). *Geriatric communication disorders*. Austin, TX: Pro-Ed.

Multiple Sclerosis.   A neurological diseases in which the white matter of the central nervous system is demyelinated; sometimes extending to gray matter; associated with weakness, incoordination, and visual disturbances; commonly associated with dysarthria.

Mutational Falsetto.   Continuation of prepubertal voice after attaining puberty; voice is high-pitched; see Voice Disorders.

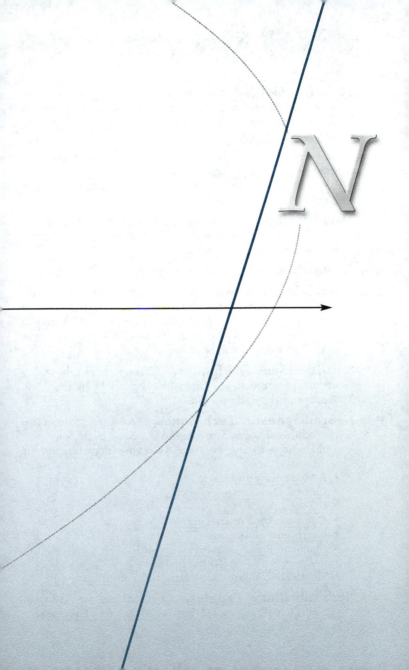

Narrative Skills.   A language skill in describing events in a sequential, chronologically correct, and logically consistent manner; for assessment procedures, see Language Disorders in Children

Nasal Emission.   Audible escape of air through the nose during speech, especially during the production of voiceless plosives and fricatives; often found in speakers with cleft palate.

Nasendoscope.   A mechanical device used to examine internal organs illuminated by a fiberoptic tube inserted through the nose; see Endoscopy.

Nephritis.   Disease of the kidneys due to various causes.

Neural Anastomosis.   Connecting a branch of an undamaged nerve to a damaged nerve; a surgical treatment for certain dysarthric clients; a branch of the intact XIIth cranial nerve may be connected to the damaged VIIth cranial nerve to restore function and appearance.

Neuritic (Senile) Plaques.   Clumps of degenerating neurons; present in the brains of Alzheimer's patients and some normal elderly persons.

Neurodiagnostic Techniques.   A variety of medical procedures designed to diagnose neural pathology; see alphabetical listing for the following neurodiagnostic techniques:
- B-Mode Carotid Imaging
- Carotid Phonoangiograph
- Cerebral Angiography
- Computerized Axial Tomograph
- Electroencephalogram (EEG)
- Magnetic Resonance Imaging (MRI)
- Positron Emission Tomography (PET)
- Single-Photon Emission Computed Tomography (SPECT)

Neurofibrillary Tangles.   Twisted and tangled neurofibrils; a basic neuropathology of Alzheimer's Disease.

Neurofibromatosis. A familial developmental neurologic disorder involving muscles, bone, and skin; characterized by pedunculated soft tumors all over the body; a condition that puts children at risk of developmental delay, including communication delay or disorder.

Neurogenic Fluency Disorders. Somewhat varied problems of fluency that have a demonstrated neurologic basis; also known as *neurogenic stuttering or acquired stuttering*; often associated with aphasia; may be associated with apraxia of speech; may be associated with strokes in the absence of aphasia; to be distinguished from stuttering of early childhood onset (developmental) with no gross neuropathology; reemergence of stuttering in a person who had stuttered but who was fluent for years until the onset of the neurologic condition also has been included in this category; may be persistent or transient.

Etiology
- Strokes (with or without aphasia)
- Head trauma
- Extrapyramidal diseases, especially Parkinson's disease
- Tumor
- Dementia, especially dialysis dementia
- Drugs prescribed for asthma and depression
- Bilateral brain damage (often resulting in persistent neurogenic stuttering)
- Multiple lesions of a single hemisphere (often resulting in transient neurogenic stuttering)

Symptoms
- Neurologic symptoms consistent with the underlying neurologic diseases or trauma
- Onset of stuttering in later years, often in older people
- Repetitions of medial and final syllables in words
- Repetition of words and phrases
- Prolongation of sounds
- Dysfluent production of function words

Neurogenic Fluency Disorders

- Dysfluencies even in imitated speech
- Frozen articulatory positions (possibly, silent prolongations)
- Pauses, revisions, and incomplete phrases
- Rapid speech rate in some cases
- Lack of the adaptation effect
- Problems in copying and drawing
- Problems in copying block designs
- Problems in sequential hand positions
- Associated motor behaviors (e.g., facial grimacing and foot stamping)
- Problems in tapping out rhythms
- Such other problems as dysphagia, seizures, and paresis or paralysis
- Other symptoms that are typically associated with Aphasia, Apraxia of Speech, Traumatic Brain Injury, and other clinical conditions
- Lack of improvement in stuttering under shadowing or unison speaking

Assessment Objectives/General Guidelines

- To assess all aspects of neurogenic communication disorder
- To assess the types and frequency or dysfluencies
- To take note of associated motor behaviors

Case History/Interview Focus

- See **Case History** and **Interview** under Standard/Common Assessment Procedures
- See also Stuttering
- Onset of the medical condition
- Onset of the fluency problem subsequent to the onset of the medical problem
- Detailed history to document normal fluency during early childhood days or if early stuttering was documented, regained normal fluency until the late onset of neurogenic stuttering

Assessment

- Assess associated Aphasia, Apraxia of Speech, Dementia, or other neurogenic communication disorder

Neurogenic Fluency Disorders

- Assess types and frequency of dysfluencies; see Stuttering
- Assess associated motor behaviors; see Stuttering
- Assess variability in stuttering; see Stuttering

Related/Medical Assessment Data

- Study the medical history of the client
- Obtain neurologic reports

Standard/Common Assessment Procedures

- Complete the Standard/Common Assessment Procedures

Diagnostic Criteria

- Clear evidence of a neurologic disease, trauma, or toxicity
- Neurological symptoms consistent with the underlying condition
- Late onset of fluency problems and convincing information suggesting lack of stuttering of childhood onset
- Specific characteristics listed

Differential Diagnosis

- See Stuttering for differential diagnostic guidelines
- Distinguish dysfluencies that are not attributable to word retrieval problems from those that are (ready recall of names and words; quick writing of names; but dysfluent production of the words)
- Stuttering may show the adaptation effect in patients with extrapyramidal diseases

Prognosis

- Variable, depending on the underlying neurologic disease or trauma

Recommendations

- Treatment to improve fluency
- See the cited sources and *PGTSLP* for details

Helm-Estabrooks, N. (1986). Diagnosis and management of neurogenic stuttering. In K. O. St. Louis (Ed.), *The atypical stutterer* (pp. 193–217). New York: Academic Press.

Rosenbek, J. C. (1984). Stuttering secondary to nervous system damage. In R. F. Curlee & W. H. Perkins (Eds.), *Nature and treatment of stuttering* (pp. 31–48). Austin, TX: Pro-Ed.

Nonfluent Aphasias.   Several syndromes of aphasia all characterized by markedly reduced speech fluency; associated with more anterior cerebral lesions; see Aphasia for a general description of etiology, symptoms, and assessment procedures; see Aphasia: Specific Types for a description of the following major nonfluent aphasias: Broca's aphasia, transcortical motor aphasia, and global aphasia; also see Fluent Aphasias.

Nonpenetrating (Closed-Head) Injury.   A head injury in which the skull may or may not be fractured or lacerated and the Meninges remain intact; see Traumatic Brain Injury.

Nonverbal Oral Apraxia.   Difficulty in executing oral movements that are typically involved in speech when given commands; disturbed volitional movements of oral structures; due to lesions in various cerebral structures including the frontal and central opercula and anterior portions of the insula; may coexist with Apraxia of Speech.

Norms.   Average (mean) performance of a typical group of persons on a selected test in its standardization process; frequently established with the method of cross-sectional sampling of a group of children; most common problems are small sample size and limited sampling of behaviors measured; frequently used in selecting treatment targets.

Nuclear Agenesis (or Aplasia).   The same as Moebius syndrome (see Syndromes Associated With Communicative Disorders)

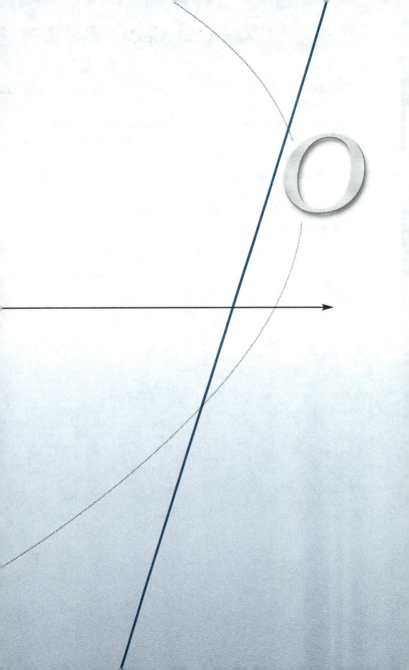

Occipital Alexia. The same as alexia without agraphia; see <u>Alexia</u>.

Oculo-Auriculo-Vertebral Dysplasia. The same as Goldenhar syndrome (see <u>Syndromes Associated With Communicative Disorders</u> .

Open-Head Injury. The same as <u>Penetrating Head Injury</u>; see <u>Traumatic Brain Injury</u>.

Orofacial Examination. See <u>Standard/Common Assessment Procedures</u>.

O

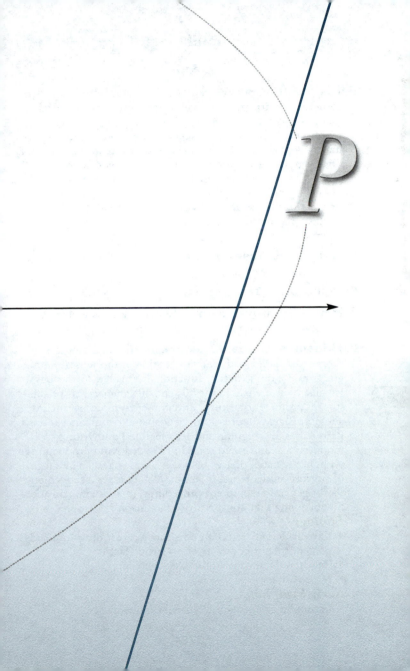

Palilalia.   Compulsive repetition of words and phrases; sometimes with progressively faster rate and decreasing loudness; sound-syllable repetitions are not characteristic; more likely in spontaneous speech than in reading and automatic speech; more likely at the end of utterances; may be observed at the beginning of utterances, but rarely in the middle; associated with many neurological diseases including Parkinson's disease, Pick's disease, Alzheimer's disease, traumatic lesions of the basal ganglia, multiple sclerosis, posttraumatic encephelopathy, and progressive supranuclear palsy.

Paradigm of Assessment.   An overall philosophy or viewpoint of assessment.

Paraphasias.   Unintended word or sound substitutions.

Parietal-Temporal Alexia.   The same as alexia with agraphia; see Alexia.

Parkinson's Disease.   A progressive neurologic syndrome associated with depigmentation of the substantia nigra, a midbrain structure functionally related to the basal ganglia; typical onset in the 50s and 60s; there is loss of ability to produce or store dopamine; symptoms include Tremor, Rigity, depression, visuospatial disturbances, and Bradykinesia; irregular and less legible handwriting; soft, monotonous, and rapid speech; crowded word productions without the usual pauses between phrases; results in a form of subcortical dementia in about 40% of cases; see Dementia for general assessment procedures; in addition, consider the following that are specific to Parkinson's disease:
Etiology
- Varied factors; idiopathic in most cases; drug induced, postencephalitic, and arteriosclerotic factors
- Reduced dopamine in the basal ganglia
- Neuronal loss
Early Symptoms
- Immobility or slow movement (bradykinesia)

Parkinson's Disease

- Tremor, often the pill-rolling type
- Rigidity
- Mask-like face
- Disturbed gait, posture, and equilibrium

Advanced Symptoms
- Deterioration in memory skills
- Deterioration in problem-solving skills
- Deterioration in reasoning skills
- Flat affect
- Depression
- Loss of speech-language functions correlated to the degree of cognitive loss (unlike in patients with Alzheimer's disease)
- Better preserved language functions (compared to other forms of dementia)
- Motor speech disorders, hypokinetic dysarthria; see Dysarthria: Specific Types
- Writing problems
- Weak and breathy voice
- Abnormal pitch, rate, and loudness
- Inappropriate periods of silence
- Slowness of response

Case History/Interview Focus
- See **Case History** and **Interview** under Standard/Common Assessment Procedures
- Document the changes in cognition, general behavior, emotional responding, and communication skills

Ethnocultural Considerations
- See Ethnocultural Considerations in Assessment

Assessment
- Assess speech, language, memory, cognition (including orientation and confusion)
- Follow the procedures described under Dementia
- Follow the procedures described under hypokinetic dysarthria; see Dysarthria: Specific Types

Parkinson's Disease

Standardized Tests
- Consider using standardized tests described under Dementia and Dysarthrias

Related/Medical Assessment Data
- Integrate available medical, neurological, psychological, behavioral, and diagnostic medical laboratory findings with the results of communication assessment

Standard/Common Assessment Procedures
- Complete the Standard/Common Assessment Procedures

Diagnostic Criteria
- Basic diagnosis of Parkinson's disease with the listed neuromotor symptoms
- Dementia and Dysarthrias

Differential Diagnosis
- Differentiate Parkinson's disease from such other diseases as Huntington's disease, Wilson's disease, and progressive supranuclear palsy that are associated with subcortical dementia
- See **Differential Diagnosis** under Dementia

Prognosis
- More favorable for patients with tremor
- Degenerative, irreversible disease

Recommendations
- Communication treatment in the early stages
- Management and coping strategies in later stages
- Family counseling and management strategies
- See the cited sources and *PGTSLP* for details

Bayles, K. A., & Kaszniak, A. W. (1987). *Communication and cognition in normal aging and dementia.* Austin, TX: Pro-Ed.

Cummings, J. L., & Benson, D. F. (1983). *Dementia: A clinical approach.* Boston: Butterworth.

Brookshire, R. H. (1997). *An introduction to neurogenic communication disorders* (5th ed.). St. Louis, MO: Mosby Year Book.

Lubinski, R. (1991). *Dementia and communication.* Philadelphia: B. C. Decker.

Ripich, D. N. (1991). *Geriatric communication disorders.* Austin, TX: Pro-Ed.

P

Penetrating (Open-Head) Injury.   An injury in which the skull is perforated or fractured and the <u>Meninges</u> are torn or lacerated; see <u>Traumatic Brain Injury</u>.

Peristalsis.   Constricting and relaxing movements of a tubular structure (such as the pharynx) to move its contents (such as food in the pharynx); pharyngeal peristalsis may be disordered in patients with <u>Dysphagia</u>.

Perseveration.   Tendency to persist with the same response even though the stimulus has changed; often seen in patients with brain injury.

Phonological Disorders.   Errors of articulation, especially systematic errors on multiple phonemes that form patterns based on <u>Phonological Processes</u>; see <u>Articulation and Phonological Disorders</u> for a description of disorders and their assessment.

Phonological Knowledge.   A child's presumed understanding of the phonological rules of his or her language; an approach to assessing and treating phonological disorders in children; proposed by M. Elbert and J. Gierut and further developed and researched by Gierut and associates; based on the assumption that sound productions reflect children's knowledge of phonological rules of the adult system; recommends that assessment include procedures to estimate phonological knowledge of the child; the greater the consistency of correct productions in varied contexts, the higher the level of phonological knowledge and vice versa; unique among phonological approaches in combining phonological analysis with behaviorally oriented, structured treatment using the paired-stimuli method; assessment places heavy emphasis on conversational speech samples; includes assessment of production of phonemes in minimal-pairs.

Assess Phonological Knowledge
• Obtain a representative, continuous, conversational speech sample

- use the techniques of evoking speech described under <u>Articulation and Phonological Disorders</u>
- tape record the entire speech sample
- ensure that the conversational speech sample includes most if not all sounds
- Sample spontaneous single-word productions
  - use pictures or objects and have the child name them
  - when the child fails to respond, name the stimulus item and re-present the same item later
  - evoke all target English sounds
  - evoke all sounds in all word positions (initial, medial, and final)
  - sample each sound in several different words to assess consistency of productions
  - sample each word more than once to assess variability in production
  - use the Gierut (1985) protocol for this purpose
- Assess production of sounds in minimal pairs
  - sample production of minimal pairs (cat/bat)
  - use the Gierut (1985) protocol for this purpose
- Assess production of morphophonemic alternations
  - sample morphophonemic alternations (e.g., dog/doggie; run/running) to assess whether the child is using sounds contrastively
  - use the Gierut (1985) protocol for this purpose
- Analyze the assessment data
  - phonetically transcribe the sample and identify the level of phonological knowledge
  - a sound produced correctly in all word positions and in all morphemes suggests Type 1 knowledge (most knowledge because of no errors; productions of sounds are adult-like); no phonological rules apply
  - a sound produced correctly in all word positions and in all morphemes with an occasional error suggests Type 2 knowledge (adult-like except for an occasional error, such as deletion of the sound in word final posi-

tion; a phonological rule—final consonant deletion rule in this case—applies

- a sound produced correctly in all positions but consistently incorrectly in a few specific words suggests Type 3 knowledge for that sound; "fossilized" forms account for the error
- a sound produced correctly in all morphemes but only in some positions (e.g., word initially) but consistently incorrectly in other position or positions (e.g., word medially and finally) suggests Type 4 knowledge
- a sound produced correctly only in some morphemes and in some positions suggests Type 5 knowledge
- a sound produced incorrectly in all morphemes and in all positions suggests Type 6 knowledge (the least knowledge because of the most consistent errors)
- classify sounds that are (1) always correctly produced; (2) almost always correctly produced with an occasional error; (3) almost always correctly produced with some fossilized and consistent errors; (4) words produced correctly but only in some word positions and incorrectly and consistently in other positions; (5) words produced correctly only in some words and in some positions and incorrectly in other words and positions; and (6) sounds that are consistently misarticulated in all words and word positions
- identify the rules that seem to account for the error patterns

Recommendations

- Recommend treatment beginning with sounds that reflect least knowledge and ending with those that reflect greater degrees of knowledge
- Note that the treatment is begun on the sounds that are most consistently misarticulated
- See the cited sources and *PGTSLP* for details

Elbert, M., & Gierut, J, (1986). *Handbook of clinical phonology*. San Diego, CA: College-Hill Press.

Phonological Processes

Gierut, J. A. (1985). *On the relationship between phonological knowledge and generalization learning in misarticulating children*. Doctoral dissertation, Indiana University, Bloomington, IN.

Phonological Processes. Multiple ways in which children simplify adult production of speech sounds; simplifications usually result in a loss of phonemic contrast; based on the assumption that multiple errors reflect the operation of certain phonological rules and that the problem is essentially phonemic, not phonetic; originally proposed as explanatory concepts in that processes explain error patterns; as explanatory concepts, presumed to be psychologically real; presumed psychological reality questioned by others; an alternative view is that the processes are ways of describing and categorizing errors without necessarily explaining them; assessed through a representative sample of conversational speech; computerized assessment programs available; see Articulation and Phonological Disorders for more detailed description of errors that characterize different processes and their assessment procedures; major processes include the following:

Assimilation Processes. A group of phonological processes in which productions of dissimilar phonemes sound more alike; major assimilation processes include:

- *Devoicing*: Substitution of a voiceless final sound for a voiced (e.g., /k/ for /g/ in final positions)
- *Devoicing of final consonants*: Substitution of a voiceless final consonant for a voiced (e.g., /t/ for /d/)
- *Labial assimilation*: Substitution of a labial sound for a nonlabial (e.g., /b/ for /d/)
- *Nasal assimilation*: Substitution of a nasal consonant for a non-nasal (e.g., /n/ for /d/)
- *Nasalization of vowels*: Nasal resonance on vowels that are adjacent to nasal sounds; nasal resonance on any vowel regardless of adjacency
- *Prevocalic voicing*: Substitution of a voiced sound for voiceless sound preceding a vowel (e.g., /b/ for /p/ in prevocalic positions)

Phonological Processes

- *Velar assimilation*: Substitution of a velar consonant for a nonvelar (e.g., /g/ for /d/)

Syllable Structure Processes: Processes that change the syllable structures; includes the deletion processes; major deletion processes include:

- *Cluster reduction:* One or more consonants are deleted in a cluster of consonants (e.g., *bu* for *blue*)
- *Diminutization*. Addition of [i] (e.g., *plati* for *plate*) or a consonant and [i] to the target word (e.g., *nodi* for *no*)
- *Epenthesis*. Insertion of an unstressed vowel, usually the schwa (e.g., bəlu for blue)
- *Initial consonant deletion:* Omission of an initial consonant of a syllable (e.g., *ink* for *sink*)
- *Final consonant deletion:* Omission of a final consonant (e.g., *goo* for *good*)
- *Medial consonant deletion:* noted infrequently
- *Reduplication:* Repetition of a syllable, resulting in substitution of one for another (e.g., *wawa* for *water*); may be classified as an assimilation process
- *Syllable deletion:* omission of a syllable, usually an unstressed one (e.g., *medo* for *tomato*)

Substitution Processes. A group of phonological processes in which one class of sounds is substituted for another; major substitution processes include:

- *Depalatalization:* Substitution of an alveolar fricative for a palatal fricative or an affricate (e.g., *su* for *shoe*)
- *Denasalization:* Substitution of an oral consonant for a nasal consonant (e.g., /d/ for /n/)
- *Gliding:* Substitution of a glide for a liquid (e.g., /w/ for /r/)
- *Stopping:* Substitution of a stop for a fricative or an affricate (e.g., /p/ for /f/)
- *Velar fronting:* Substitution of an alveolar for a velar (e.g., /t/ for /k/)
- *Vocalization:* Substitution of a vowel (often [o]) for a syllabic liquid (e.g., *bado* for *bottle*)

P

Bernthal, J. E., & Bankson, N. W. (1998). *Articulation and phonological disorders* (4rd ed.). Englewood Cliffs, NJ: Prentice-Hall.

Bleile, K. M. (1995). *Manual of articulation and phonological disorders.* San Diego, CA: Singular Publishing Group.

Creaghead, N. A., Newman, P. W., & Secord, W. A. (1989). *Assessment and remediation of articulatory and phonological disorders* (2nd ed.). Columbus, OH: Merrill.

Elbert, M., & Gierut, J. (1986). *Handbook of clinical phonology.* San Diego, CA: College-Hill Press.

Lowe, R. J. (1994). *Phonology: Assessment and intervention applications in speech pathology.* Baltimore: Williams & Wilkins.

Peña-Brookes, A., & Hegde, M. N. (2000). *Assessment and treatment of articulation and phonological disorders in children.* Austin, TX: Pro-Ed.

Stoel-Gammon, C., & Dunn, C. (1985). *Normal and disordered phonology in children.* Austin, TX: Pro-Ed.

Pick's Disease.   A progressive neurologic disease associated with a gradual decrease in brain mass, especially in the temporal and frontal lobes; no known causes for the decreased brain mass; similar to Alzheimer's disease in its effects (but not in histopathology); results in cortical dementia (as does Alzheimer's disease); language symptoms grossly similar to those of Alzheimer's disease; see Dementia for general assessment procedures; in addition, consider the following that are specific to Pick's disease:

Etiology
• No known causes

Early Symptoms
• Behavioral changes
• Intellectual disturbances
• Deterioration in social behavior
• Uninhibited behavior (e.g., inappropriate sexual jokes, offensive comments)
• Repetitive, meaningless behavior (e.g., repeatedly folding napkins and putting them away)
• Impaired judgment and insight
• Excessive eating and weight gain

Pick's Disease

Advanced Symptoms
- Intellectual deterioration
- Naming problems
- Circumlocution
- Echolalia and verbal stereotypes
- Meaningless repetition of phrases
- Impaired confrontation naming
- Impaired comprehension of spoken and printed material
- Muteness
- Total disorientation and confusion

Case History/Interview Focus
- See **Case History** and **Interview** under Standard/Common Assessment Procedures
- Document the changes in cognition, general behavior, emotional responding, and communication skills

Ethnocultural Considerations
- See Ethnocultural Considerations in Assessment

Assessment
- Assess speech, language, memory, cognition (including orientation and confusion)
- Follow the procedures described under Dementia

Standardized Tests
- Consider using standardized tests described under Dementia and Dysarthrias

Related/Medical Assessment Data
- Integrate available medical, neurological, psychological, behavioral, and diagnostic medical laboratory findings with the results of communication assessment

Standard/Common Assessment Procedures
- Complete the Standard/Common Assessment Procedures

Diagnostic Criteria
- Basic diagnosis of Pick's disease with the listed symptoms; See Dementia for additional information

Differential Diagnosis
- Differentiate Pick's disease from Alzheimer's disease; see **Differential Diagnosis** under Dementia

Prognosis
- Degenerative, irreversible disease

Recommendations
- Communication treatment in the early stages
- Management and coping strategies in later stages
- Family counseling and management strategies
- See the cited sources and *PGTSLP* for details

Bayles, K. A., & Kaszniak, A. W. (1987). *Communication and cognition in normal aging and dementia.* Austin, TX: Pro-Ed.

Brookshire, R. H. (1992). *An introduction to neurogenic communication disorders* (4th ed.). St. Louis, MO: Mosby Year Book.

Cummings, J. L., & Benson, D. F. (1983). *Dementia: A clinical approach.* Boston: Butterworth.

Lubinski, R. (1991). *Dementia and communication.* Philadelphia: B. C. Decker.

Ripich, D. N. (1991). *Geriatric communication disorders.* Austin, TX: Pro-Ed.

Phytanic Acid.   A fatty acid concentrated in dairy products; excessively stored in tissue or plasma of patients with Refsum syndrome (see Syndromes Associated With Communicative Disorders).

Polydactyly.   A genetic anomaly characterized by supernumerary toes or fingers; found in several genetic syndromes; see Laurence-Moon syndrome and oro-facial-digital syndrome type 11 (see Syndromes Associated With Communicative Disorders).

Polyneuritis.   Simultaneous inflation of several peripheral nerves; part of some genetic syndromes including Refsum syndrome (see Syndromes Associated With Communicative Disorders).

Positron Emission Tomography (PET).   A neurodiagnostic procedure based on computed tomography; measures differential metabolic rates in different areas of the brain; patient is injected with a radioactive substance which spreads throughout the brain; amount of radioactivity is then scanned; differences in the amount of radioactivity suggest different rates of cerebral metabolism; lower than the normal metabolic rate suggests neuropathology; used in diagnosing neuropathology associated with communication disorders, including aphasia.

Posterior Isolation Syndrome.   The same as transcortical sensory aphasia (see Aphasia: Specific Types).

Pragmatic Language Skills.   Aspects of appropriate language use in naturalistic communicative contexts; targets of language assessment; include such skills as topic initiation, topic maintenance; and turn taking (see Language Disorders in Children).

Preauricular Tags.   Rudimentary appendage of auricular tissue on the face, often at the corner of mouth and toward the ear; part of certain genetic syndromes; see Goldenhar syndrome (see Syndromes Associated With Communicative Disorders).

Primary Progressive Aphasia.   Aphasia due to degenerative neurologic disease of insidious onset and slow progression of symptoms; also known as slowly progressive aphasia; possibly affecting the left perisylvian region of the brain; minimal or no generalized cognitive impairment; language symptoms resemble those of Broca's aphasia and may include apraxia of speech; use assessment procedures described under Aphasia and Apraxia of Speech.

Prognosis.   A professional judgment made about the future course of a disorder or disease under specified conditions; a conditional statement of best judgment given certain facts; a predictive statement about what might happen under different circumstances; highly dependent on individual variations; in the case of communication disorders, such factors as the physiological course of an underlying disease, health of the client, severity of the disorder, time of intervention, intensity and quality of treatment offered, consistency with which the treatment is received, family support and participation in the treatment process, the client's motivation to work hard in and outside the clinical setting, social reinforcement for maintaining the treatment gains, among other variables, influence the final outcome and hence the prognostic statement.

Progressive Supranuclear Palsy (PSP).   A degenerative disease of the brainstem basal ganglia, and cerebellum; in its early stages, resembles Parkinson's disease; includes paralysis of the upward gaze (ophthalmoplegia); gait and balance problems; frequent falling; neck rigidity; mixed dysarthria and dysphagia in early stages; cortical stuttering or palilalia associated with frontal atrophy; aphonia; slowly developing dementia.

Prosopagnosia.   Difficulty in recognizing familiar faces; voice may help recognize the face; includes difficulty in matching known person's pictures with names; a possible symptom of Right Hemisphere Syndrome.

Pseudodementia.   Psychiatric depression that mimics the symptoms of dementia including slowness of movement, forgetfulness, disorientation, and attentional deficits; more rapid progression of symptoms, patient complaint about memory problems, and a history of psychiatric problems, among others, help distinguish dementia from pseudodementia in depressed patients.

Ptosis.   Drooping or retrogression of an organ or part; drooping of the upper eyelid as seen in Noonan syndrome (see Syndromes Associated With Communicative Disorders).

Pulmonary Stenosis.   Narrowing of the opening between the pulmonary artery and the right ventricle.

Pure Alexia.   The same as alexia without agraphia, see Alexia.

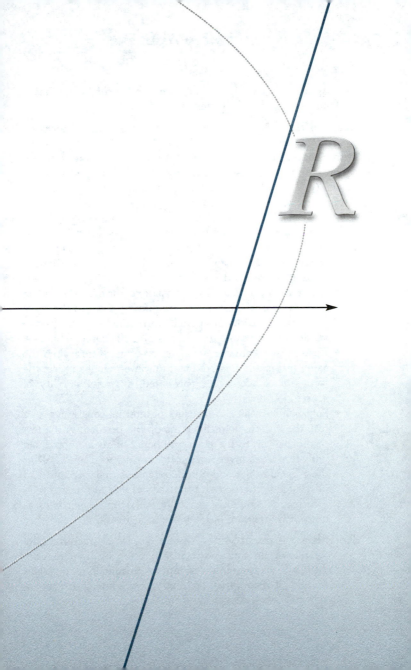

Receptive Aphasia.   The same as Wernicke's aphasia; see Aphasia: Specific Types.

Reliability.   Consistency with which the same event is repeatedly measured; consistency of scores or values across repeated testing or measurement means the same; a criterion for selecting assessment procedures; described here are the types of reliability that are important in selecting a standardized test; select a test that reports adequate reliability of at least one kind; most reliability measures are expressed in terms of a correlational coefficient; the higher the correlational coefficient, the greater the reliability; see *PGTSLP* for *interobserver* and *intraobserver reliability* of measures that are not based on standardized tests.

- Alternate form reliability: Consistency of measures when two forms of the same test are administered to the same persons; also known as parallel form reliability; needs two versions of the same test that sample the same behaviors.
- Test-retest reliability: Consistency of measures when the same test is administered to the same persons twice; the two sets of scores are correlated; suggests stability of scores over time.
- Split-half reliability: A measure of internal consistency of a test; the responses to the items on the first half of the test or those given to the even-numbered items are correlated with responses given to the items on the second half or those given to the odd-numbered items; to derive this kind of reliability, the first and the second half of a test should measure the same skill; generally overestimates reliability as it does not measure stability of scores over time.

Retinitis Pigmentosa.   An eye disease characterized by progressive retinal atrophy and migration of pigmentation; night blindness is an initial symptom; results in gradual loss of peripheral vision; may be inherited in some cases; associated with several genetic syndromes.

Right Hemisphere Syndrome.   A syndrome of brain injury in the right cerebral hemisphere and its consequences; may be caused by cerebrovascular accidents, tumors, head trauma, or various neurologic diseases; associated with perceptual, attentional, emotional, and communicative deficits; varying degrees of functional involvement depending on the site, nature, and extent of damage; associated with communication disorders in about 50% of cases; lower level of education and cortical lesions (rather than subcortical lesions) increase the chances of communication disorders; the relation between specific communication disorders and right hemisphere poorly understood

Etiology
- Generally, the same neuropathological factors affect both the left and right hemispheres
- Cerebrovascular accidents
- Tumors
- Head trauma
- Various neurological diseases

Perceptual, Attentional, and Other Behavioral Deficits
- Left hemisphere neglect or left-sided neglect; most severe and consistent neglect associated with right hemisphere damage; the patient may:
  - fail to perceive the stimuli on the left when both right and left sides are stimulated
  - need specific instruction to attend to stimuli on the left
  - may use only the right-sided pockets or right-sided drawers
  - fail to perceive left-sided tactile and perceptual stimuli in the absence of sensory deficits
  - copy only a right side of a geometric design (e.g., crowding all the numbers of a clock into the right half of the circle)
  - read only the right half of a printed page and complain that what is read does not make sense

R

Right Hemisphere Syndrome

- bump into things on the left side
- deny the existence of paralyzed left body parts or claim that they belong to someone else
- fail to localize stimuli on the left side
- fail to give margin on the left side while writing
- have difficulty in recognizing faces (Prosopagnosia); voice may help recognition; difficulty in matching known persons' pictures with names; associated more often with posterior right hemisphere damage
- fail to recognize stimuli the patient constantly dealt with (e.g., a carpenter may fail to recognize his hammer)
- recover from left-sided neglect a few weeks or months post-onset
- Disorientation
  - disorientation is common during the immediate postonset period
  - disorientation to time and space
  - disorientation to familiar faces (facial recognition problems)
- Constructional impairment
  - difficulty in constructing block designs
  - problems in reproducing two-dimensional stick figures
  - problems in drawing or copying geometric designs
  - omission of components in constructing designs or copying figures
- Affective deficits
  - difficulty in experiencing emotions only if the limbic system also is involved
  - more frequently, difficulty in expressing emotions
  - difficulty in recognizing emotional expressions of other people
  - difficulty in using tone, prosody, facial expressions, and context as cues to specific emotions
- Denial of illness
  - indifference to problems the patient acknowledges
  - minimize the consequence of problems that are acknowledged

R

- deny the existence of physical problems (e.g., paralysis of an arm)
- Impaired inference
  - difficulty drawing inferences from logical premises or situations
- Impaired reasoning, planning, organizing, and problem-solving skills
  - difficulty in planning such activities as shopping or vacationing
  - difficulty in organizing such activities as parties
  - difficulty in planning a meal
- Problems in logical reasoning
  - difficulty in identifying absurd statements
  - justification of absurd statements with bizarre reasons
  - problems in logical reasoning
- Other behavioral deficits
  - depression in some patients
  - impulsive and uninhibited behavior
  - distractibility
  - delayed response

Communication Disorders

- Prosodic problems; often cited; however, there is some conflicting evidence about these problems
  - monotonous speech lacking in intonation in most patients
  - emotionally flat speech in some patients; knowing that their speech does not convey emotional tones, use specific verbal expressions ("I am upset with you" or "I am sad about that")
  - hypermelodic speech in some patients (high pitch and pitch variability)
- Inappropriate and anomalous speech
  - confabulation
  - inappropriate humor
  - excessive and rambling speech that does not make much sense

R

Right Hemisphere Syndrome

- Problems in distinguishing significant from irrelevant information
  - irrelevant details when telling a story
  - unimportant details while talking
- Problems in comprehending implied meanings
  - concerned with literal meaning of messages
  - unable to interpret proverbs, idiomatic expressions, figures of speech, and metaphors
- Problems in integrating information
  - difficulty in comprehending a story when sentences are presented on separate cards
- Problems in speech pragmatics
  - recall isolated and unimportant details of stories
  - lack of sequence or event relationships in narration
  - irrelevant comments while narrating an event
  - poor eye contact with listeners
  - topic maintenance problems
  - failure to take turns or yield to others in conversation because of excessive talk
  - impulsive responses
  - failure to engage in such conversational repair strategies as clarifying statements when the listener does not understand and asking for clarification when a speaker's statements are unclear
- Auditory comprehension of language
  - difficulty in comprehending language in some cases
- Word-retrieval problems
  - naming problems especially naming categories (e.g., may name each flower separately, but not say "flowers")
- Reading and writing problems
  - left neglect dyslexia (reading only the right portion of a printed page)
  - reading comprehension problems
  - motor writing problems (e.g., repetition of letters) and spatial agraphia (e.g., poor spacing, crowding of words)

- Dysarthria
  - weak production of consonants
  - somewhat similar to hypokinetic dysarthria

Assessment Objectives/General Guidelines

- To evaluate the perceptual and attentional deficits associated with right hemisphere syndrome
- To assess communication disorders associated with the syndrome
- To support or justify a diagnosis of right hemisphere syndrome
- To identify the strengths and deficits that help plan treatment

Case History/Interview Focus

- See **Case History** and **Interview** under Standard/Common Assessment Procedures
- Document the onset and recovery from stroke or other clinical condition

Ethnocultural Considerations

- See Ethnocultural Considerations in Assessment

Assessment: Perceptual and Attentional Deficits

- Assess left-sided neglect and attentional deficits by a variety of tasks (most of which may be parts of standardized tests), observations of the patient during interview and assessment, and interview of family members:
  - draw small circles, dots, squares, or lines on a sheet of paper, randomly spaced, and ask the patient to cross out all of them; note that the patient with left neglect will cross out only the stimuli on the right half of the page
  - draw horizontal lines on a sheet of paper and ask the patient to draw vertical lines through all of them to divide them into two equal halves; note that a patient with left neglect will divide the line such that the left portion will be longer than the right side
  - observe the patient for evidence of neglect (e.g., the patient may forget to comb the hair on the left side of the head)

- ask the patient to describe his or her problems on the left side of the body; note the patient may deny the existence of a paralyzed left limb
- ask the family about evidence of neglect (e.g., bumping into things or persons on the left)
- interview hospital staff about evidence of neglect
- touch both the arms simultaneously and ask the patient to report sensation; note that the patient may report sensation only on the right side (even if the left has no sensory problems)
- ask the patient to write a paragraph or copy a paragraph; note the distribution or organization of writing on the page for evidence of neglect
- ask the patient to cross out a specific letter when the target letters are printed along with nontarget letters on a sheet of paper; count the number of correctly crossed out letters and their location for evidence of inattention, neglect, or both
- Assess disorientation
  - ask such questions as "where are you now?" and "where is your home?" to assess spatial orientation
  - ask questions about time, date, month, and the year
  - use assessment data relative to facial recognition to assess orientation to human faces
- Assess constructional impairment
  - ask the client to copy a block design of the kind found in nonverbal intelligence tests
  - arrange a matchstick figure on the desk and ask the client to copy it
  - ask the client to draw or copy the face of a clock; note the crowding of all numbers on the right half of the circle
  - ask the client to copy printed figures and designs; note the omission of details
- Assess affective deficits
  - observe the client for evidence of difficulty in expressing emotions (e.g., does the patient show facial expressions consistent with verbal expressions?)

- demonstrate different facial expressions of emotions and ask the client to identify them (e.g., identifying a happy or a sad face)
- show pictures of faces that clearly depict contrasting emotions and ask the patient to name the emotional experience
- show pictures that express contrasting emotions and ask the patient to match them with appropriate printed words (e.g., "happy" or "sad")
- observe the patient as you talk for evidence of difficulty in using prosodic features to surmise emotional expression
- Assess denial of illness
  - ask various questions about the patient's problems and evaluate the responses for evidence of denial (e.g., "do you have problems of writing now?"; "why are you here in the hospital?"; "what kinds of tasks are difficult for you now?") and take note of the answers that might suggest denial of obvious problems
  - interview family members of the patient's denial of physical or behavioral problems
  - judge the patient's level of motivation for assessment or treatment; low motivation may suggest denial
  - observe whether the patient makes attempts at self-correction; lack of such attempts may suggest denial
- Assess impaired inference
  - tell a brief story and ask the patient to describe its moral or message and its implied meaning
  - tell a few proverbs and ask the patient to say what they mean (e.g., "what does it mean to say that a stitch in time saves nine?")
  - tell a few metaphors and ask the patient to say what they mean (e.g., "what does it mean when you say the problem was nipped in the bud?")
  - tell a joke without its punchline and ask the patient to complete it
  - show pictures that show absurdities and ask the patient what is wrong with them and why (e.g., a picture of a cat chasing a dog)

R

- place a variety of objects on the table and ask the patient to classify them according to similarities and differences; take note of errors to evaluate difficulty in abstraction and inferencing
- Assess impaired reasoning, planning, organizing, and problem-solving skills
  - ask the patient to describe how he or she would plan a shopping trip
  - ask the client to describe how he or she would plan a brief vacation
  - ask the patient to describe steps involved in organizing a birthday party
  - ask the client to describe how he or she would plan a meal for a few guests
- Assess problems in logical reasoning
  - present a series of logical and absurd statements and ask the patient to sort them
  - ask the patient to explain why a statement is absurd
  - use other assessment data (e.g., those related to impaired inference, discourse cohesion, and sequencing events in story telling) to make judgments about logical reasoning skills
- Assess other behavioral deficits
  - ask the family members or hospital staff about signs of depression (e.g., lack of interest in food or visitors)
  - obtain psychological or psychiatric reports on depression and other behavioral problems
  - interview family members or caretakers about impulsive and uninhibited behavior (e.g., emotional outbursts or inappropriate jokes); observe and take note of these behaviors during the interview and assessment
  - observe the client's speed of responses, concentration on various assessment tasks, and distractibility

Assessment: Communication Disorders

- Take a conversational speech sample
- Assess prosodic problems

- note any prosodic deviations (e.g., rate variations, monopitch and monoloudness, and equal or inappropriate stress patterns)
- take note of hypermelodic speech
- ask the patient to imitate an intonational pattern of a modeled sentence; note deviations in intonational patterns including variations in stress and pitch
- note the expression of emotionality in speech
- Assess inappropriate and anomalous speech
  - record all inappropriate responses to questions, anomalous responses, meaningless or irrelevant comments
  - document inappropriate humor
  - take note of rambling speech
  - take note of potential of obvious confabulation
  - question the family members and other caregivers about inappropriate and anomalous speech, off-color jokes, confabulations, and rambling and meaningless speech
- Assess problems in distinguishing significant from irrelevant information
  - tell a story and ask the patient to retell it
  - note insignificant details retold and missing important details
  - note missing background information in story retelling or in narrating events and experiences
- Assess problems in comprehending implied meanings
  - use the same or similar tasks involved in assessing impaired inference
  - note the degree to which the client states or summarizes literal versus implied and unstated meanings, conclusions, and consequences
- Assess problems in integrating information
  - present a short story the sentences of which are written on separate cards
  - ask questions about the story
  - use procedures described under Assess Impaired Inference and Assess Impaired Reasoning, Planning, Orga-

nizing, and Problem Solving Skills to evaluate integration of information

- evaluate continuity, cohesion, and logical sequencing of events evident in discourse that might suggest problems in integrating and sequencing information
- Assess problems in speech pragmatics
  - evaluate eye contact during discourse
  - note the number of times the patient interrupts you
  - note the number of times the patient fails to yield to you when you try to speak
  - note excessive talking
  - initiate a topic of conversation and assess whether the patient maintained it for a reasonable amount of time
  - note irrelevant, tangential, or inappropriate comments, jokes, and interruptions
  - note how often the patient complies with requests for clarification of statements he or she makes
  - make some ambiguous statements and note how often the patient asks for clarification
- Assess auditory comprehension of language
  - assess auditory comprehension of speech during the interview
- Assess word-retrieval problems
  - note naming difficulties the patient exhibits
  - note other word-retrieval problems as evidenced by pauses and word substitutions that suggest word-retrieval problems
- Assess reading and writing problems
  - obtain as much detailed information as possible on premorbid reading and writing skills and interests and involvement in these activities
  - make a more detailed assessment of literacy skills only if they are important to the patient
  - reanalyze assessment data pertaining to neglect and attention to evaluate their role in reading and writing deficits (e.g., ignoring the left side of the printed page while reading and drawing only the right side of a picture)

- have the patient read a paragraph or two and ask questions about the material to assess reading comprehension
- assess functional reading skills including reading a medical prescription, restaurant menu, and daily newspaper
- ask the patient to write a paragraph and analyze it for errors (e.g., repetition of letters, poor letter formation, and spacing)
- assess functional writing skills by having the patient write as you dictate a message and a set of directions
- Assess dysarthria
  - assess the production of speech sounds from the speech sample; analyze the pattern of errors
  - note any phonatory deviations that might be present

Standardized Tests

- Administer selected subtests of a test of Aphasia; in addition, consider administering one or more of the following:

Test	Purpose
Mini Inventory of Right Brain Injury (P. A. Pimental & N. A. Kingbury)	To assess visual-perceptual skills, higher language function, affect, and general behavior
Right Hemisphere Language Battery (K. L. Bryan)	To assess comprehension of metaphors, implied meanings, humor, and other language functions
Test of Visual Neglect (M. L. Albert)	To assess visual neglect through crossing out lines drawn on a sheet
Revised Token Test (M. M. McNeil & T. E. Prescott)	To assess auditory comprehension of spoken commands through token manipulations
Behavioral Inattention Test (B. A. Wilson, J. Cockburn, & P. Halligan)	To assess unilateral visual neglect

R

Right Hemisphere Syndrome

Related/Medical Assessment Data
- Integrate available medical, neurological, psychological, behavioral, and diagnostic medical laboratory findings with the results of communication assessment

Standard/Common Assessment Procedures
- Complete the Standard/Common Assessment Procedures

Diagnostic Criteria
- History and medical evidence consistent with right hemisphere injury, especially strokes, tumors, or head trauma
- More pronounced perceptual and affective disorders than specific language disorders
- More pronounced communication disorder than specific loss of language functions

Differential Diagnosis
- Differentiate right hemisphere syndrome from aphasia typically caused by left hemisphere pathologies
- Use the following grid to distinguish right hemisphere syndrome and aphasia (adapted from Hegde, 1998):

Right Hemisphere Syndrome or Aphasia?

Right Hemisphere Syndrome	Aphasia
Only mild problems in naming, fluency, auditory comprehension, reading, and writing	Significant or dominant problems in naming, fluency, auditory comprehension, reading, and writing
Left-sided neglect	No left-sided neglect
Denial of illness	No denial of illness
Speech is often irrelevant, excessive, rambling	Speech is generally relevant
Often lack of affect	Generally normal effect
Possibly, impaired recognition of familiar faces	Intact recognition of familiar faces
Rotation and left-sided neglect	Simplification of drawings

(continued)

Right Hemisphere Syndrome

(continued)

Right Hemisphere Syndrome	Aphasia
More prominent prosodic defect	Less prominent prosodic defect
Inappropriate humor	Appropriate humor
May retell only nonessential, isolated details (no integration)	May retell the essence of a story
Understands only literal meanings	May understand implied meanings
Pragmatic impairments more striking (eye contact, topic maintenance, etc.)	Pragmatic impairments less striking
Though possessing good language skills, communication is very poor	Though limited in language skills, communication is often good
Pure linguistic deficits are not dominant	Pure linguistic deficits are dominant

Note: Right hemisphere damage in the few individuals whose right hemisphere is dominant for language results in aphasia, and for the same etiologic factors.

Prognosis
• Variable, depending on neuropathology and severity of deficits
• More severe initial symptoms suggest less favorable prognosis
• Smaller and unilateral lesions suggest more favorable prognosis

Recommendations
• Treatment to improve communication and cognitive and perceptual functioning
• See the cited sources and *PGTSLP* for details

Brookshire, R. H. (1997). An *introduction to neurogenic communication disorders* (5th ed.). St. Louis, MO: Mosby Year Book.

405

Hegde, M. N. (1998). A *coursebook on aphasia and other neurogenic language disorders* (2nd ed.). San Diego, CA: Singular Publishing Group.

Tompkins, C. A. (1995). *Right hemisphere communication disorders: Theory and management.* San Diego, CA: Singular Publishing Group.

Rigidity.   Stiffness of muscles and joints.

Robin Sequence.   The same as Pierre-Robin syndrome; see <u>Syndromes Associated With Communicative Disorders</u>.

R

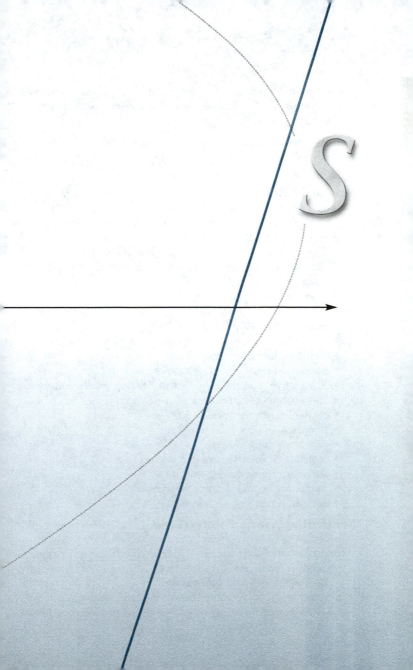

S

Sanfilippo Syndrome

Sanfilippo Syndrome. A type of mucopolysaccharidosis syndrome (see Syndromes Associated With Communicative Disorders).

Scheie Syndrome. A type of mucopolysaccharidosis syndrome (see Syndromes Associated With Communicative Disorders.

Semantic Relations. Theoretical and abstract relational meanings attributed to word combinations; categories into which children's early productions may be assigned; categories that may be used in assessing children's language disorders; usefulness questioned because of the argument that these abstract relations may not be empirical for children; include the following:

- Nomination: *this car*; *that doll*
- Agent-Object: *daddy hammer* (Daddy is hammering); *mommy cook* (Mommy is cooking)
- Agent-Action: *mommy run* (Mommy is running)
- Action-Object: *kick ball*; *hit nail*
- Modifier-Head: *big ball*; *more juice*
- X + Dative: *give Bobby* (give it to Bobby); *kiss mommy*
- X + Locative: *ball box* (ball is in the box)
- Nonexistence: *no truck*; *no baby*
- Recurrence: *more juice*; *more jump*
- Notice: *see this*; *hi Kermit*
- Instrumental: *cut scissors* (cut it with scissors)
- Attribution: *red car*; *big ball*
- Rejection: *no milk* (I don't want milk)
- Denial: *not hungry*; *not sleepy*

Sequential Motion Rate (SMR). A measure of rapid movement of articulators from one articulatory position to the other; the same as the Diadochokinetic Rate; the typical procedure is to ask the client to "say 'puh-tuh-kuh-puh-tuh-kuh-puh-tuh-kuh-puh-tuh-kuh' for as long as you can and as rapidly and as steadily as you can"; of diagnostic value in assessing motor speech disorders; a routine measure in most assessment procedures because it helps assess the structural and functional integrity of the lips, jaw, and the tongue; related to alternating motion rates; usually, SMRs follow AMRs; for procedures and analysis, see Alternating Motion Rates (AMRs).

Single-Photon Emission Computed Tomography (SPECT). A neurodiagnostic method that evaluates the amount of blood flowing through a structure; also known as regional cerebral blood flow (rCBF); helps assess cerebral metabolism; the patient inhales xenon 133, a radioactive gas that immediately spreads throughout the cerebral hemispheres and enters the bloodstream; a scanner detects radiation uptake in cerebral blood; a computer calculates the amount of blood flow in given regions and displays variations in blood flow in different colors; helpful in diagnosing cerebral lesions associated with various neuropathologies causing communication disorders.

Sly Syndrome. A type of mucopolysaccharidosis syndrome (see Syndromes Associated With Communicative Disorders .

Speech, Language, and Motor Development. General guidelines on assessing speech, language, and motor development in infants, toddlers, and children; use them only as guidelines as individual differences in development are significant; guidelines are most useful in making broad judgments when the deviation is marked; less useful when subtle deviations need to be documented; many of the guidelines, especially at higher age levels, are vague and difficult to evaluate.

0–6 Months
Speech and Language Skills
❑ Repeats the same sounds;
❑ Frequently coos, gurgles, and makes pleasure sounds;
❑ Uses a different cry to express different needs;
❑ Smiles when spoken to;

❏ Recognizes voices;
❏ Localizes sound by turning head;
❏ Listens to speech;
❏ Uses the phonemes /b/, /p/, and /m/ in babbling;
❏ Uses sounds or gestures to indicate wants.

Motor Skills
❏ Smiles;
❏ Rolls over from front to back and back to front;
❏ Raises head and shoulder from a face-down position;
❏ Sits while using hands for support;
❏ Reaches for objects with one hand but often misses;
❏ Blows bubbles on lips;
❏ Visually tracks people and objects;
❏ Watches own hands.

7–12 Months

Speech and Language Skills
❏ Understands *no* and *hot*;
❏ Responds to simple requests;
❏ Understands and responds to own name;
❏ Listens to and imitates some sounds;
❏ Recognizes words for common items (e.g., cup, shoe, juice);
❏ Babbles using long and short groups of sounds;
❏ Uses a song-like intonation pattern when babbling;
❏ Uses a large variety of sounds in babbling;
❏ Imitates some adult speech sounds and intonation patterns;
❏ Uses speech sounds rather than only crying to get attention;
❏ Listens when spoken to;
❏ Uses sound approximations;
❏ Begins to change babbling to jargon;
❏ Uses speech intentionally for the first time;
❏ Uses nouns almost exclusively;
❏ Has an expressive vocabulary of 1 to 3 words;
❏ Understands simple commands.

Motor Skills
❏ Crawls on stomach;
❏ Stands or walks with assistance;

S

❏ Attempts to feed self with a spoon;
❏ Rises to a sitting position;
❏ Attempts to imitate gestures;
❏ Uses smooth and continuous reaches to grasp objects;
❏ Sits unsupported;
❏ Drinks from a cup;
❏ Pulls self up to stand by furniture;
❏ Holds own bottle;
❏ Plays ball with a partner;
❏ Has poor aim and timing of release when throwing;
❏ Enjoys games like peek-a-boo and pat-a-cake;
❏ Uses a primitive grasp for writing, bangs crayon rather than writes;
❏ Cooperates with dressing, puts foot out for shoe, and places arms through sleeves.

13–18 Months

Speech and Language Skills

❏ Uses adult-like intonation patterns;
❏ Uses echolalia and jargon;
❏ Uses jargon to fill gaps in fluency;
❏ Omits some initial consonants and almost all final consonants;
❏ Produces mostly unintelligible speech;
❏ Follows simple commands;
❏ Receptively identifies 1 to 3 body parts;
❏ Has an expressive vocabulary of 3 to 20 or more words (mostly nouns);
❏ Combines gestures and vocalization;
❏ Makes requests for more of desired items.

Motor Skills

❏ Points to recognized objects;
❏ Runs but falls frequently;
❏ Imitates gestures;
❏ Removes some clothing items (e.g., socks, hat);
❏ Attempts to pull zippers up and down.

S

Speech, Language, and Motor Development

19–24 Months
Speech and Language Skills
- ❏ Uses words more frequently than jargon;
- ❏ Has an expressive vocabulary of 50–100 or more words;
- ❏ Has a receptive vocabulary of 300 or more words;
- ❏ Starts to combine nouns and verbs;
- ❏ Begins to use pronouns;
- ❏ Maintains unstable voice control;
- ❏ Uses appropriate intonation for questions;
- ❏ Is approximately 25–50% intelligible to strangers;
- ❏ Answers "what's that?" questions;
- ❏ Enjoys listening to stories;
- ❏ Knows 5 body parts;
- ❏ Accurately names a few familiar objects.

Motor Skills
- ❏ Walks without assistance;
- ❏ Walks sideways and backwards;
- ❏ Uses pull toys;
- ❏ Strings beads;
- ❏ Enjoys playing with clay;
- ❏ Picks up objects from the floor without falling;
- ❏ Stands with heels together;
- ❏ Walks up and down stairs with help;
- ❏ Jumps down a distance of 12 inches;
- ❏ Climbs and stands on chair;
- ❏ Rotates head while walking;
- ❏ Reaches automatically with primary concern on manipulation of object;
- ❏ Inserts key into lock;
- ❏ Stands on one foot with help;
- ❏ Seats self in a child's chair;
- ❏ Makes a tower 3 cubes high.

2–3 Years
Speech and Language Skills
- ❏ Speech is 50–75% intelligible;
- ❏ Understands *one* and *all*;

Speech, Language, and Motor Development

- ❏ Verbalizes toilet needs (before, during, or after act);
- ❏ Requests items by name;
- ❏ Points to pictures in a book when named;
- ❏ Identifies several body parts;
- ❏ Follows simple commands and answers simple questions;
- ❏ Enjoys listening to short stories, songs, and rhymes;
- ❏ Asks 1- to 2-word questions;
- ❏ Uses 3- to 4-word phrases;
- ❏ Uses some prepositions, articles, present progressive verbs, regular plurals, contractions, and irregular past tense forms;
- ❏ Uses words that are general in context;
- ❏ Continues use of echolalia when difficulties in speech are encountered;
- ❏ Has a receptive vocabulary of 500–900 or more words;
- ❏ Has an expressive vocabulary of 50–250 or more words (rapid growth during this period);
- ❏ Exhibits multiple grammatical errors;
- ❏ Understands most things said to him or her;
- ❏ Frequently exhibits repetitions—especially pronouns and initial syllables of words;
- ❏ Speaks with a loud voice;
- ❏ Increases range of pitch;
- ❏ Uses vowels correctly;
- ❏ Consistently uses initial consonants (although some are misarticulated);
- ❏ Frequently omits medial consonants;
- ❏ Frequently omits or substitutes final consonants;
- ❏ Uses approximately 27 phonemes;
- ❏ Uses auxiliary *is* including the contracted form;
- ❏ Uses some regular past tense verbs, possessive morphemes, pronouns, and imperatives.

Motor Skills

- ❏ Walks with characteristic toddling movements;
- ❏ Begins developing rhythm;
- ❏ Walks up and down stairs alone;

- ❏ Jumps off floor with both feet;
- ❏ Balances on one foot for one second;
- ❏ Walks on tip-toes;
- ❏ Turns pages one by one, or two to three at a time;
- ❏ Folds paper roughly in half on imitation;
- ❏ Builds a tower of 6 cubes;
- ❏ Scribbles;
- ❏ Uses a palmar grip with writing tools;
- ❏ Paints with whole arm movements;
- ❏ Steps and rotates body when throwing;
- ❏ Drinks from a full glass with one hand;
- ❏ Chews food;
- ❏ Undresses self.

3–4 Years

Speech and Language Skills

- ❏ Understands object functions;
- ❏ Understands differences in meanings (stop-go, in-on, big-little);
- ❏ Follows 2- and 3-part commands;
- ❏ Asks and answers simple questions (who, what, where, why);
- ❏ Frequently asks questions and often demands detail in responses;
- ❏ Produces simple verbal analogies;
- ❏ Uses language to express emotion;
- ❏ Uses 4 to 5 words in sentences;
- ❏ Repeats 6- to 13-syllable sentences accurately;
- ❏ Identifies objects by name;
- ❏ Manipulates adults and peers;
- ❏ May continue to use echolalia;
- ❏ Uses up to 6 words in a sentence;
- ❏ Uses nouns and verbs most frequently;
- ❏ Is conscious of past and future;
- ❏ Has a 1,200–2,000 or more word receptive vocabulary;
- ❏ Has a 800–1,500 or more word expressive vocabulary;

Speech, Language, and Motor Development

- ❑ May repeat self often, exhibiting blocks, disturbed breathing, and facial grimaces during speech;
- ❑ Increases speech rate;
- ❑ Whispers;
- ❑ Masters 50% of consonants and blends;
- ❑ Speech is 80% intelligible;
- ❑ Sentence grammar improves, although some errors still persist;
- ❑ Appropriately uses *is*, *are*, and *am* in sentences;
- ❑ Tells two events in chronological order;
- ❑ Engages in long conversations;
- ❑ Uses some contractions, irregular plurals, future tense verbs, and conjunctions;
- ❑ Consistently uses regular plurals, possessives, and simple past tense verbs.

Motor Skills

- ❑ Kicks ball forward;
- ❑ Turns pages one at a time;
- ❑ Learns to use blunt scissors;
- ❑ Runs and plays active games with abandonment;
- ❑ Rises from squatting position;
- ❑ Balances and walks on toes;
- ❑ Unbuttons but cannot button;
- ❑ Holds crayon with thumb and fingers, not fist;
- ❑ Uses one hand consistently for most activities;
- ❑ Traces a square, copies a circle, and imitates horizontal strokes;
- ❑ Puts on own shoes, but not necessarily on the correct foot;
- ❑ Rides a tricycle;
- ❑ Builds a tower of 9 cubes;
- ❑ Alternates feet while walking up and down stairs;
- ❑ Jumps in place with both feet together;
- ❑ Uses a spoon without spilling;
- ❑ Opens doors by turning the handle.

Speech, Language, and Motor Development

4–5 Years

Speech and Language Skills

❑ Imitatively counts to 5;
❑ Understands concept of numbers up to 3;
❑ Continues understanding of spatial concepts;
❑ Recognizes 1 to 3 colors;
❑ Has a receptive vocabulary of 2,800 or more words
❑ Counts to 10 by rote;
❑ Listens to short, simple stories
❑ Answers questions about function;
❑ Uses grammatically correct sentences;
❑ Has an expressive vocabulary of 900–2,000 or more words;
❑ Uses sentences of 4 to 8 words;
❑ Answers complex 2-part questions;
❑ Asks for word definitions;
❑ Speaks at a rate of approximately 185 words per minute;
❑ Reduces total number of repetitions;
❑ Enjoys rhymes, rhythms, and nonsense syllables;
❑ Produces consonants with 90% accuracy;
❑ Significantly reduces number of persistent sound omissions and substitutions;
❑ Frequently omits medial consonants;
❑ Speech is usually intelligible to strangers;
❑ Talks about experiences at school, at friends' homes, and so forth;
❑ Accurately relays a long story;
❑ Pays attention to a story and answers simple questions about it;
❑ Uses some irregular plurals, possessive pronouns, future tense, reflexive pronouns, and comparative morphemes in sentences.

Motor Skills

❑ Runs around obstacles;
❑ Pushes, pulls, and steers wheeled toys;
❑ Jumps over 6-inch-high object and lands on both feet together;
❑ Throws ball with direction;

S

- ❑ Balances on one foot for 5 seconds;
- ❑ Pours from a pitcher;
- ❑ Spreads substances with a knife;
- ❑ Uses toilet independently;
- ❑ Skips to music;
- ❑ Hops on one foot;
- ❑ Walks on a line;
- ❑ Uses legs with good strength, ease, and facility;
- ❑ Grasps with thumb and medial finger;
- ❑ Releases objects with precision;
- ❑ Holds paper with hand when writing;
- ❑ Draws circles, crosses, and diamonds;
- ❑ Descends stairs without assistance;
- ❑ Carries a cup of water without spilling;
- ❑ Enjoys cutting and pasting.

5–6 Years

Speech and Language Skills

- ❑ Names 6 basic colors and 3 basic shapes;
- ❑ Follows instructions given to a group;
- ❑ Follows 3-part commands;
- ❑ Asks *how* questions;
- ❑ Answers verbally to *hi* and *how are you*?;
- ❑ Uses past tense and future tense appropriately;
- ❑ Uses conjunctions;
- ❑ Has a receptive vocabulary of approximately 13,000 words;
- ❑ Names opposites;
- ❑ Sequentially names days of the week;
- ❑ Counts to 30 by rote;
- ❑ Continues to drastically increase vocabulary;
- ❑ Reduces sentence length to 4 to 6 words;
- ❑ Reverses sounds occasionally;
- ❑ Exchanges information and asks questions;
- ❑ Uses sentences with details;
- ❑ Accurately relays a story;
- ❑ Sings entire songs and recites nursery rhymes;
- ❑ Communicates easily with adults and other children;

S

❏ Uses appropriate grammar in most cases.

Motor Skills

❏ Walks backward heel-to-toe;
❏ Does somersaults;
❏ Cuts on a line with scissors;
❏ Prints a few capital letters;
❏ Cuts food with a knife;
❏ Ties own shoes;
❏ Builds complex structures with blocks;
❏ Gracefully rollerskates, skips, jumps rope, and rides a bicycle;
❏ Competently uses miniature tools;
❏ Buttons clothes, washes face, and puts toys away;
❏ Reaches and grasps in one continuous movement;
❏ Catches a ball with hands;
❏ Makes precise marks with crayon, confining marks to a small area.

6–7 Years

Speech and Language Skills

❏ Names some letters, numbers, and currencies;
❏ Sequences numbers;
❏ Understands left and right;
❏ Uses increasingly more complex descriptions;
❏ Engages in conversations;
❏ Has a receptive vocabulary of approximately 20,000 words;
❏ Uses a sentence length of approximately 6 words;
❏ Understands most concepts of time;
❏ Recites the alphabet;
❏ Counts to 100 by rote;
❏ Uses most morphologic markers appropriately;
❏ Uses passive voice appropriately.

Motor Skills

❏ Enjoys strenuous activities like running, jumping, racing, gymnastics, playing chase, and tag games;
❏ Shows reduced interest in writing and drawing;
❏ Draws a recognizable *man*, *tree*, and *house*;

S

❑ Draws pictures that are not proportional;
❑ Uses adult-like writing, but it is slow and labored;
❑ Runs lightly on toes;
❑ Walks on a balance beam;
❑ Cuts out simple shapes;
❑ Colors within lines;
❑ Indicates well-established right- or left-handedness;
❑ Dresses self completely;
❑ Brushes teeth without assistance;
❑ Follows advanced rhythms.

From K. G. Shipley, & J. G. McAfee, *Assessment in speech-language pathology: A resource manual* (pp. 32-40). San Diego, CA: Singular Publishing Group. Copyright © 1992 Singular Publishing Group, Inc. Used by permission.

Sound Level Meter. An instrument to assess vocal loudness; important components include the microphone and a voltmeter; magnifies and converts the acoustic signals into electrical signals and displays sound pressure in decibels; the microphone is placed about 1 meter from the mouth; note that the loudness of voice measured on a sound level meter may not represent vocal loudness in natural settings.

Spasmodic Dysphonia. A hyperfunctional voice disorder of uncertain etiology; may be classified into *adductor and abductor spastic dysphonia*; the adductor type is more common and the abductor type somewhat controversial; characterized in most cases by severe overadduction of vocal folds and strained or choked-off voice quality; phonation may be impossible; in other cases, characterized by sudden abduction of folds and resulting aphonia; earlier, thought to be psychogenic; currently, most experts now favor a neurologic explanation although this, too, is debated; possibly of heterogeneous etiology as evidence of neurologic involvement may be present or absent across patients; affects mostly adults, typical onset in the late 30s; more common in females (about 57% of the cases); diagnosis assisted by neurologic examination though it may not rule out spastic dysphonia; prognosis with voice therapy has been discouraging; see <u>Voice Disorders</u> for assessment.

Specific Language Impairment (SLI). Language disorders in children who are otherwise normal although some may have subtle cognitive deficits; different language skills may be somewhat differentially affected; pragmatic skills may be better than syntactic and morphological skills; a diagnosis made on negative grounds (such other factors as mental retardation or neurologic deficits do not explain the disorder); some believe that SLI suggests limited language skills with no pathology; other experts believe that SLI is not truly specific to language and that there are significant cognitive deficits; the very presence of this diagnostic category debated; see <u>Language Disorders in Children</u> for assessment procedures; note some unique aspects of SLI in this section.

Etiology
- Unknown
- Possibly, higher familial incidence suggesting the importance of genetic factors
- Possibly, cognitive deficits in some, but not all children who exhibit SLI; whether they are serious enough to account for the language problems is debatable
  - attentional deficits
  - tendency toward hyperactivity
  - difficulty interpreting rapidly sequenced auditory or visual stimuli
  - disturbed symbolic play
  - impaired reasoning skills
  - impaired touch perception
  - deficient object classification skills

Language Characteristics
- Generally, the same characteristics as described under <u>Language Disorders in Children</u>
- Possibly, uneven language profile in children with SLI (similar to language profiles of children with Down syndrome)

- Generally better pragmatic skills than syntactic and morphologic skills
- Deficient prelinguistic behaviors in toddlers who later exhibit SLI (greater use of gestures, difficulty in exhibiting mutual attention involving an adult, and less complex babbling)

Assessment Objectives/General Guidelines

- Generally, the same as those described under Language Disorders in Children

Case History/Interview Focus

- Generally, the same as those described under Language Disorders in Children

Ethnocultural Considerations

- Ethnocultural Considerations in Assessment

Assessment

- Assess semantic skills
- Assess morphologic skills
- Assess syntactic skills
- Assess pragmatic skills
- Use procedures described under Language Disorders in Children

Standardized Tests

- Use selected standardized tests of language described under Language Disorders in Children

Related/Medical Assessment Data

- Obtain psychological reports on cognitive functioning, behavioral deficits including attentional problems
- Obtain any medical evaluation reports that are relevant to communication assessment

Educational Assessment Data

- Obtain any educational assessment data that help evaluate the educational demands made on the child

Standard/Common Assessment Procedures

- Complete the Standard/Common Assessment Procedures

Spondylitis

Diagnostic Criteria
- Significant language problems in the absence of sensory deficits, neurological impairment, and psychiatric disorders that could account for the problems

Differential Diagnosis
- Differentiate from children who have language disorders along with mental retardation, hearing impairment, neurological disorders, and autism; see <u>Language Disorders in Children</u> for details

Prognosis
- Most children improve with systematic treatment although the possibility of persistent deficits exists

Recommendations
- Language treatment to be initiated as early as possible
- Parent training in language stimulation at home, especially in the case of infants and toddlers
- Integration of language treatment with academic activities in school-age children
- Behavioral or psychological treatment in the case of children who have significant problems besides language problems
- See *PGTSLP* for details

Spondylitis. Inflammation of one or more of the vertebrae; see <u>Refsum Syndrome.</u>

Standard/Common Assessment Procedures

Assessment techniques used across disorders of communication; include case history, hearing screening, interview, orofacial examination, and speech and language sampling.

Case History. Detailed information on the client, the communication disorder, the family, health, education, occupation, and related matters that helps understand the client and his or her disorder; a common assessment procedure across disorders; relative emphasis on different aspects depends on the nature of the disorder and the age of the client; information collected through a printed case history form and interview of the client, the family members, or both; obtain information on the following; select the relevant items depending on the age of the client:

- Identifying information: Obtain the client's names, date of birth, address, telephone, parents' name, ages, education and occupation; names, address, and telephone number of the referring professional or person and of the client's physician; any other information the particular clinical or educational setting requires
- Whether on a printed form or during interview, ask such questions as the following, note that some of the questions are alternative ways of getting the same information; modify the wording to suit the age and education of the client, the parents, or both; skip questions that are not relevant for a particular client
- The client's or parents' description of the disorder
  - What do you think is your (your child's) communication problem?
- How would you describe your (your child's) speech problem (voice problem, language problem)?
  - onset and development of the disorder
  - when did the problem (voice problem, stuttering, language difficulties) begin; or, when did you first notice the problem?
  - what were the early signs of the problem? Can you describe them? Can you imitate them?
  - what were the circumstances under which you first noticed the problem? Were there any special circumstances surrounding the onset of the problem? Did anything special happen around the time the problem was first noticed? What do you think is the cause of the disorder?
  - how did the problem progress? Did the problem (the stuttering, hoarseness, memory problems, language production) change over time? How did it change? Did it become progressively worse? Did it fluctuate? How did

it fluctuate over time? Did you see any pattern in its change? What kind of pattern?

- Prior assessment and treatment of the disorder
  - did you see any specialists? Who did you see? Could you supply the name and the telephone number of the professional you saw? Could we contact the professional to get reports?
  - what did the professional recommend? Did you follow-up on the recommendation?
  - did you (the child) receive treatment? What kind of treatment? Can you describe what you did in a session? What were you asked to do? What were the results? Did the problem (stuttering, articulation problem, language difficulties, hoarseness) improve? How much did it improve? Did the improvement last? For how long? Why do you think the improvement did not last? Did the problem return suddenly or gradually?
- Family constellation and communication
  - how many brothers and sisters do you (does the child) have?
  - what language (or languages) do you speak at home? What is your (your child's) primary language? Second language? Do you (does the child) speak, read, and write the second language well? How well?
  - is there any family history of communication problems? What kinds of problems? Who has them? For how long? Has it improved? Was it treated? If so, with what results? What is the current status of the problem in the relative?
  - how does the child communicate with other members of the family? Words and phrases? Sentences? Gestures?
  - how does the child communicate with peers? How does the child play with others? How do they get along with each other?
- Prenatal and birth history (mostly in case of children)

Standard/Common Assessment Procedures

- what was the mother's health during pregnancy? Any major illnesses? Accidents? Medications? Any evidence of maternal substance abuse during pregnancy?
- full term or premature? Any birth complications? What type of delivery (head first, feet first, breech, Cesarean)?
- what was the birth weight of the child?
- Medical history
  - did the child (did you) have any illness during the early childhood years? What kinds of illnesses?
  - what kinds of medical and surgical treatment did you (or your child) have?
  - are you (is your child) on any medications? What kinds? Any negative side effects?
- Developmental history
  - when did the child crawl, sit, stand, walk, feed self, and dress self? Were there any feeding problems? How would you describe the child's physical development? If not normal, what were the problems?
  - did you notice any signs of hearing loss? What kinds of problems or signs did you notice?
  - how would you describe your child's speech and language development? When did the child babble? Say first words? Use phrases? Produce sentences? Were you or were you not concerned about speech and language development? Why were you concerned?
- Educational history
  - what grade is the child is in? How has the child done academically? Did the child receive special educational services? What kinds of services? How did the child do? Did he or she benefit from the program? How did the child's communication problem affect his or her academic performance? What were the reactions of teachers?
  - what level of education have you completed? How was your academic performance? How did your communication problem affect your academic performance?
- Occupational history

- what is your current occupation? What do you do on your job? How does your communication problem affect your job performance?
- what is your relationship with your colleagues? With your supervisors? How do they react to your communication problem? Are you concerned about their reactions?
- do you think you cannot get a job because of your communication problem? Why do you think so?
- what is your occupational goal in seeking treatment now?

Hearing Screening. Quick procedures to determine whether a person needs to be evaluated by an audiologist or can be assumed to have normal hearing.

- Screen the hearing of all clients you assess
- Use a screening procedure adopted at your clinical site as the procedures vary
- Generally, screen hearing at 20 or 25 dB HL for 500, 1000, 2000, and 4000 Hz; for 500 Hz, screen at 25 dB HL
- Screen younger children at 15 dB HL for 500, 1000, 2000, and 4000, and 8000 Hz
- Make sure the ambient noise in the screening situation is acceptable
- Refer the client who fails your screening test to an audiologist for a complete hearing evaluation

Interview. A face-to-face contact with the client, the parents, or both to obtain additional information, to get information given on the printed case history form clarified or expanded, to get familiarized with the client and family, and to make initial observations of the client and the family.

- Note that the same questions specified under **Case History** may be asked during the interview; however, information deemed satisfactory on the case history form may not be reexamined during the interview
- Before starting the interview, study the filled-out case history form; note areas that need to be addressed during the interview

- Note the client's ethnocultural background; if necessary, review information on the particular ethnocultural characteristics of interaction, language use, expected level of ease with which information can be gathered, special precautions to be taken, and so forth; see <u>Ethnocultural Considerations in Assessment</u>

- Go over the case history form and ask questions about unclear information or information that needs to be expanded

- Listen well, offer comments to suggest that you understand and appreciate what the clients or family members say; do not give specific advice at this time; do not criticize or contradict; record their responses verbatim when appropriate (e.g., description of the disorder, prior treatment procedure, comments of colleagues or teachers, statements regarding causes and effects of the disorder)

Orofacial Examination. An examination of the oral and facial structures to evaluate their structural and functional integrity from the standpoint of speech production; helps identify or rule out obvious structural abnormalities that may require medical attention; an important standard/common assessment procedure; use the following format from Shipley and McAfee (1992) to complete the assessment:

Orofacial Examination Form

Name: _____ Age: _____ Date: _____

Examiner: _____

Instructions: Check and circle each item noted.

Include descriptive comments in the right-hand margin.

Evaluation of Face   **Comments**

__ symmetry: normal/droops on right/droops on left _____

__ abnormal movements: none/grimaces/spasms _____

__ mouth breathing: yes/no _____

__ other: _____

427

Standard/Common Assessment Procedures

Evaluation of Jaw and Teeth
Tell client to open and close mouth.

__ range of motion: normal/reduced

__ symmetry: normal/deviates to right/deviates to left

__ movement: normal/jerky/groping/slow/asymmetrical

__ TMJ noises: absent/grinding/popping

__ other:
Observe dentition:

__ occlusion (molar relationship): normal/neutroclusion
   (Class I)/distoclusion (Class II)/mesioclusion (Class III)

__ occlusion (incisor relationship): normal/overbite/ un-
   derbite/crossbite

__ teeth: all present/dentures/teeth missing (specify) ____

__ arrangement of teeth: normal/jumbled/spaces/mis-
   aligned _____

__ hygiene: _____

__ other: _____

Evaluation of Lips
Tell client to pucker.

__ range of motion: normal/reduced _____

__ symmetry: normal/droops bilaterally/droops

__ right/droops left _____

__ strength (press tongue blade against lips):

__ normal/weak _____

__ other: _____
Tell client to smile.

__ range of motion: normal/reduced

__ symmetry: normal/droops bilaterally/droops

__ right/droops left _____

__ other: _____
Tell client to puff cheeks and hold air.

__ lip strength: normal/reduced _____

__ nasal emission: absent/present other: _____

__ other: _____

Evaluation of Tongue

__ surface color: normal/abnormal (specify) _____

__ abnormal movements: absent/jerky/spasms/writhing/

  fasciculations _____

__ size: normal/small/large _____

__ frenum: normal/short _____

__ other: _____
Tell client to protrude the tongue.

__ excursion: normal/deviates to right/deviates to left ____

__ range of motion: normal/reduced _____

__ speed of motion: normal/reduced _____

__ strength (apply opposing pressure with tongue blade):

  normal/reduced _____
Tell client to retract tongue.

__ excursion: normal/deviates to right/deviates to left ____

__ range of motion: normal/reduced _____

__ speed of motion: normal/reduced other: _____
Tell client to move tongue tip to the right.

__ excursion: normal/incomplete/groping _____

__ range of motion: normal/reduced _____

___ strength (apply opposing pressure with tongue blade):

normal/reduced other: _____

Tell client to move the tongue tip to the left.

___ excursion: normal/incomplete/groping _____

___ range of motion: normal/reduced _____

___ strength (apply opposing pressure with tongue blade):

normal/reduced _____

Tell client to move the tongue tip up.

___ movement: normal/groping: _____

___ range of motion: normal/reduced other: _____

Tell client to move the tongue tip down.

___ movement: normal/groping: _____

___ range of motion: normal/reduced other: _____

Observe rapid side-to-side movements.

___ rate: normal/reduced/slows down progressively _____

___ range of motion: normal/reduced on left/reduced on

right _____

___ other: _____

Evaluation of Pharynx

___ color: normal/abnormal _____

___ tonsils: absent/normal/enlarged _____

___ other: _____

Evaluation of Hard and Soft Palates

___ color: normal/abnormal _____

___ rugae: absent/present _____

___ arch height: normal/high/low _____

___ arch width: normal/narrow/wide _____

__ growths: absent/present (describe) _____

__ fistula: absent/present (describe) _____

__ clefting: absent/present (describe) _____

__ symmetry at rest: normal/lower on right/lower on left

_____

__ gag reflex: norma/absent/hyperactive/hypoactive _____

__ other: _____

Tell client to phonate using /a/.

__ symmetry of movement: normal/deviates right/devi-
ates left _____

__ posterior movement: present/absent/reduced
__ lateral movement: present/absent/reduced _____

__ uvula: normal/bifid/deviates right/deviates left _____

__ nasality: absent/hypernasal _____

__ other: _____

Summary of Findings: _____

_____

_____

From K. G. Shipley & J. McAfee (1992). *Assessment in Speech-Language Pathology: A resource manual* (pp. 87–90). San Diego, CA: Singular Publishing Group. Copyright © 1992 Singular Publishing Group, Inc. Used by permission.

Speech and Language Sample. Primary means of assessing speech and language production; an audio-recorded sample of speech and language from a child or an adult; more naturalistic than the results of standardized tests; contrived or manipulated to varying extents to evoke specific constructions; ideally, conversational speech between a client and his or her caregiver on the one hand and the client and the clinician on the other; often involves stimuli designed to evoke conversational speech; when the concern is speech production, may be described as a speech sample, and when the concern is language, may be described as a language sample; in either case, the goal is to obtain a representative sample of a person's speech and language functions; because connected speech is important for phonological analysis, a language sample may be just as important for assessing articulation and phonological disorders; many basic procedures of evoking speech and language are the same; however, the primary concern is on language structures in the case of clients with language disorders and speech sound production in single words and connected speech in the case of clients with articulation and phonological disorders; see Language Disorders in Children for procedures that focus on language structures and Articulation and Phonological Disorders for procedures that focus on connected speech production; physical stimuli, questions, and topics of conversation need to be modified to suit the age and the ethnocultural background of the client.

- Tape record the entire speech and language sample
- Record in stereo for a more dynamic range
- Obtain 50 to 100 utterances; expect to spend about 30 minutes
- Observe carefully and take notes on the context of utterances that may not be clear from the audiotaped sample
- Use a quiet room and avoid noisy stimulus materials
- Carefully select stimuli that are appropriate for the client's age, education, occupation, and ethnocultural background
- In the case of adults, use pictures and objects only when necessary; in most cases, engage them in conversation
  - use pictures and objects in the case of adults with neurogenic communication disorders
  - use natural conversation in the case of adults with stuttering and voice disorders
  - judge the necessity of physical stimulus materials in the case of adult clients who are mentally retarded;

select stimuli carefully to match the adult client's level of functioning

- In the case of children, use a variety of stimulus materials to evoke and sustain conversation
  - have the parents bring a few of the child's favorite toys
  - in the case of younger children, use toys, objects, pictures, pretend situations, role playing, storytelling and story retelling, and such other devices to evoke speech and language structure
  - engage the older child in conversational speech; use appropriate stimulus materials as found necessary
  - in the case of most children, first have the mother, father, or any accompanying family member and the child interact with each other; let them interact in their usual manner; supply soft toys and toys that can be assembled and disassembled; supply picture books the child prefers; consider the child's interests and ethno-cultural background in selecting stimulus materials; observe from the one-way mirror and take notes
  - next, engage the child in communicative interaction using the same stimulus materials the family member used; if necessary, add new stimulus materials
  - use a bag or box that conceals materials to induce curiosity and questioning; pull something out of the container to surprise the child and thus to sustain the child's interest in talking
- Do not talk all the time, but do talk enough to make it a natural conversation between you and the client
- Listen carefully
- Do not make it a session of interrogation
- Let the client initiate conversation; tolerate some periods of silence to encourage speech initiation
- Repeat what you think the child just said when the child's speech is not clear
- Let the client initiate new topics; give hints of new topics (e.g., "what about this?" or "you want to talk about _____?")

S

- Let the client continue to talk on a topic; do not interrupt the client
- Do not ask yes/no questions; ask open-ended questions
- Ask questions that evoke single-word responses when it is important (e.g., "what is this?" or "what color is this?"); ask questions that evoke phrases and sentences when this is needed (e.g., "what did you do last weekend?" or "tell me about your friends")
- Use both simple and complex sentences to see the effects on the client's speech, especially in the case of children
- Encourage conversation after picture description as the former tends to evoke more complex language from children
- Evoke single-word productions to assess vocabulary and speech sound productions;
- Evoke conversation with a variety of strategies
- Evoke specific language structures of interest by designing task-specific procedures; see Language Disorders in Children
- Have the child tell a story by looking at picture cards; see Articulation and Phonological Disorders for procedures
- Ask the child to narrate a story
- Tell a story and ask the child to retell it
- Role play activities (cooking, shopping, planning a picnic)
- See Language Disorders in Children and Articulation and Phonological Disorders for all procedural details
- Obtain a home sample; ask the parents to observe your interaction with the child and have them repeat at home
- Repeat language sampling before beginning treatment
- Supplement language sampling with standardized tests if preferred
- Supplement language sampling with base rates established before treatment
- Transcribe the entire sample for analysis; identify the speakers involved (e.g., C for the clinician, M for the mother, CL for the client)
- Mark utterance endings with a slash (/)
- Number all utterances and obtain a total count

- Make further analysis as dictated by the purpose of speech and language sampling; see <u>Language Disorders in Children</u> and <u>Articulation and Phonological Disorders</u> for all procedural details
- Use a computerized method of transcript analysis if preferred

Strabismus.   A visual disorder in which the two eyes do not focus together; one eye deviates from the other either inwardly (convergent strabismus) or outwardly (divergent strabismus).

Stridency.   A voice disorder characterized by an unpleasant, shrill, and metallic-sounding voice; caused by excessive pharyngeal constriction and an elevated larynx.

Stroboscopy.   An instrument that helps assess structures in motion and hence used to assess vibratory patterns of vocal folds; used in combination with an endoscope or laryngeal mirror; involves flashing light at varying frequencies into the larynx; when the light flash rates are the same as the frequency of vocal fold vibration, the vibrating folds are seen as static structures (an optical illusion); the laryngeal image is a composite of samples of different cycles; when the light is flashed at frequencies that differ from the fold vibratory cycles, the motions appear to slow down; used in assessing various structural and functional aspects of vocal folds including fundamental frequency, the health of the folds, different phases of vibration, the degree of contact between the two folds, and symmetry of movement of the two folds.

Stuttering.   A speech problem generally regarded as a disorder of fluency and rhythm; a disorder with no universally agreed-on definition; a disorder of primarily early childhood onset; generally, clinicians have little or no difficulty diagnosing stuttering, especially in adults, but have difficulty measuring it reliably; definitions vary; some definitions are descriptions of observable behaviors, whereas others are descriptions of covert processes, and still others are descriptions of presumed etiological factors with very little reference to symptoms or behaviors; dysfluencies play some role in most if not all definitions or their descriptive expansions; some definitions include only certain kinds of dysfluencies (e.g., part-word repetitions and speech sound prolongations); other definitions include all kinds of dysfluencies; still other definitions mention moments or events of stuttering with no description of observable behaviors; some definitions do not specify a quantitative criterion for dysfluencies for a diagnosis of stuttering; other definitions specify a quantitative criterion (e.g., a 5% or a 10% dysfluency rate); many clinicians diagnose stuttering based on excessive amounts of dysfluencies, excessive durations of dysfluencies, unusually fast tempo of dysfluencies, and unusual amount of muscular effort associated with dysfluencies and the act of speaking; may be associated with avoidance of certain words and speaking situations, experience of negative emotions and expression of negative verbalizations about him- or herself and about listeners; the final diagnosis based on multiple factors including the types, amounts, and the characteristics of dysfluencies, avoidance and negative emotions, and struggle and tension associated with dysfluent speech production; more common in males than in females; prevalence rate about 1% in the general population; the lifetime incidence (persons who have stuttered at least once and for some time) is higher (between 5 and 10%); the earliest age of reported onset is about 18 months; new cases replace spontaneously recovered cases throughout childhood; incidence rate declines as children grow older; may coexist with another fluency disorder, Cluttering.

Etiology

The causes of stuttering are not clearly understood; studies of persons who stutter and differential prevalence rates in specific subpopulations have suggested various factors as have variations in stuttering within and across individuals; in general, etiology remains somewhat speculative and theoretical.

Stuttering

- Genetic factors, or more likely, genetic predisposition; suggested by:
  - higher familial incidence of stuttering
  - greater concordance rate in monozygotic (identical) twins than in ordinary siblings
  - interaction between gender and familial incidence (highest familial incidence with a female stutterer in the family)
- Neurophysiologic factors; suggested by:
  - subtle abnormality in the electrical activity of the brain in some individuals (who stutter)
  - atypical cerebral language processing in some individuals
  - subtle and variable problems in neuromotor control of speech musculature (including the laryngeal mechanism) in some individuals
  - subtle central auditory processing problems in some individuals
  - elevated autonomic nervous system activity in some individuals
- Environmental contingencies; suggested by:
  - higher concordance rate in dizygotic (fraternal) twins than in ordinary siblings
  - demonstrated stimulus control of stuttering (e.g., variations in stuttering frequency related to audience size, punishment effect, adjacency effect, consistency effect, adaptation effect, chorus reading, shadowing, discriminative stimuli associated with prior increase or decrease in stuttering, among others)
- Multiple factors; suggested by:
  - lack of a single, convincing etiologic factor
  - studies that clearly show the influence of genetic, neurophysiologic, and environmental factors on the prevalence of stuttering and on the frequency of stuttering in individual clients

Description of Stuttering
- Dysfluencies: Most clinicians describe some or all forms of dysfluencies as a part of their description of stuttering; forms include:

S

Stuttering

- Repetitions
  - → sound/syllable repetitions or part-word repetitions ("t-t-t- time"; "sa-sa-saturday"; "abou-abou-about")
  - → word repetitions: monosyllabic or multisyllabic (I-I-I will go with you"; "his cousin-cousin came today")
  - → phrase repetitions ("how is-how is-how is it done?")
- Prolongations
  - → sound prolongations ("Ssssssoup, please"; "Mmm-mommy")
  - → silent prolongations or articulatory postures without voicing (a silent period with a tensed articulatory posture for the initial sound in saying a word such as "Bob")
- Broken words
  - → silent intervals within words ("g-(silent pause)-oing")
- Interjections
  - → sound/syllable interjections ("he was um going to do it")
  - → word interjections ("I can well do it")
  - → phrase interjections ("It is you know-you know well done")
- Pauses
  - → excessively long silent intervals at inappropriate loci in speech ("I was [long pause] going to tell you")
- Revisions
  - → productions that retain the same idea but with word changes ("I will take a cab—bus")
- Incomplete phrases
  - → productions that suggest that the speaker dropped the idea he or she was going to express ("I was going to—but let me just say this")
- Associated motor (nonverbal) behaviors (mostly associated with dysfluencies or stutterings)
  - rapid and tensed eye blink
  - tensed and prolonged shutting of the eyelids

- rapid upward, downward, or lateral movement of the eyes
- knitting of the eyebrows
- nose wrinkling
- nose flaring
- pursing or quivering of the lips
- tongue clicking and other noises
- teeth clenching, grinding, and clicking
- tension in facial muscles
- wrinkling of the forehead
- clenched jaw or jerky or slow or tensed movement of the jaws
- jaw openings or closings that are unrelated to target speech production
- tension in chest, shoulder, and neck muscles; including twitching and extraneous movements
- head movements including turns, shakes, jerks, and lateral, upward, and downward movements
- tensed and jerky hand movements including fist clenching and hand wringing
- tensed and jerky arm movements including banging on the thighs or pressing against the sides of the abdomen
- tensed and jerky leg movements including kicking
- tensed and jerky foot movements including grinding, pressing, rubbing, or circular movements on the floor
- generally tensed body postures
- Avoidance
  - avoidance of speaking situations (e.g., speaking on the telephone, ordering in restaurants, buying at a counter, speaking to a group)
  - avoidance of certain conversation partners (e.g., strangers, authority figures, persons of the opposite gender)
  - avoidance of certain words (because of sound-specific difficulties) as indicated by word substitutions and circumlocutions
  - avoiding talking as much as possible (reduced verbal output)

S

- depending on others to communicate (e.g., having a spouse or a friend order at restaurants)
- Negative emotional reactions
  - verbally expressed feelings of tension or anxiety associated with speaking
  - verbally expressed feelings of frustration due to difficulty in expressing oneself
  - verbally expressed feeling (or a sense) of loss of control over the speech mechanism or over fluent production
  - verbally expressed feelings of helplessness
  - negative verbal expressions about oneself
  - negative verbal expressions about certain listeners
  - description of lack of self-confidence in speaking situations
  - anxious or dreaded expectation of stuttering on certain words and in certain speaking situations (expectancy)
- Breathing abnormalities
  - attempts at speaking on limited or shallow inhalation
  - attempts at speaking during exhalation
  - running out of air at the end of phrases and sentences
  - apparent efforts to squeeze the air out of lungs to continue talking
  - inhalations and exhalations interrupting each other
  - impounding of inhaled air with a sudden closure of the glottis and apparent attempts to speak while the air is impounded
  - dysrhythmic respiration
  - audible inhalation, exhalation, or both
  - difficulty in maintaining an even airflow throughout an utterance

Assessment Objectives/General Guidelines
- To assess the types and frequency of dysfluencies or stutterings in conversational speech and oral reading
- To assess associated motor behaviors
- To assess variability in stuttering across speaking situations
- To assess avoidance and negative emotional reactions

- To use the assessment data to make a diagnosis of stuttering
- To suggest treatment options

Case History/Interview Focus

- See **Case History** and **Interview** under <u>Standard/Common Assessment Procedures</u>
- Concentrate on the onset and course of stuttering; the client's avoidance and emotional reactions

Ethnocultural Considerations

- See <u>Ethnocultural Considerations in Assessment</u>

Assessment

- Assess frequency and types of dysfluencies or stutterings
  - conversational speech with the clinician
    - → take an extended conversational speech sample
    - → in the case of young children, have toys, books, objects, and other materials to evoke speech; see Speech and Language Sample under <u>Standard/Common Assessment Procedures</u>
    - → in the case of adults, use the interview for this purpose as well
    - → tape record the speech sample for later analysis of dysfluencies or stutterings
    - → take note of associated motor behaviors
    - → if you are trained or you want to train yourself to do it reliably, count dysfluencies as you interview the client; until the reliability of your measures are established, consider repeated counting of dysfluencies on the tape as the more reliable measure (see Analysis of Assessment Data for additional suggestions)
  - conversational speech with a family member
    - → ask the accompanying family member to engage the client in conversation
    - → in the case of children, let the parent or other family member use toys, pictures, objects, and story books to stimulate and maintain conversation for about 10 minutes

→ audiotape the conversation for later analysis of dysfluencies
- oral reading sample
    → select a printed passage that is appropriate for the client's age, education, cultural background, and general interest
    → have the client read it aloud in his or her usual manner
    → tape record the oral reading for later analysis of dysfluencies or stutterings
    → count the number and types of dysfluencies as the client reads if you are trained to do that reliably or you wish to train yourself to do that reliably
    → if you wish to count dysfluencies during the session, have a copy of the printed passage in front of you and mark dysfluencies on the page itself; until the reliability of your measures are established, consider counting of dysfluencies from repeated listening of the tape as the more reliable measure
- Assess speech, language, and voice
    - Use the conversational speech for making clinical judgments about speech, language, and voice
        → note errors of articulation
        → note the client's use of language including grammatic, syntactic, and pragmatic structures; note limitations or deviations
        → note voice quality, intensity, loudness, and resonance characteristics
        → make a detailed assessment of articulation and phonological disorders, language disorders, and voice disorders if clinical judgment indicates a need
- Assess associated motor behaviors
    - note that, for most clinical purposes, it is sufficient to describe associated motor behaviors and make judgments about their general frequency levels (e.g., frequent nose wrinkling, an occasional foot tapping); systematic counting may be necessary only for research purposes

S

→ take notes during the interview and oral reading on all the associated motor behaviors

→ give clear and specific descriptions of them

→ prepare a checklist of the behaviors listed previously and use it

- Assess avoidance behaviors
  - note that most avoidance behaviors are self-reported by the client
  - explore avoidance behaviors during interview
  - ask the client to make a list of sounds or words that are especially difficult
  - ask the client to make a hierarchy of most difficult (e.g., speaking to boss) to least difficult (speaking to a close friend) speaking situations
  - ask the client to expand and refine the difficult sounds/words list and the hierarchy of situations during the next few days and give them back to you on the next visit
  - note word substitutions, circumlocutions, and easy and fluent repetitions that are followed by severe dysfluencies (such repetitions may be attempts at avoiding or postponing ensuing dysfluencies)
  - ask the family members or friends who accompany the client to describe avoidance reactions they have observed
- Assess frequency and types of dysfluencies in nonclinical situations
  - at home
    → ask the client or a family member to audiotape three conversational samples over the following few days and submit them for evaluation
    → ask the family member to watch your method of recording the conversational speech sample
    → in the case of children, ask the parents to use your method of recording a speech sample
  - at school

- → obtain verbal report from teachers about the amount and types of dysfluencies the client exhibits in the classroom
- → have the teacher audiotape a brief conversational speech sample and submit for analysis
- → have the teacher audiotape the client's conversation with a peer and submit for analysis
- → have the teacher audiotape a reading sample and submit for analysis
- at work
  - → if practical, have the client audiotape a sample of conversation with a colleague
  - → note that such assignments often are more readily completed when treatment is started, a good working relationship is established, and you have convinced the client about their necessity and importance
- Assess the overall rate of speech
  - use the speech sample to assess the rate
  - take at least three 2-minute samples from the total speech sample; select one sample from the beginning, one from the middle, and one more from the final portion of the interview
  - with a digital stopwatch, calculate the number of words/syllables spoken per minute
  - discount pauses
- Assess the articulatory rate
  - use the three 2-minute samples selected from the larger sample
  - discount all dysfluencies or stuttering including pauses that exceed 2 seconds
  - count the number of syllables produced per minute to obtain the articulatory rate
- Assess variability in stuttering and establish reliability of measures
  - obtain verbal reports from the client about variability in stuttering across different situations and over time

- obtain verbal reports from family members regarding variability in stuttering across time and situations
- compare the frequency of dysfluencies produced at home with the frequency obtained in the clinic
- if the clinic and the home samples are widely discrepant, repeat both; question the client, family members, or both to evaluate the representativeness of the amount of dysfluencies exhibited in all speech and reading samples
- Assess fluency characteristics
  - use the recorded speech sample for this assessment
  - determine the longest fluent utterance (measured in words or syllables)
  - determine the most frequently occurring fluent interval (measured in seconds or minutes)
  - determine the most frequently occurring fluent response (measured in words or syllables)
- Assess negative emotional reactions
  - during interview, explore the various negative emotional reactions listed earlier; ask the client to describe his or her feelings about speech, speaking situations, listeners, and him- or herself
  - administer *Brutten's Behavior Assessment Battery*, which includes *Speech Situation Checklist* and *Communication Attitude Test* to assess negative emotions and attitudes associated with stuttering
  - administer the S-Scale (the original by R. L. Erickson and the modified version by G. Andrews & J. Cutler)
  - ask the spouse, parents, or other family members about negative emotions the client typically expresses
- Assess breathing abnormalities
  - note all breathing abnormalities exhibited during the assessment session
  - note all the different kinds of dysfluencies with which specific breathing abnormalities may be associated
- Assess Adaptation Effect and Consistency Effect

S

- have the client read a printed passage aloud five times in succession (e.g., the Rainbow Passage for adults and Arthur the Young Rat for children)
- count the number of dysfluencies separately for each reading trial
- chart the frequency of dysfluencies across oral readings; note the degree of adaptation
- on a copy of the passage, mark the words stuttered during each of the five oral readings; note the words or loci on which stuttering was repeated twice, thrice, four times, and five times
- make a list of words and sounds on which stuttering was most consistent
- make a list of words and sounds on which stuttering was least consistent (i.e., stuttered only once; most adapted)
- use the data to identify words on which stuttering is most and least likely
- Assess stimulability (potential treatment probes)
  - ask the client to reduce the speech rate dramatically; model a slow rate with continuous phonation; note the effects on dysfluencies
  - ask the client to initiate sounds softly and gently; note the effects on dysfluencies
  - ask the client to inhale and exhale a small amount of air before starting to speak; model the behaviors; note the effects on dysfluencies
  - try such other treatment contingencies as time-out or response cost to evaluate their potential usefulness

Related/Medical Assessment Data

- Integrate any medical information of relevance with your assessment data; if there is evidence of neurologic involvement, investigate this further and re-examine the age of onset; consider the possibility of neurogenic stuttering (not stuttering of early childhood onset)
- Integrate educational and occupational information with your assessment data

- Integrate any information available on central auditory functioning with your assessment data

Standard/Common Assessment Procedures

- Complete the <u>Standard/Common Assessment Procedures</u>

Analysis of Assessment Data

- Analyze all speech and oral reading samples for the frequency and types of dysfluencies or stutterings
- List the types of dysfluencies and their frequencies separately for each sample
- Count the number of words in a speech or reading sample
- Calculate either the percent dysfluency rate or the number of dysfluencies per 100 words spoken or read (percent dysfluency rate = number of dysfluencies divided by the total number of words spoken or read and multiplied by 100)
- Measure durations of at least 15 longest dysfluencies and 15 shortest dysfluencies to give a range of durations
- Note that the following kinds of dysfluencies are especially difficult to measure and that you need to train yourself to measure them reliably:
  - pauses (tendency is to ignore them)
  - different types of dysfluencies that are clustered, combined, or produced in rapid succession
  - interjections (tendency is to ignore them)
  - word repetitions (tendency is to ignore them)
  - any dysfluency that is extremely brief, fleeting, and softly produced
  - silent prolongations on audiotapes (tendency is to not recognize them as silent prolongations and to consider them as insignificant pauses)
- Summarize the associated motor behaviors, avoidance behaviors, negative emotional reactions, and situational variability in stuttering
- If desired, rate the severity of stuttering; consider using the Stuttering Severity Instrument by G. Riley

Diagnostic Criteria

- Use one of several primary diagnostic criteria:

- an operationally defined excessive amount of dysfluencies when all types of dysfluencies are counted (e.g., 5% dysfluency rate)
- part-word repetitions, sound prolongations, and broken words at less than 5% of the words spoken because of lower social threshold of tolerance for these dysfluency types (perhaps only 3%)
- clinically judged excessive duration of dysfluencies when neither of the first two criteria is met
- Consider other assessment data in conjunction with the primary diagnostic criteria:
  - rapidity of dysfluencies
  - the number of repetition units in an instance of part-word and word repetitions
  - tension and effort associated with dysfluencies
  - associated motor behaviors
  - negative emotional experiences associated with speech and speaking situations
  - avoidance of speaking situations, certain conversational partners, and sounds and words

Differential Diagnosis
- Differentiate stuttering from normally fluent speech
  - use one of the diagnostic criteria specified above to diagnose stuttering
  - use associated features of stuttering to support a diagnosis of stuttering
- Differentiate stuttering from cluttering on the basis of:
  - overall symptom complex: stuttering being a fluency disorder and cluttering being more than a fluency disorder
  - rate of speech: excessively fast in cluttering, which is not a distinguishing feature of stuttering
  - indistinct articulation, possibly due to excessively fast rate of cluttering, which is not a distinguishing feature of stuttering
  - disorganized language in some individuals with cluttering, which is not a characteristic of stuttering
  - awareness of the problem; high in people who stutter and low in those who clutter

Stuttering

- speaking under stress: possibly better in people who clutter and worse in those who stutter
- speaking while relaxed: possibly worse in people who clutter and better in those who stutter
- giving short answers: possibly better in people who clutter and worse in those who stutter
- reading a well-known text: possibly worse in people who clutter and better in those who stutter
- reading an unknown text: possibly better in people who clutter and worse in those who stutter
- concern about speech: little or none in people who clutter and much, to the extent of being fearful, in people who stutter
- motivation for therapy: generally poor in people who clutter and generally good in people who stutter
- Differentiate stuttering of childhood onset (SCO) from neurogenic stuttering (NG) on the basis of:
  - age of onset: stuttering during early childhood and neurogenic stuttering in later years, often in older people
  - neurologic symptoms: prominent in NG and absent or extremely subtle in SCO
  - repetitions of medial and final syllables in words: rarely if ever in SCO but may be observed in NG
  - dysfluent production of function words: less common in older children and adults with SCO and may be more common in NG
  - etiology: largely unknown and no specific cause detected in most cases with SCO but the presence of such neurologic-medical conditions as stroke, tumors, traumatic brain injury, parkinsonism, dialysis dementia in NG
  - adaptation effect: may be absent or less pronounced in NG than in SCO
  - problems in copying and drawing: may be a distinguishing feature of NG, but not SCO
  - problems in copying block designs: may be a distinguishing feature of NG, but not SCO
  - problems in sequential hand positions: may be a distinguishing feature of NG, but not SCO

- problems in tapping out rhythms: may be a distinguishing feature of NG, but not SCO

Prognosis

- Prognosis for improved fluency is good with systematic treatment
- Maintenance of fluency is good with systematic follow up and periodic booster treatment
- Early intervention is especially effective

Recommendations

- Treatment for all clients and at all age levels when a diagnosis of stuttering is made
- See the cited sources and *PGTSLP* for details

Bloodstein, O. (1995). *A handbook on stuttering.* San Diego, CA: Singular Publishing Group.

Conture, E. G. (1990). *Stuttering* (2nd ed.). Englewood Cliffs, NJ: Prentice-Hall.

Culatta, R., & Goldberg, S. A. (1995). *Stuttering therapy: An integrated approach to theory and practice.* Needham Heights, MA: Allyn & Bacon.

Curlee, R. F., & Perkins, W. H. (Eds.). (1984). *Nature and treatment of stuttering: New directions.* San Diego, CA: College-Hill Press.

Peters, T. J., & Guitar, B. (1991). *Stuttering: An integrated approach to its nature and treatment.* Baltimore, MD: Williams & Wilkins.

Silverman, F. H. (1996). *Stuttering and other fluency disorders.* Needham Heights, MA: Allyn & Bacon.

Van Riper, C. (1982). *The nature of stuttering* (2nd ed.). Englewood Cliffs, NJ: Prentice-Hall.

Substitution Processes.   See <u>Phonological Processes</u>.

Supratentorial Level.   An anatomical division of brain that includes the externally visible frontal, temporal, and occipital lobes along with basal ganglia, thalamus, hypothalamus, and olfactory (I) and optic (II) cranial nerves.

Synchondroses.   The union of two bones by cartridge; a characteristics of some genetic syndromes.

Syndactyly.   Fusion of fingers or toes; a genetic defect; found in such syndromes as Apert syndrome and orofacial-digital syndrome (see <u>Syndromes Associated With Communicative Disorders</u>.

Syndrome.   A constellation of signs and symptoms that are associated with a morbid process.

Syndromes Associated With Communicative Disorders.   Syndromes that affect the normal acquisition of speech and language; varied etiology as specified under each syndrome; the following are among the more frequently described syndromes associated with communicative disorders; in assessing a client with a suspected syndrome:

- Use the <u>Common/Standard Assessment Procedures</u>; pay special attention to orofacial examination, and hearing screening and audiological assessment
- During the interview, concentrate on the family history and familial incidence of communicative disorders and related genetic syndromes
- Use assessment procedures described under <u>Language Disorders in Children</u> and <u>Articulation and Phonological Disorders</u>; administer selected tests described under these and other entries
- Use other procedures as found necessary (e.g., procedures described under <u>Stuttering</u>, <u>Voice Disorders</u>)
- Obtain medical records and work with the team serving the child
- Integrate your findings with those of other specialists
- Make periodic assessment to document positive or negative changes

Alport Syndrome.   A genetic syndrome that affects kidney functions and causes hearing loss and speech and language problems; more severe and more rapidly progressing symptoms in males.

Etiology
- Autosomal dominant inheritance in most cases

- X-linked inheritance in some cases.

Physical Symptoms
- Nephritis (kidney disease) begins early in childhood
- Kidney failure in some cases, requiring kidney transplantation

Speech, Language, and Hearing
- Articulation disorders; progressive deterioration in articulatory skills, especially in males
- Bilateral, sensorineural, progressive hearing loss starts around age 10; more commonly in males

Diagnostic Criteria
- A constellation of listed symptoms
- Consider variations in syndrome manifestations

Prognosis
- Generally poor for males, better for females
- A probable 50% transmission rate from the affected person

Recommendations
- Early communication treatment with aural rehabilitation for males
- Somewhat later communication treatment and aural rehabilitation for females, as indicated by periodic reassessment

Apert Syndrome. A genetic syndrome whose dysmorphology includes cranial Synostosis, Syndactyly of hands and feet, midfacial Hypoplasia, Strabismus, hearing loss, and speech problems.

Etiology
- Possibly, spontaneous autosomal dominant mutations
- Limited parent-to-child transmission because of low reproductive capacity

Physical Symptoms
- Syndactyly; typically, second, third, and fourth digits may be fused
- Cranial synostosis resulting in smaller anterior-posterior skull diameter, flat frontal and occipital bones, and high forehead

- Increased intracranial pressure and compensatory growth in cranial structures
- Midfacial hypoplasia (incomplete development) with a small nose
- Arched and grooved hard palate
- Conductive hearing loss in some individuals
- Class III malocclusion
- Irregularly placed teeth
- Thickened alveolar process
- Long or thickened soft palate
- Cleft of the hard palate in 25 to 30% of the cases

Speech, Language, and Hearing
- Tendency toward hyponasality
- Forward carriage of the tongue
- Articulation disorders involving mostly alveolar consonants (e.g., /s/ and /z/) and labial dental sounds (e.g., /f/ and /v/)
- Language skills dependent on intellectual and hearing levels
- High incidence of conductive hearing loss

Diagnostic Criteria
- Constellation of listed symptoms; consider variations in syndrome manifestations

Prognosis
- Better with early surgical intervention for cranial, facial, and oral abnormalities than with delayed intervention
- A probable 50% transmission rate from the affected person

Recommendations
- Early surgical intervention to facilitate communication treatment
- Communication treatment with an emphasis on articulation training
- Aural rehabilitation as found necessary

Bronchio-Oto-Renal Syndrome. A genetic syndrome characterized by malformations of the auricle, bronchial fistulas or cysts, and abnormalities of the kidneys; associated with hearing loss and resulting speech language problems.

Etiology
- Autosomal dominant syndrome
- Varied expression in individuals

Physical Symptoms
- Bronchial fistulas or cysts
- Hypoplasia of kidneys, anomalies of the collecting system, or both
- Outer ear anomalies including preauricular pits
- Narrow or malformed external auditory canal
- Displaced or malformed auditory ossicles
- Fused or unconnected stapes
- Hypoplastic apex of the cochlea

Speech, Language, and Hearing
- Conductive, sensorineural, or mixed hearing loss
- Articulation disorders associated with hearing loss
- Possible language delay depending on the age of onset of hearing loss
- A high incidence of hearing loss in children of individuals with this syndrome

Diagnostic Criteria
- A constellation of listed symptoms; consider variations in syndrome manifestations

Prognosis
- Varies with the severity and complexity of symptom expression
- More favorable in cases of late onset of hearing loss and mild kidney problems
- More favorable with early initiation of aural rehabilitation

Recommendations
- Early communication treatment with aural rehabilitation for males
- Somewhat later communication treatment and aural rehabilitation for females, as indicated by periodic reassessment

Cornelia de Lange Syndrome. A congenital syndrome characterized by microcephaly, mental retardation, and severe speech and language problems; also known as de Lange Syndrome and Brachman-de Lange Syndrome.

Etiology
- Not well understood, possibly heterogeneous
- Thought to occur sporadically
- Possibly, autosomal dominant inheritance in some cases
- Chromosomal abnormalities in a few cases

Physical Symptoms
- Retarded physical growth
- Brachycephaly
- Low-set ears
- Bushy eyebrows that meet at the midline
- Coarse, shaggy, and excessive hair growing low in the forehead and neck
- Webbed neck
- Small nose, upward-tilted nares
- Down turned upper lip
- Flat hands with short, tapering fingers

Speech, Language, and Hearing
- Possible sensorineural hearing loss
- Hoarse voice
- Severe articulation disorders
- Severe language disorders associated with mental retardation

Diagnostic Criteria
- A constellation of listed symptoms; consider variations in syndrome manifestations

Prognosis
- Varies with the degree of mental retardation; often poor because of generally severe mental retardation

Recommendations
- Early speech-language treatment

Cri du Chat Syndrome. An autosomal chromosome disorder that tends to be associated with mental retardation and speech-language problems; the infant's cry may resemble that of a cat (hence the name).

Etiology
• Absence of the short arm of the fifth chromosome (known as 5p)

Physical Symptoms
• Low-set ears
• Narrow oral cavity
• Laryngeal hypoplasia

Speech, Language, and Hearing
• Articulation disorders
• Language disorders associated with mental retardation

Diagnostic Criteria
• A constellation of listed symptoms; consider variations in syndrome manifestations

Prognosis
• Varies with the severity and complexity of symptom expression
• More favorable in cases of less severe mental retardation

Recommendations
• Early communication treatment

Crouzon Syndrome. A genetic syndrome characterized by cranial and midface abnormalities, ocular hypertelorism, strabismus, hearing loss, and speech-language problems.

Etiology
• Autosomal dominant syndrome
• Varied expression in individuals

Physical Symptoms
• Craniosynostosis (fusion of the cranial suture, especially that of the coronal)
• Hypoplasia of the midface, maxilla, or both; small maxillary structure
• Sphenoethmoidal Synchondroses
• Ocular hypertelorism (eyes that are far apart)
• "Parrot-like" nose

- Facial asymmetry and tall forehead
- Malocclusion Class III in some cases
- Highly arched palate
- Shallow oropharynx
- Long and thick soft palate
- Brachycephaly (short cranial diameter from front to back)

Speech, Language, and Hearing

- Conductive hearing loss in one third to one half of individuals with the syndrome, possibly due to abnormalities of the ear
- Articulation disorders associated with hearing loss and abnormalities of palatal oral cavity structures
- Hyponasality
- Possible language disorders depending on hearing loss and cognitive deficits

Diagnostic Criteria

- A constellation of listed symptoms; consider variations in syndrome manifestations

Prognosis

- Varies with the severity and complexity of symptom expression
- More favorable in cases of early orofacial surgery and early intervention for communication deficits

Recommendations

- Early communication treatment with aural rehabilitation as needed

Down Syndrome. A genetic syndrome resulting from one of the common chromosomal abnormalities; associated with varying degrees of mental retardation and communication deficits.

Etiology

- Extra whole number chromosome 21, resulting in 47, rather than the normal 46 chromosomes
- Increased risk of Trisomy 21 with advanced maternal age
- Predisposition to Alzheimer's disease

Physical Symptoms
- Generalized hypotonia
- Flat facial profile
- Small ears
- Small nose
- Small chin
- Short front-to-back cephalic dimension (Brachycephaly)
- Midface Dysplasia
- Shortened oral and pharyngeal structures
- Narrow and high arched palate
- Relatively large, fissured tongue which tends to protrude
- Short neck with excess skin on back of it
- Hyperflexible joints
- Cardiac malformations in about 40% of cases
- Epicanthal folds
- Short fingers

Speech, Language, and Hearing
- Conductive hearing loss in many cases and sensorineural hearing loss in some cases
- Delayed language and language disorders; syntactic and morphologic features especially deficient; relatively better vocabulary
- Hypernasality and nasal emission
- Breathier voice
- Articulation disorders

Diagnostic Criteria
- A constellation of listed symptoms; chromosomal test for Trisomy 21; variations in syndrome manifestations to be considered

Prognosis
- Varies with the severity and complexity of symptom expression
- More favorable in cases of less severe mental retardation and early, comprehensive medical and educational intervention

Recommendations
- Early communication treatment

Ectrodactyly-Ectodermal Dysplasia-Clefting Syndrome (EEC Syndrome). A genetic syndrome that affects the development of ectodermal and mesodermal tissue; associated with clefts of the lip and palate; association of mental retardation is infrequent.

Etiology
- Autosomal dominant inheritance with variable and sometimes incomplete expression

Physical Symptoms
- Ectrodactyly
- Ectodermal Dysplasia including sparse hair and scanty eyebrows, absence of lashes, dystrophied nails, Hypodontia and Microdontia
- Cleft lip and palate (more common) or cleft lip only (less common)
- Absent sweat glands, predisposing the individual to heat stroke

Speech, Language, and Hearing
- Mild to moderate conductive loss in some cases
- Sensorineural hearing loss reported, but not well documented
- Speech and resonance problems if the repairs of the clefts are delayed
- Potential language problems associated with hearing loss
- Potential articulation disorders associated with hearing loss
- Potential compensatory articulatory strategies associated with cleft palate

Diagnostic Criteria
- A constellation of listed symptoms; ultrasonographic data if available; variations in syndrome manifestations to be considered

Prognosis
- Better with prompt surgical treatment for the clefts

- Prolonged medical and orthopedic treatment prospects

Recommendations

- Early communication treatment designed to rehabilitate a child with cleft palate and hearing loss, if present

Fetal Alcohol Syndrome. A congenital syndrome in which the prenatal and postnatal growth is affected because of maternal alcoholism during pregnancy; associated with physical abnormalities and mental retardation.

Etiology

- Embryonic exposure to 1 or 2 ounces of absolute alcohol per day for some effects
- Embryonic exposure of more than 2 ounces a day for more severe effects

Physical Symptoms

- Microcephaly
- Maxillary Hypoplasia
- Posterior rotation of the ears
- Prominent forehead and mandible
- Short palpebral (eyelid) fissures
- Thin upper lip
- Hypoplastic Philtrum
- Epicanthal Folds
- Microphthalmia
- Severe growth retardation
- Cleft palate
- Heart anomalies
- Small teeth with faulty enamel
- Kidney disorders

Speech, Language, and Hearing

- Hearing loss not characteristic of the syndrome
- Disorders of articulation
- Aggravated speech and resonance problems if clefts are present and their repairs are delayed
- Potential compensatory articulatory strategies associated with cleft palate

- Language disorders including deficits in syntactic, semantic, and pragmatic aspects of language
- Learning disabilities associated with language problems
- Limited fluency
- Voice problems

Diagnostic Criteria
- A constellation of listed symptoms
- History of maternal alcoholism or binge drinking
- Variations in syndrome manifestations to be considered

Prognosis
- Dependent on the degree of mental retardation, time of surgical treatment for the clefts, and time speech-language treatment is initiated

Recommendations
- Early communication treatment

Fragile X Syndrome. An X-linked genetic syndrome; caused by a chromosomal abnormality; associated with mental retardation, which is more severe in the male than in the female.

Etiology
- A fragile site on the long arm of the X chromosome

Physical Symptoms
- Large, long, and poorly formed pinna
- Big jaw
- Enlarged testes
- High forehead

Speech, Language, and Hearing
- Hearing loss not characteristic of the syndrome
- Jargon
- Perseveration
- Echolalia
- Inappropriate language, more often in the male
- Talking to oneself, more often in the male
- Lack of nonverbal means of communication that normally accompany speech
- Voice problems

- Articulation disorders

Diagnostic Criteria
- A constellation of listed symptoms
- Cytogenetic diagnostic data supporting the fragile X site
- Variations in syndrome manifestations to be considered

Prognosis
- Dependent on the degree of mental retardation and time speech-language treatment is initiated
- Heterozygous female carriers may not be affected or may only exhibit mild mental retardation

Recommendations
- Early communication treatment

Goldenhar Syndrome. A genetic syndrome characterized by oculoauriculovertebral dysplasia; rarely associated with mental retardation; also called *facio-auriculo vertebral syndrome, first and second branchial arch syndrome,* and *hemifacial microsomia.*

Etiology
- Often, sporadic occurrence with no family history
- When a parent is affected, autosomal dominant inheritance is suspected

Physical Symptoms
- Hemifacial Microsomia mostly due to an underdeveloped mandible
- Hypoplastic or dysfunctional facial, masticatory, and palatal muscles
- Cleft-like lateral extension of the mouth
- Microtia
- Preauricular Tags
- Vertebral Dysplasia, typically in the cervical region
- High arched palate
- Cleft palate, cleft lip, and congenital heart and kidney diseases in a few cases

Speech, Language, and Hearing
- Conductive hearing loss in several, sensorineural loss in a few; more often unilateral
- Possibly, disorders of articulation

S

- Resonance problems if clefts are present and their repairs are delayed
- Possibly, language disorders

Diagnostic Criteria

- A constellation of listed symptoms
- Variations in syndrome manifestations to be considered

Prognosis

- Dependent on the severity of manifestation and prompt surgical intervention for facial deformities, including cleft palate if present

Recommendations

- Early communication treatment

Laurence-Moon Syndrome. A genetic syndrome characterized by polydactyly, retinitis pigmentosa, hypogonadism, obesity, and mental retardation; also known as *Laurence-Moon-Biedl syndrome, Bardet-Biedl syndrome,* and *Laurence-Moon-Bardet-Biedl syndrome.*

Etiology

- Autosomal recessive inheritance
- Ophthalmologic disease
- Potential kidney diseases

Physical Symptoms

- Spastic paraplegia
- Vision problems due to retinitis pigmentosa; initial difficulty in night vision
- Retarded sexual development (hypogonadism)
- Extra fingers, toes, or both (polydactyly)
- Obesity

Speech, Language, and Hearing

- Hearing loss not common; conductive or sensorineural loss in a few cases
- Delayed language and language disorders
- Hypernasality
- Breathy voice
- Articulation disorders
- Motor control problems

Diagnostic Criteria
- A constellation of listed symptoms; variations in syndrome manifestations to be considered

Prognosis
- Varies with the severity and complexity of symptom expression
- More favorable in cases of less severe mental retardation and early, comprehensive medical and educational intervention

Recommendations
- Early communication treatment

Moebius Syndrome. A genetic syndrome characterized by congenital bilateral facial palsy; mild mental retardation observed in 10 to 15% of the affected individuals; infrequent association of hearing loss.

Etiology
- Heterogeneous causation
- Agenesis or Aplasia of the motor nuclei of the cranial nerves
- Sporadic occurrence in most cases
- Autosomal dominant inheritance in some cases

Physical Symptoms
- Involvement of facial and hypoglossal nerves; also, trigeminal in some cases
- Bilabial paresis and weak tongue control for lateralization, elevation, depression, and protrusion
- Unilateral or bilateral paralysis of the abductors of the eye
- Upper face affected more than the lower face
- Limited strength, range, and speed of movement of articulators
- Feeding problems in infancy
- Mask-like face
- Eyelids that may not fully close

Speech, Language, and Hearing
- Hearing loss not a characteristic of the syndrome

- Conductive hearing loss noted in a few cases
- Delayed language in some cases, especially in children with frequent hospitalization
- Articulation disorders ranging from mild to severe; bilabial, linguadental, and lingua-alveolar sounds affected more than the others

Diagnostic Criteria
- A constellation of listed symptoms; consider varied expression of the syndrome

Prognosis
- Varies with the severity and complexity of symptom expression
- Varies with the degree, quality, and time of intervention for communication deficits
- More favorable if fewer cranial nerves are affected

Recommendations
- Early communication treatment

Mucopolysaccharidoses (MPS) Syndromes. A group of syndromes characterized by excessive storage of complex carbohydrates in the body, progressive mental retardation, clouding of the corneas, skeletal dysplasia, thick coarse hair and bushy eyebrows, hearing loss, large tongue, anomalies of the hand, flat nasal bridge, and Hypertelorism; varieties include Hunter syndrome, Hurler syndrome, Maroteau-Lamy syndrome, Morquio syndrome, Sanfilippo syndrome, and Scheie syndrome; known for its extremely variable clinical expression.

Etiology
- Autosomal recessive inheritance in all varieties except for Hunter syndrome
- X-linked recessive inheritance in case of Hunter syndrome

Physical, Mental, and Auditory Symptoms
- *Hunter Syndrome:* Symptoms similar to Hurler Syndrome except for the following: less severe symptoms; X-linked inheritance; absence of corneal clouding;

slower progression of symptoms; and higher survival rate; some form of hearing loss in about 50% of the cases; also called MPS II

- **Hurler Syndrome:** Coarse facial features, clouded corneas, skeletal dysplasia, thick and coarse hair, enlargement of viscera, and bushy eyebrows; anomalies of the middle ear; large tongue, depressed nasal bridge; short fingers and short broad hands; short neck and trunk; severe and progressive mental retardation; conductive hearing loss in most cases; the most severe of the MPS syndromes; death often in the second decade of life; also called MPS I-H.

- **Maroteaux-Lamy Syndrome:** Similar to Hurler syndrome except for normal or near-normal intelligence; mild forms similar to Scheie syndrome; chronic otitis media; hearing impairment in cases of severe expression of the syndrome; also called MPS VI.

- **Morquio Syndrome:** The most distinguishing feature is dwarfism due to bone dysplasia; short neck and trunk; extremely mild corneal clouding; progressive and mixed or sensorineural hearing loss; also called MPS IV.

- **Sanfilippo Syndrome:** Similar to Hurler syndrome, though milder somatic symptoms; enlarged head; somewhat aggressive; rapid mental deterioration resulting in dementia; hearing impairment in 10% of the cases; death usually before age 20; also called MPS III.

- **Scheie Syndrome:** A milder form of Hurler syndrome; hence, difficult to diagnose before age six; no significant mental retardation; normal stature and life expectancy, hearing impairment in 20% of the cases; also called MPS I-S.

Speech and Language

- Little specific information available on the various forms of MPS; communication deficits vary depending on the severity of symptoms, presence and degree of mental retardation and hearing loss, and associated physical symptoms; both speech and language disorders to be expected based on these variables

Diagnostic Criteria
- A constellation of listed symptoms
- Biochemical test results
- Consider varied expression of the syndrome

Prognosis
- Varies with the severity and complexity of symptom expression
- Varies with the degree, quality, and time of intervention for communication deficits
- More favorable in less severely affected cases and less severe forms of MPS

Recommendations
- Early communication treatment

Noonan Syndrome. A genetic syndrome characterized by congenital heart disease, facial and skeletal anomalies, cryptorchidism, and mental retardation (in 50 to 60% of the cases).

Etiology
- Autosomal Dominant inheritance suspected
- Multifactorial inheritance suggested
- Nearly half free from heart diseases

Physical Symptoms
- Heart diseases, often Pulmonary Stenosis
- Short stature
- Hypertelorism
- Ptosis of the eyelids
- Epicanthal Folds
- Webbed neck
- Low-set, large, and posteriorly rotated ears

Speech, Language, and Hearing
- Hearing loss not characteristic of the syndrome; some with conductive or sensorineural loss
- Articulation Problems

467

- Delayed language development; limited expressive language skills
- Hypernasality

Diagnostic Criteria
- A constellation of listed symptoms
- To be distinguished from Turner syndrome, Prader-Willi syndrome, and fetal alcohol syndrome because of their apparent similarity
- Variations in syndrome manifestations to be considered

Prognosis
- Varies with the severity and complexity of symptom expression
- More favorable in cases of less severe mental retardation and early, comprehensive medical and educational intervention

Recommendations
- Early communication treatment

Oro-Facial-Digital Syndrome Type II. A genetic syndrome characterized by cranial, facial, lingual, palatal, and digital anomalies; also called Mohr syndrome.

Etiology
- Autosomal Recessive inheritance

Physical Symptoms
- Brachydactyly
- Clinodactyly
- Polydactyly
- Syndactyly
- Bilateral reduplication of the big toe (hallux)
- Midline partial tongue cleft
- Lobate tongue with nodules
- Midline cleft lip
- Broad or bifid nasal tip
- Mandibular Hypoplasia
- Microtia and external auditory canal atresia in some cases

Speech, Language, and Hearing
- Conductive hearing loss

- Language delay depending especially on the intellectual level
- Articulation problems related to mandibular and lingual abnormalities and hearing loss

Diagnostic Criteria

- A constellation of listed symptoms; variations in syndrome manifestations to be considered

Prognosis

- Varies with the severity and complexity of symptom expression
- More favorable in cases of less severe oro-facial anomalies and early surgical treatment for possible clefts, mandibular anomalies, and lobulation of the tongue

Recommendations

- Early communication treatment

Oto-Palatal-Digital Syndrome. A genetic syndrome characterized by otologic, palatal, and digital anomalies; associated with hearing loss and mild mental retardation.

Etiology

- Possibly, X-linked semidominant inheritance

Physical Symptoms

- Cleft palate
- Short and broad finger tips
- Congenital malformations of the ossicular chain
- Short fingers

Speech, Language, and Hearing

- Bilateral conductive loss in many cases
- Otitis media
- Speech problems associated with cleft palate and conductive hearing loss
- Delayed language associated with mental retardation

Diagnostic Criteria

- A constellation of listed symptoms; variations in syndrome manifestations to be considered

Prognosis

- Varies with the severity and complexity of symptom expression

- More favorable in cases of less severe mental retardation, less severe cleft palate, early surgical treatment, and early, comprehensive medical and educational intervention

Recommendations

- Early communication treatment

Pendred Syndrome. A genetic syndrome characterized by congenital, bilateral, sensorineural hearing loss and Goiter in middle childhood; mental retardation in some cases.

Etiology

- Autosomal Recessive inheritance

Physical Symptoms

- Enlarged thyroid (goiter)
- Hypothyroidism in early years
- Delayed skeletal maturation

Speech, Language, and Hearing

- Bilateral, mild to profound sensorineural hearing loss; profound loss in many cases; progressive in some
- Severe delay in language acquisition
- Language disorders associated with significant hearing loss
- Articulation disorders

Diagnostic Criteria

- A constellation of listed symptoms; variations in syndrome manifestations to be considered

Prognosis

- Varies with the severity and complexity of symptom expression
- More favorable in cases of less severe hearing loss, and comprehensive medical and educational intervention

Recommendations

- Early communication treatment

Pierre-Robin Syndrome. A genetic syndrome characterized by Mandibular Hypoplasia, Glossoptosis, and cleft of the soft palate; in some cases this syndrome may be a part of Stickler syndrome.

Etiology
- Autosomal Recessive inheritance in most cases
- Autosomal Dominant inheritance suspected if the syndrome is a part of the Stickler syndrome.
- Sporadic occurrence in isolated cases

Physical Symptoms
- Mandibular Hypoplasia
- Glossoptosis (downward displacement of the tongue)
- Cleft of the soft palate in most cases; typically not associated with the cleft of the lips
- Velopharyngeal incompetence
- Deformed pinna, low-set ears, and temporal bone and ossicular chain deformities

Speech, Language, and Hearing
- Unilateral or bilateral conductive hearing loss associated with otitis media and cleft palate
- Delayed language and language disorders
- Hypernasality and nasal emission
- Articulation disorders and hypercompensatory articulatory behaviors

Diagnostic Criteria
- A constellation of listed symptoms; variations in syndrome manifestations to be considered

Prognosis
- Varies with the severity and complexity of symptom expression
- More favorable in cases of less severe hearing loss, early surgical intervention for the cleft, and with early, comprehensive medical and educational intervention

Recommendations
- Early communication treatment

Prader-Willi Syndrome. A genetic syndrome characterized by Hypotonia, slow motor development, small hands and feet, underdeveloped genitals, almond-shaped eyes, obesity due to insatiable appetite, and mental retardation in most but not all cases.

Etiology
- <u>Autosomal Dominant</u> inheritance is suspected
- Deletion in the region of the long arm of chromosome 15 (15q11–15q13) in some cases

Physical Symptoms
- Low muscle tone and resulting early feeding difficulties
- Failure to thrive initially
- Obesity after the first year
- Excessive eating
- Underdeveloped genitals

Speech, Language, and Hearing
- Hearing loss not a typical characteristic
- Delayed language and language disorders
- Articulation disorders ranging from mild to severe, resulting in unintelligible speech
- Nasal air emission

Diagnostic Criteria
- A constellation of listed symptoms; variations in syndrome manifestations to be considered

Prognosis
- Varies with the severity and complexity of symptom expression
- More favorable in cases of less severe mental retardation and early, comprehensive medical and educational intervention

Recommendations
- Early communication treatment

Refsum Syndrome. A genetic syndrome characterized by progressive sensorineural hearing loss, cerebellar ataxia, chronic <u>Polyneuritis</u>, and <u>Retinitis Pigmentosa</u>.

Etiology
- <u>Autosomal Recessive</u> inheritance
- Biochemical imbalance involving excessive storage of <u>Phytanic Acid</u> in tissue or plasma

Physical Symptoms
- Chronic inflammation of the peripheral nerves (Polyneuritis)
- Pigmentary degeneration of the retina
- Night blindness
- Disturbed balance (cerebellar ataxia)
- Heart diseases in about 50% of the cases
- Skeletal abnormalities including Spondylitis and Kyphoscoliosis in about 75% of the cases

Speech, Language, and Hearing
- Slowly progressive sensorineural hearing loss that begins during the second or the third decade of life in 50% if the cases
- Articulation disorders associated with acquired hearing loss
- Dysarthria if the facial muscles are involved
- Hypernasality and nasal emission
- Harsh voice
- Variable pitch and loudness
- Altered rate of speech and stress patterns

Diagnostic Criteria
- A constellation of listed symptoms; variations in syndrome manifestations to be considered

Prognosis
- Generally poor because of the progressive nature of the syndrome; however, varies with the severity and complexity of symptom expression

Recommendations
- Early communication treatment

Stickler Syndrome. A genetic syndrome characterized by facial deformities, ophthalmologic problems, musculoskeletal deficiencies, Pierre-Robin sequence including cleft palate or submucous cleft, and hearing impairment; intelligence within normal limits.

Etiology
- Autosomal Dominant inheritance

Physical Symptoms
- Cataracts or retinal detachments
- Severe myopia
- Arthropathy (joint diseases, including juvenile rheumatoid arthritis)
- Hypotonia
- Prominent ankle, knee, and wrist bones
- Long and thin legs and hands
- Midface Hypoplasia
- Micrognathia
- Cleft palate, submucous cleft, or bifid uvula
- Auricular malformations in 10 to 12% of the cases

Speech, Language, and Hearing
- Feeding, sucking, and swallowing problems in infancy
- Bilateral conductive hearing loss in many cases and sensorineural loss in a few
- Language problems associated with hearing loss and Cleft Palate
- Hypernasality and nasal emission associated with clefts Articulation disorders associated with Cleft Palate

Diagnostic Criteria
- A constellation of listed symptoms; extreme variations in syndrome manifestations to be considered

Prognosis
- Varies with the severity and complexity of symptom expression
- More favorable in cases of less severe expression and early, comprehensive medical and educational intervention

Recommendations
- Early communication treatment

Treacher Collins Syndrome. A genetic syndrome characterized by mandibulofacial Dysostosis, hearing impairment, cleft or velopharyngeal incompetence, dental problems, external ear malformations; mental retardation not a typical characteristic.

Etiology
- Autosomal Dominant inheritance
- Spontaneous mutation in some cases

Physical Symptoms
- Underdeveloped facial bones including mandibular Hypoplasia (small chin) and malar (cheek) Hypoplasia
- Dental malocclusion and Hypoplasia
- Downwardly slanted palpebral fissures
- Coloboma of the lower eyelid
- Stenosis or Atresia of the external auditory canal
- Malformations of the pinna
- Preauricular ear tags
- Middle and inner ear malformations
- High hard palate
- Cleft palate in about 30% of the cases; submucus cleft in some cases
- Short or immobile soft palate
- Sucking and swallowing problems in infancy

Speech, Language, and Hearing
- Congenital, bilateral, conductive hearing loss in many cases and sensorineural loss in some
- Language disorders typically associated with hearing impairment; syntactic and morphologic features may be especially deficient
- Hypernasality and nasal emission in cases with clefts and velopharyngeal incompetence
- Articulation disorders consistent with hearing loss and gross oral structural deviations

Diagnostic Criteria
- A constellation of listed symptoms; variations in syndrome manifestations to be considered

Prognosis
- Varies with the severity and complexity of symptom expression
- More favorable in cases of early medical management of facial and oral anomalies and early, comprehensive medical and educational intervention

S

Recommendations
- Early communication treatment

Turner Syndrome. A genetic syndrome characterized by defective gonadal differentiation, congenital edema (swelling) of neck, hands, or feet; webbing of the neck, and low posterior hair line; mental retardation in only 10% of the cases; occurs only in the female; a similar syndrome that occurs in both males and females is called *Noonan syndrome.*

Etiology
- A missing X chromosome in most cases
- Structural abnormality of an X chromosome in some cases

Physical Symptoms
- Ovarian abnormality resulting in amenorrhea (absence of menstruation) and infertility
- Congenital swelling of the foot, neck, and hands
- Cardiac defects
- Webbing of the neck (excess skin over the neck)
- Low posterior hairline
- Broad chest with widely spaced nipples
- Cubitus valgas (elbows bent outward or away from the midline)
- Dysplastic nails
- Pigmented skin lesions
- Narrow maxilla and palate
- Micrognathia (abnormally small lower jaw)
- Maxillary Hypoplasia
- Anomalies of the auricle including low-set, elongated, and cup-shaped ears; thick earlobes
- High arched palate
- Cleft palate in some cases
- Evidence of right hemisphere dysfunction

Speech, Language, and Hearing
- Sensorineural hearing loss in many cases; rarely congenital; usually noticed after the 10th year

- Middle ear infection during infancy and early childhood; conductive hearing loss in some cases
- Language disorders consistent with hearing impairment
- Articulation disorders consistent with hearing impairment
- Possible auditory processing, visual, spatial, and attentional problems

Diagnostic Criteria
- A constellation of listed symptoms; variations in syndrome manifestations to be considered

Prognosis
- Varies with the severity and complexity of symptom expression
- More favorable in cases of early, comprehensive medical and educational intervention

Recommendations
- Early communication treatment

Usher Syndrome. A genetic syndrome characterized by Retinitis Pigmentosa and nonprogressive congenital hearing loss; disturbed gait in many cases; mental retardation in some cases; 50% of individuals who are deaf and blind may have this syndrome.

Etiology
- Autosomal Recessive inheritance in most cases
- X-linked in rare cases

Physical Symptoms
- Night blindness in early childhood
- Limited peripheral vision as the visual problems worsen
- Eventual blindness
- Cochlear abnormalities

Speech, Language, and Hearing
- Sensorineural hearing loss; consistent with cochlear pathology in most cases; related to central auditory pathology in some
- Language disorders consistent with hearing impairment

- Hypernasality and nasal emission
- Articulation disorders consistent with hearing impairment

Diagnostic Criteria

- A constellation of listed symptoms
- To be differentiated from other syndromes with retinitis pigmentosa and congenital hearing loss (e.g., Refsum syndrome and Laurence-Moon-Biedl syndrome)

Prognosis

- Poor (blindness and hearing loss are permanent)
- Better rehabilitative potential with communication treatment

Recommendations

- Early communication treatment

Van der Woude Syndrome. A genetic syndrome characterized by lower lip pits and cleft lip with or without cleft palate.

Etiology

- Autosomal Dominant inheritance

Physical Symptoms

- Pits or cysts of the lower lip in all cases
- Cleft lip and cleft palate in many cases

Speech, Language, and Hearing

- Otitis media and conductive hearing loss associated with cleft palate
- Language disorders consistent with hearing loss
- Hypernasality and nasal emission associated with cleft palate
- Articulation disorders consistent with hearing loss

Diagnostic Criteria

- A constellation of listed symptoms; variations in syndrome manifestations to be considered
- To be distinguished from isolated cleft lip

Prognosis

- Varies with the severity and complexity of symptom expression

- More favorable in cases of less severe clefts and early and effective medical management and educational intervention

Recommendations
- Early communication treatment

Waardenburg Syndrome, Type I and Type II. Type I is a genetic syndrome characterized by wide bridge of the nose caused by lateral displacement of inner (nasal) canthi, pigmentary disturbances; hearing impairment in about 25% of the cases; Type II is a genetic syndrome characterized by cranial and facial anomalies, brachydactyly, cleft palate, and cardiac defects; hearing impairment in about 50% of the cases.

Etiology
- Autosomal Dominant inheritance (Type I)
- Autosomal Recessive inheritance (Type II)

Physical Symptoms, Type I
- Lateral displacement of the inner (nasal) Canthi, causing wide bridge of the nose
- Pigmentary anomalies including white forelock, Heterochromia irides, Vitiligo, and white eyelashes
- Medial flare of eyebrows
- Cochlear anomalies

Physical Symptoms, Type II
- Acrocephaly
- Orbital and facial deformities
- Brachydactyly
- Mild Syndactyly of soft tissue
- Cleft Palate
- Hydrophthalmos
- Cardiac malformations in some cases

Speech, Language, and Hearing
- Congenital unilateral or bilateral sensorineural hearing loss; more common in Type II than in Type I; may vary from mild to profound

- Language disorders consistent with congenital hearing impairment; syntactic and morphologic features especially deficient
- Hypernasality and nasal emission, especially with the presence of cleft palate
- Articulation disorders consistent with hearing impairment and compensatory articulatory gestures consistent with cleft palate
- Early feeding and swallowing problems consistent with cleft palate

Diagnostic Criteria

- A constellation of listed symptoms; variations in syndrome manifestations to be considered

Prognosis

- Varies with the severity and complexity of symptom expression
- More favorable in cases of less severe hearing loss and early, comprehensive medical and educational intervention coupled with a strong aural rehabilitation program

Recommendations

- Early communication treatment

Dorland's Illustrated Medical Dictionary (28th ed.). (1994). Philadelphia: W. B. Saunders.

Jung, J. H. (1989). *Genetic syndromes in communication disorders.* Austin. TX: Pro-Ed.

Shprintzen, R. J. (2000). *Syndrome identification for speech-language pathology.* San Diego: Singular Thomson Learning.

Syntactic Aphasia. The same as Wernicke's aphasia (see <u>Aphasia: Specific Types</u>).

Synostosis. Fusion of bones that are normally separate.

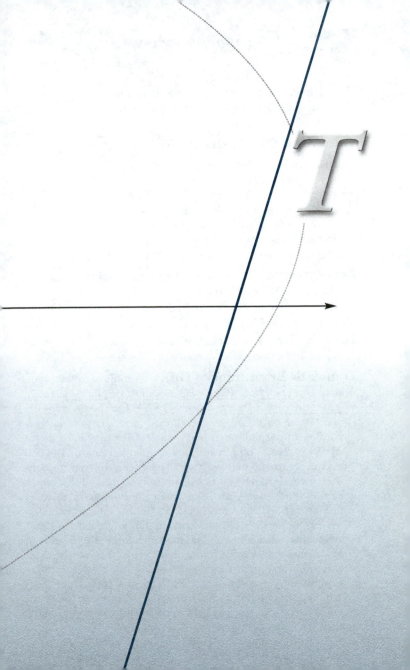

Taybi Syndrome.   The same as oto-palatal-digital syndrome (see <u>Syndromes Associated With Communicative Disorders</u>).

Third Alexia.   The same as frontal alexia; see <u>Alexia</u>.

Thrombosis.   Disease process leading to blood clot formation in larger arteries of the body; due to accumulation of fat and other materials, arteries harden and restrict the movement of blood, thus encouraging clot formation; clots then cut off blood supply to areas beyond their location; these clots remain at their point of origin; cerebral thrombosis is a frequent cause of stroke and resulting <u>Aphasia</u>.

Tomography.   A computerized radiographic method of taking pictures of different planes of body structures; a method of scanning brain structures; useful in neurodiagnostics; see <u>Computerized Axial Tomograph</u>.

Tongue Thrust.   A deviant swallow in which the tongue is pushed forward against the central incisors.

Traumatic Brain Injury (TBI).   An injury to the brain; may be <u>Penetrating (Open-Head) Injury</u> or <u>Nonpenetrating (Closed-Head) Injury</u>; in causing TBI, either the head moves and hits an object or an object moves and hits the head; according to hospital emergency room records, the incidence of TBI is about 200 per 100,000 people; kills about 100,000 a year; up to 100,000 who survive suffer from various consequences; leading cause of death for people under 35 years of age; third-leading cause of death (cardiovascular diseases and cancer are numbers 1 and 2); the prevalence is higher among males than females; risk of TBI is greater for those who have had a history of it and for children 4 to 5 years of age and those over 75; more than two thirds of TBI cases suffer minor injuries that do not result in loss of consciousness; main symptoms of major TBI include restlessness, irritation, disorientation to time and place, disorganized and inconsistent responses; impaired memory, attention, reasoning, drawing, naming, and repetition; also known as craniocerebral trauma.

Two Main Varieties

- Penetrating brain injuries, also known as open-head injuries
  - the skull is fractured or perforated
  - the meninges are torn or lacerated
  - *note that some experts consider the injury penetrating when the skull is fractured*
- Nonpenetrating brain injuries, also known as closed-head injuries
  - the skull may or may not be fractured or lacerated
  - the meninges remain intact
  - *note that some experts consider the injury nonpenetrating only when the skull also is intact*

Etiology

- **Penetrating Brain Injury**
  - bullets and other high velocity projectiles that strike the head
  - automobile accidents, blow to the head, and such other low velocity impacts when they produce a concentrated impact on a small area of the skull
  - falls
  - assaults
  - sports-related accidents
- **Nonpenetrating Brain Injury**
  - mostly the same factors that cause penetrating brain injury, except that they do not tear or lacerate the meninges
  - the head suffers various kinds of impacts

Neurophysiological Consequences of TBI

- **Penetrating Brain Injury**
  - injury to tissue on both sides of the projectile tract
  - the skull may be fractured or perforated with high velocity projectiles
  - the skull is more likely to be fractured (not perforated) with low velocity impacts

- foreign substance (hair, skin, and bone fragments) may be carried into the brain by the projectile
- secondary infection due to the foreign materials in the brain
- possibly death, especially in case of brainstem injury
- **Nonpenetrating Brain Injury**
  - no entry of foreign substances into the brain because of intact meninges
  - indirect damage to the brain and the brainstem
  - abrasions (scrapes) of the brain tissue
  - lacerations (cuts) of the brain tissue
  - contusions (bruises) of the brain tissue
  - shearing (tearing) of the brain tissue
  - impression trauma (skull deformation at the point of impact)
  - coup injuries (trauma at the point of impact)
  - contrecoup injuries (injury to the brain tissue on the opposite side of the impact)
  - injury to various brain tissues as they rub against the bony projections of the base of the skull as the brain moves inside the skull because of the impact
- **General Effects**
  - loss of consciousness, the duration depending on the severity of the injury; may vary between a few seconds to many days or months
  - slow or sudden recovery from consciousness
  - brief loss of consciousness in case of concussion or minor head injury with quick regaining of consciousness followed by headache, neckache, backache, blurred vision, fatigue, sleep disturbances, and so forth; subtle but long physical and cognitive effects in some cases
  - interrupted respiration and lower blood pressure and heart rate
  - traumatic hematoma (accumulation of blood in the brain due to hemorrhage, often as a result of automobile accidents)

- epidural hematoma (accumulation of blood between the dura matter and the skull)
- subdural hematoma (accumulation of blood between the dura and the arachnoid), a more frequent cause of death
- increased intracranial pressure due to accumulation of fluid in the brain (blood, water, or cerebrospinal fluid)
- ischemic brain damage (injury to brain tissue; even death of the tissue) due to lack of oxygen caused by reduced or interrupted blood supply

Initial Symptoms of TBI

- On regaining consciousness, the patient may exhibit:
  - inconsistency
  - disorganization
  - disoriented to time and place
  - confused, slow, or inappropriate speech
  - restlessness
  - irritability
  - inattentive behavior, distractible behavior
  - cognitive impairments including loss of memory, judgment, and abstract reasoning skills
  - generally poor control over emotional responses
  - aggressive behaviors (in some cases)
  - anxiety (in some patients)
  - socially inappropriate behavior
  - slow reaction time
  - paranoia in some cases
  - lack of self-appraisal of deficits
  - lack of purposeful behavior
  - lack of self-care skills, needing constant supervision and assistance
  - stepwise recovery (periods of little or no improvement alternated with rapid improvement)

Recovery From the Early Symptoms

- Gradual improvement in most of the symptoms, including:
  - clearing up of confusion

T

- improved orientation to space and time
- improved social awareness
- improved control over emotional responses
- more appropriate responses to simple questions
- slow re-emergence of some of the self-care skills, although still needing assistance and supervision
- more purposeful
- re-emergence of purposeful behavior
- progressively more independent functioning in routine situations
- Some symptoms, although showing signs of abatement, may still be present:
  - irritability, restlessness, shorter attention span, poor control over emotions, aggressive tendencies, impulsivity, slow reaction time, and most of the listed cognitive deficits

Subsequent and More Persistent Symptoms

- Emotional and social problems; as the recovery continues, the patient may experience:
  - depression after the initial recovery, possibly due to an awareness of physical and cognitive deficits; however, depression may be unrelated to the degree of impairment
  - feelings of helplessness or hopelessness
  - social withdrawal
  - suicidal tendencies in some cases
  - lower threshold of tolerance for noise
  - impulsivity
- Cognitive deficits; these are among the more persistent in TBI; may be more or less subtle; including:
  - poor judgment
  - memory deficits (amnesia for events prior to or subsequent to the trauma; pretraumatic amnesia or posttraumatic amnesia)
  - problem-solving skills
  - abstract reasoning
  - distractibility

- inattention
- slower reaction time
- Visual and perceptual deficits
  - problems in drawing
  - visual-spatial deficits
  - construction impairment
  - attentional deficits
- Communication problems; generally less pronounced than attentional, cognitive, emotional, and general behavioral deficits
  - dysarthria, especially in patients with brainstem or cerebellar involvement
  - dysarthria may range from mild articulatory problems (especially imprecise consonants) to severely unintelligible speech
  - dysarthria may be of mixed variety; other types also reported
  - reduced rate of speech
  - apraxia of speech
  - initially, confused language
  - aphasic-like symptoms in initial stages that tend to clear up
  - bizarre, inappropriate, incoherent, and paraphasic language in severely confused patients
  - mutism or aphonia in some extreme cases
  - problems in auditory comprehension of spoken language
  - persistent word-finding problems
  - nearly normal or normal syntactic features in mostly recovered patients
  - impaired pragmatic features of language including difficulty in conversational turn taking and topic management (problems in initiation, maintenance, expansion, and shifting)
  - prosodic impairments including difficulty in monitoring rate, pitch, and vocal loudness

T

- residual spelling errors in writing
- generally ineffective communicative attempts
- generally, significant recovery of many of the communicative skills within the first 2 months; continued improvement for up to 1 year; residual pragmatic deficits and word-finding problems
- Related problems
  - dysphagia
  - persistent physical disabilities including limited or impaired use of hands and limbs and visual or other sensory deficits

Assessment Objectives/General Guidelines

- To assess the communication deficits associated with TBI
- To evaluate the strengths and limitations that might help in planning treatment
- To evaluate communicative deficits in relation to cognitive, sensory, and physical deficits
- To evaluate the need for augmentative and alternative modes of communication
- Make an initial, brief assessment at the bedside; make detailed assessment as soon as the patient's condition permits
- Give frequent breaks from assessment tasks as the patient with TBI is likely to get tired soon; complete the assessment in more than one session, if necessary
- Repeat selected portions of assessment as the patient's condition improves
- Continue to assess the patient during treatment

Case History/Interview Focus

- See **Case History** and **Interview** under Standard/Common Assessment Procedures
- Document TBI and its details

Ethnocultural Considerations

- See Ethnocultural Considerations in Assessment

Traumatic Brain Injury (TBI)

Assessment

- Make a brief and initial bedside evaluation; create your own procedure of the kind described below or administer a standardized test:
  - assess simple responses to verbal commands; for example, ask the patient to:
    - → "Open your eyes"
    - → "Move your feet"
    - → "Wiggle your toes"
    - → "Nod your head"
    - → "Raise your hand"
    - → "Move your fingers"
  - assess the presence or absence of verbal responses; note the speed, relevance, and appropriateness of all responses given; note whether the patient:
    - → can say "Hi"
    - → gives only single-word responses; and if so the kinds of words produced
    - → can use sentences; and if so, the types of sentences
    - → responds spontaneously; and if so, note the types and length of utterance spontaneously produced
    - → responds only to questions and commands
    - → responds only nonverbally, but appropriately
    - → tries to respond nonverbally, but not successfully
    - → shows no signs of a response of any kind
  - assess simple memory skills and basic orientation; note whether the stimuli have to be repeated; ask the patient such questions as:
    - → "How old are you?"
    - → "What is your name?"
    - → 'What is your [wife's, husband's, mother's, father's] name?"
    - → "Where do you live?"
    - → "What do you do?"
    - → "Where are you now?"
    - → "What time is it?"

T

→ "What day is it?"
→ "What year is it?"
→ "What month is it?"
→ "Can you count to ten?"
→ "Can you recite the days of the week?"

- Assess cognitive deficits; wait until the patient's initial symptoms subside
  - assess memory deficits
    → question the patient about events prior to brain injury to assess pretraumatic amnesia
    → ask such questions as "where were you when the accident happened?" "what were you doing when the accident happened?" and "where were you going when the accident happened?"
    → question the patient about events subsequent to brain injury to assess posttraumatic amnesia
    → ask such questions as "how long have you been in the hospital?" "what did you eat for breakfast this morning?" "who visited you this afternoon?" and "what did you do after lunch today?"
    → have the client read a list of words and ask him or her to recall as many words as possible
    → have the client read the list repeatedly and, by requesting interspersed recall, assess the number of trials needed to learn the list in meeting a performance criterion such as 90% accuracy
    → assess recognition by presenting a list of words that contains previously shown words and new words that were not shown and ask the patient to point to the ones previously presented
    → read a paragraph aloud to the patient and immediately ask questions about the content
    → read a paragraph aloud to the patient and ask questions about the content after a delay of about 20 to 30 minutes
    → ask the patient to read a short paragraph repeatedly and assess repeatedly to find out the number of

readings necessary to meet a criterion such as 90% recall
- → administer a standardized test such as the *Wechsler Memory Scale—Revised*
- → obtain neuropsychological reports for more detailed assessment of memory functions
- → take note of errors and analyze the patient's strategies (e.g., repeating only the last few words of a list or a read paragraph; repeating the same words; intrusion of novel or nontarget words)
- assess attention span and distractibility
  - → observe the patient during assessment and interview
  - → note lack of attention as evidenced by the need to repeat instructions, need to represent test items, need to repeatedly give alerting stimuli (e.g., "look at me," "look at this picture")
  - → ask the patient to repeat clusters of two, three, four, five, six and seven digits to assess memory span for digits
  - → ask the patient to repeat sentences of varying length to assess the attention span for words
  - → note response to extraneous stimuli such as people passing by and noise to assess distractibility
  - → note fatigue during assessment and how fast it sets in
- assess reaction time
  - → note the speed of response to questions
  - → take note of the speed of response when spontaneous speech is offered
  - → make a judgment about the reaction time
- Assess visual and perceptual deficits
  - assess visuospatial, drawing, and constructional deficits
    - → ask the patient to copy selected, simple line drawings that you present
    - → ask the patient to copy geometric figures
    - → ask the patient to draw a face, a cup, a pencil, and such other common items from memory

T

→ ask the patient to copy a block design
→ ask the patient to copy a stick figure
- Assess communication problems
  - assess dysarthria; if necessary, determine its type
    → initially, observe speech sound production as the patient talks; note articulatory problems
    → when feasible, record a conversational speech sample
    → analyze the sample for the kinds of speech sound problems; take note especially of imprecise consonant productions
    → administer selected tests described under Dysarthrias
    → use the additional assessment procedures described under Dysarthrias
    → if a particular type of dysarthria seems a likely diagnosis, use the assessment procedures described under specific types of dysarthria
    → rate severity of dysarthria following the guidelines given under Dysarthrias
  - assess the rate of speech
    → measure the speech rate in segments of multiple speech samples
    → calculate the number of words or syllables spoken per minute
  - assess apraxia of speech
    → use the recorded conversational speech sample to assess apraxia of speech
    → assess the imitative and spontaneous production of syllables, words, phrases, and sentences that are described under Apraxia of Speech
    → make an orofacial examination
    → determine the presence of oral apraxia; use the procedures described under Apraxia of Speech
  - assess confused, bizarre, inappropriate, and incoherent language
    → assess relevance, appropriateness, and meaningfulness of answers to questions

- → evaluate extended language productions for their appropriateness and social acceptability
- → look for signs of confabulation and irrational and illogical statement
- → consider the general state of the patient (confusion and disorientation) in evaluating speech production
- assess mutism or aphonia
  - → assess reasons for lack of responses
  - → rule out motor problems that prevent expression
  - → note attempts on the part of the patient to communicate in any manner possible; such attempts negate mutism
- assess problems in auditory comprehension of spoken language
  - → note problems in auditory comprehension during interview and speech samples as evidenced by wrong responses or requests for repetitions
- assess persistent word-finding problems
  - → ask the patient to name selected common objects or pictures of objects
  - → ask the patient to name family members and friends
  - → ask the patient to point to the correct stimuli among several as you name them
  - → observe signs of word-finding difficulty in conversational speech (e.g., undue pauses, word repetitions, interjections, gestures, word substitutions, and the use of vague or general words instead of specific terms)
- assess syntactic and morphologic features informally; record a conversational speech (discourse) sample; note that they are adequate in most patients; if warranted, analyze the following:
  - → the length of typical sentences
  - → grammatic complexity of sentences
  - → transformational variety of sentences

T

- → word order and its appropriateness
- → use of such grammatic morphemes as the plural, the possessive, the present progressive, prepositions, pronouns, auxiliary verbs, copula, and so forth
- assess impaired pragmatic features of language; make judgments as you interview the client and while recording a conversational speech sample of difficulty in conversational turn taking and topic management (problems in initiation, maintenance, expansion, and shifting)
  - → judge the appropriateness of conversational turn taking; take note of the frequency of interruptions, silence when it is the patient's turn to talk; yielding to your speech attempts
  - → judge the frequency with which the patient initiates conversation or a topic of conversation; judge the adequacy of such initiations
  - → evaluate the rough duration for which the patient sustains conversation on given topics; judge the adequacy of topic maintenance, topic expansion, and topic shifting
  - → judge the adequacy of eye contact, use of gestures, facial expressions, and so forth
  - → judge the appropriateness of emotional expressions that accompany verbal expressions
- assess prosodic impairments including difficulty in monitoring rate, pitch, and vocal loudness
  - → measure speech rate and judge its appropriateness
  - → judge the appropriateness of vocal loudness
  - → judge the appropriateness of the patient's vocal pitch
  - → evaluate the patient's intonational patterns
  - → assess the patient's linguistic stress patterns
- assess the residual spelling errors in writing
  - → have the client write a paragraph on a topic of relevance
  - → have the client copy a printed paragraph

→ analyze spelling errors; take note of any other kinds of errors
- Assess related problems
  - assess dysphagia; use procedures described under Dysphagia
  - during assessment sessions, observe and take note of persistent physical and sensory disabilities
    → screen hearing and, if warranted, refer the patient to an audiologist
    → refer the client to a vision specialist

Assessment of Children With TBI

- Generally, the causes and effects are the same as those described earlier
- Assessment procedures and targets also are the same as described so far
- Consider the child's special needs in assessing the effects of TBI in children
  - assess the child's academic needs and demands
  - talk to the teachers and find out what kinds of demands are placed on the child
  - assess reading, writing, and literacy skills more thoroughly than you would in case of adults with TBI
  - if evaluated by a reading specialist, obtain the report
  - if the child is in a special educational program, assess the communication demands placed on the child within the program
  - obtain psychological reports from the school psychologist to better understand the intellectual and behavioral status of the child
  - focus on evaluating the communication deficits as described previously
  - integrate your findings with those of the special educators, teachers, and psychologists to obtain a more complete picture of the child's strengths and limitations
  - suggest a treatment plan that facilitates the child's academic achievement

T

Standardized Tests

- To assess memory, orientation, and communication skills, administer selected subtests of Aphasia; in addition, consider the following:

Test	Purpose
Glasgow Coma Scale (G. Teasdale & B. Jenette)	To make a bedside screening of general awareness and responsiveness
Galveston Orientation and Amnesia Test (H. S. Lfevin, V. M. O'Donnel, & R. G. Grossman).	To make a bedside screening of memory and orientation
Weschler Memory Scale—Revised (E. W. Russell)	To assess memory skills
Ranchos Los Amigos Scale of Cognitive Levels (C. Hagen & D. Malkamus)	To assess the cognitive and behavioral level and recovery
Communicative Abilities in Daily Living (A. L. Holland)	To assess functional communication skills

Related/Medical and Neuropsychological Assessment Data

- Patient's medical diagnosis
- Current medications and their side effects
- Current and future medical treatment plans for the patient
- Medical prognosis
- Radiologic and brain imaging data that might be integrated or correlated with speech diagnosis
- Physical rehabilitation plans that might affect communication treatment
- Audiologic findings that might be integrated with communication assessment
- Reports from neuropsychologist on cognitive impairment, intellectual functioning, and emotional and behavioral disorders or deficits

Traumatic Brain Injury (TBI)

Standard/Common Assessment Procedures
- Complete the <u>Standard/Common Assessment Procedures</u>

Analysis of Assessment Data
- Analyze and summarize the assessment data relative to physiologic and neuromotor problems
- Integrate the findings with medical-neurologic and neuropsychological assessment data to obtain a comprehensive profile of the patient's physiologic, neurologic, neuropsychological, and behavioral (including communication) performance
- Rate the severity of the disturbances noted
- Summarize the communication problems in relation to cognitive deficits

Diagnostic Criteria
- History and medical evidence of TBI
- Dominant neurophysiological consequences of TBI
- Dominance of listed cognitive deficits
- Communication deficits though relatively intact language functions; dominance of pragmatic problems
- Dysarthria

Differential Diagnosis
- Distinguish TBI from dementia: characteristics of dementia that contrast with those of TBI include gradual onset (vs. sudden onset of TBI), progressive course (vs. improving course of TBI), and symptoms and medical evidence of a degenerative neurological disease (vs. head trauma in case of TBI)
- Distinguish TBI from schizophrenia: characteristics of schizophrenia that contrast with TBI include gradual onset (vs. sudden onset of TBI), such serious thought disorders as delusions (vs. attentional and perceptual problems of TBI), no evidence of head trauma (vs. evidence of head trauma in TBI), and persistent or deteriorating mental and behavioral symptoms (vs. improving course of TBI)
- Distinguish TBI from right hemisphere syndrome: characteristics of right hemisphere syndrome that contrast

Traumatic Brain Injury (TBI)

with those of TBI include left-sided neglect (which is absent in TBI), denial of illness (not a significant symptom of TBI), and medical evidence of right hemisphere injury (vs. variable, diffuse injury in TBI)

- Distinguish TBI from aphasia with which it is most likely to be confused; use the following grid in making a differential diagnosis:

Traumatic Brain Injury or Aphasia?

Traumatic Brain Injury	Aphasia
Pure linguistic problems are not dominant	Pure linguistic problems are dominant
Grammatic errors not significant	Significant grammatic errors
Dysarthria part of the syndrome	Dysarthria not a part of the syndrome
Initially, confused language	Language not confused
Faster improvement in language	Slower improvement in language
More serious pragmatic problems	Less serious pragmatic problems
Social interaction seriously impaired	Social interaction not as seriously impaired
Initially disorganized and confused	Not disorganized or confused
Initially disoriented to time and space	Not disoriented to time and space
Responses may be inconsistent or irrelevant	Responses not inconsistent or irrelevant
Serious attentional problems including distractibility, impulsivity, poor social judgment, and lack of insight	Attentional problems not as serious

Prognosis

- Variable depending on the nature and extent of brain injury; prognostic guidelines are only suggestive and in need of stronger empirical support
- Generally good for improvement in all symptoms
- Cognitive and communication rehabilitation
- Persistent mutism after initial recovery may suggest relatively poor prognosis for more complete recovery of verbal skills
- Possibly, the longer the duration of posttraumatic amnesia, the poorer the prognosis for more complete recovery

Recommendations

- Communication treatment with an emphasis on improving dysarthria and pragmatic language disorders in the context of cognitive rehabilitation
- See the cited sources and *PGTSLP* for details

Beukelman, D. R., & Yorkston, K. M. (1991). *Communication disorders following traumatic brain injury: Management of cognitive, language, and motor impairments.* Austin, TX: Pro-Ed.

Bilger, E. D. (Ed.). (1990). *Traumatic brain injury.* Austin, TX: Pro-Ed.

Brookshire, R. H. (1997). *An introduction to neurogenic communication disorders* (5th ed.). St. Louis, MO: Mosby Year Book.

Hegde, M. N. (1998). *A coursebook on aphasia and other neurogenic language disorders* (2nd ed.). San Diego, CA: Singular Publishing Group.

Mira, M. P., Tucker, B. F., & Tyler, J. S. (1992). *Traumatic brain injury in children and adolescents.* Austin, TX: Pro-Ed.

Ylvisaker, M. (1985). *Head injury rehabilitation: Children and adolescents.* Austin, TX: Pro-Ed.

Tremor. A pattern of shaking, defined as an involuntary rhythmical movement of small amplitude.

Trisomy-21. The same as Down syndrome (see <u>Syndromes Associated With Communicative Disorders</u>).

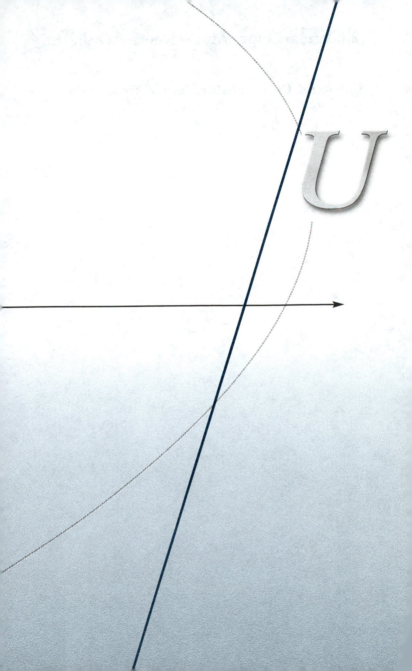

Unilateral Upper Motor Neuron Dysarthria.   See
<u>Dysarthria: Specific Types</u>.

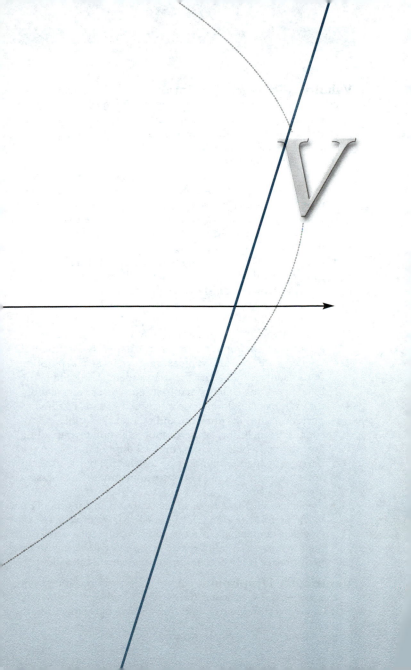

Validity. The degree to which a measuring instrument measures what it purports to measure; a criterion for test selection; may be demonstrated in many ways, resulting in different kinds of validity; see *PGSLP* for *Logical Validity* and *Empirical Validity*; validity measures of standardized tests include the following:

- Concurrent validity: The degree to which a new test correlates with an established test of known validity; too high a correlation suggests that the new test may be as valid as the old one and that the two tests are too similar, questioning the need for the new test; considered a form of criterion-related validity.

- Construct validity: The degree to which test scores are consistent with theoretical constructs or concepts; a language test, for example, that shows higher scores for older children compared to younger children is consistent with the theoretical construct that language changes (improves) with age.

- Content validity: A measure of validity of a test based on a thorough examination of all test items to determine if the items are relevant to measuring what the test purports to measure and whether the items adequately sample the full range of the skill being measured; a test of articulation, for example, should include all speech sounds in all word positions and in phrases and sentences; omission of sounds or inclusion of items not relevant to measuring articulation would reduce the validity of a test; often based on expert evaluation of test items and agreement among experts that the items are appropriate for assessing a given behavior.

- Predictive validity. The accuracy with which a test predicts future performance on a related task; for example, a test of language competence may be shown to predict academic performance; also known as *criterion-related validity*; future performance is the criterion used to evaluate the validity.

Ventricular Dysphonia. A voice disorder resulting from the use of the ventricular (false) vocal folds for phonation; possibly because the true folds have some pathology; sometimes associated with enlarged ventricular folds; ventricular folds overlap the true folds and thus dampen their vibrations; characterized by low pitch, monotone, decreased loudness, harshness, and arhythmic voicing; difficult to diagnose based only on how the voice sounds; endoscopy, X-ray, or stroboscopy essential to make a diagnosis.

Verbal Aphasia. The same as Broca's aphasia (see <u>Aphasia: Specific Types</u>).

Videofluoroscopy. A radiologic method of examining movement of internal structures and video recording the movement patterns for assessment and diagnosis; useful in assessing the functions of the velopharyngeal mechanism vocal folds, swallowing, and respiratory movement; preferred because it needs less radiation than cineradiography; X-rays are transmitted through the tissue under observation; the soft tissue is coated with barium with the help of a nasal spray; permits multiple views of the structures (e.g., frontal, lateral, base, and oblique views of the velopharyngeal mechanism) and their movements; the images are shown on a fluorescent screen; images recorded on a videotape for later examination and diagnosis.

Videofluorographic Worksheet. A detailed protocol for systematically observing and recording relevant structures, functions, symptoms, and disorders related to swallowing during videofluoroscopic studies; developed by J. A. Logemann; contains two sections: one for recording the results of liquid swallow tests and the other for recording the results of semisolid and solid food swallow tests; provides space for recording additional observations; makes a clear distinction between various swallowing disorders and their symptoms; useful in recording detailed and systematic observations during videofluoroscopic examination of patients with swallowing disorders.

Logemann, J. A. (1993). A *manual of videofluoroscopic evaluation of swallowing* (2nd ed.). Austin, TX: Pro-Ed.

Vitiligo. An anomaly of skin pigmentation that results in white patches surrounded by hyperpigmented border; part of some genetic syndromes; see Waardenburg syndrome under Syndromes Associated With Communicative Disorders).

Vocal Fold Paralysis. Laryngeal pathology resulting from damage to the branches of the vagus (Xth cranial) nerve; unilateral or bilateral paralysis of the folds; one or both the folds may be fixated in various positions; may be unilateral (more common) adductor paralysis (inability to close the folds), which is often due to trauma or accidental cutting of the recurrent laryngeal nerve; bilateral abductor paralysis, often caused by a brainstem lesion, is associated with dysarthrias; results in aphonia or dysphonia; complete neurologic examination essential for diagnosis; see Voice Disorders.

Vocal Fundamental Frequency in Males and Females. Typical vocal pitch levels of the male and female voice; various data sources suggest either the following ranges for the two genders or averages when no information on range is available; use them in evaluating the appropriateness of assessed pitch in case of clients with voice disorders:

Age (in years)	Male (Hz)	Female (Hz)
1–2	340–470	340–470
3	255–360	255–360
4–8	340–210	340–215
9–12	285–195	290–200
13	275–140	280–195
14–18	215–105	270–175
30–40	112	171–222
40–50	107	168–208
50–60	118	176–241
60–70	112	143–235
80–90	146	170–249

Vocal Hyperfunction

Vocal Hyperfunction.   Speaking with excessive muscular effort and force; vocally abusive behaviors; see <u>Voice Disorders</u> for assessment.

Vocal Nodules.   A form of laryngeal pathology resulting from vocally abusive behaviors; benign lesions of the vocal folds; generally bilateral; found at the junction of the anterior one third and posterior two thirds of the true vocal folds; symptoms may include hoarseness, harshness, periodic aphonia, frequent throat clearing, hard glottal attacks, tension, and a dry vocal tract; result of continuous vocal abuse; see <u>Voice Disorders</u>.

Voice Disorders.   Various disorders of communication related to faulty, abnormal, or inappropriate loudness, pitch, quality, and resonance; voice that does not help meet the social and occupational demands of communication; voice that deviates from expectations based on age, culture, or gender; may be associated with tension or a sense of discomfort in some cases; many descriptive terms of voice disorders lack objective definitions; classification varies across experts; many classifications confuse voice disorders (deviations of loudness, pitch, quality, and resonance) with their immediate or more or less remote causes (nodules, vocal abuse, cancer, papilloma); causes include vocally abusive behaviors resulting in laryngeal structural changes; physical trauma to the laryngeal mechanism; problems in neural control of the laryngeal mechanism due to central nervous system pathology; various physical diseases including cancer; and no apparent cause leading to the inference of faulty learning (functional disorder); may be the first and the only sign of a serious laryngeal pathology; little information on the incidence in different populations; disorders associated with nodules are the most common; those associated with edema, polyps, carcinoma, and no known laryngeal pathology occur with decreasing frequency; those associated with carcinoma and vocal fold paralysis most common in the elderly; nodules most common in males under 14 years of age and females in the age range of 25 to 45 years; people who talk excessively or those who have to talk continuously because of occupational demands are more prone to voice disorders.

Functional Aphonia. Loss of voice; inability to produce phonation (sound) for speech, phonation may be heard during coughing, laughing, or throat clearing; may be constant or intermittent; most patients communicate well with whispers and gestures; a few may be mute; some patients may speak with a faint voice with breathiness; associated factors include:

- Psychological or behavioral; sometimes described as hysterical reaction (conversion reaction); reaction to difficult life situations (acute or prolonged stress)
- Reaction to physical diseases including flu and an upper respiratory illness; possibly, temporary loss of voice due to organic causes that cease to operate although aphonia persists
- Difficulty in terminating complete voice rest following laryngeal surgery (with intact folds)

Voice Disorders of Loudness (Intensity). Socially inappropriate loudness; include the following:

- Excessively loud voice: Voice that is too loud from the standpoint of social situations; associated factors include:
  - general vocal hyperfunction (voice produced with excessive force)
  - hearing loss
  - presumably faulty learning (often referred to as functional)
- Excessively soft voice: Voice that is too soft to meet the social and occupational demands of communication; associated factors include:
  - neurological diseases (e.g., amyotrophic lateral sclerosis)

- laryngeal pathologies including vocal nodules and paralysis
- faulty learning (functional)
- Shimmer: Intensity perturbations; a cycle-to-cycle variation that exceeds 1 dB; may be described as a voice quality disorder; associated factors include:
  - possible neurologic factors
  - various organic factors

Voice Disorders of Pitch (Frequency). Voice characterized by various deviations in pitch include the following:

- Inappropriate pitch: Inappropriate in relation to the speaker's age and gender; includes falsetto or puberphonia: very high pitch in the postpubertal males and females; associated factors include:
  - faulty learning; failure to learn the new voice pattern with lower pitch
  - persistence of prepubertal vocal pattern with its high pitch
- Pitch breaks: A high-pitched voice may break lower; a low-pitched voice may break higher; may be described as a quality disorder; associated factors include:
  - developmental changes in the laryngeal mechanisms in adolescents
  - speaking at inappropriate pitch levels; consequently, voice may break an octave or two up or down in children and adults
  - vocal fatigue due to prolonged use of voice
- Lack of pitch variations: Monopitch; associated factors include:
  - vocal fold paralysis
  - neurological diseases (e.g., Parkinson's disease)
  - faulty learning (functional)
- Diplophonia: Production of double pitch; associated factors include:

- two folds vibrating at different rates because of differences in mass between the two
- vocal fold paralysis, laryngeal web, ventricular fold vibration, and aryepiglottic vibration
- faulty learning (functional)

- Jitter: Frequency perturbations; cycle-to-cycle variations in vocal intensity that exceed 1%; may be described as a voice quality disorder; associated factors include:
  - possible neurologic factors
  - faulty learning (functional)

Voice Disorders of Quality. Voice characterized by undesirable vocal qualities due primarily to faulty approximation of the vocal folds; include the following:

- Breathiness: excessive and audible air leakage associated with phonation; primary and immediate cause is a failure to achieve optimum approximation of the vocal folds; associated factors include:
  - various organic factors including nodules and polyps; paralysis of vocal cords
  - faulty learning (functional)

- Harshness: Unpleasant, strident, or rough voice; aperiodicity of laryngeal vibration; associated factors include:
  - excessive vocal effort, hard glottal attacks, and abrupt initiation of voice
  - constriction of the vocal tract
  - possible neurologic problems
  - laryngeal structural problems
  - vocal abuse and faulty learning (functional)

- Hoarseness: A grating or husky voice quality that includes voice breaks, diplophonia, low pitch, harshness, and breathiness; the most commonly observed voice disorder; may be dry hoarseness (because of lack of sufficient lubrication of the folds) or wet hoarseness (because of excessive mucous secretions on the vocal folds); associated factors include:

V

Voice Disorders

- various laryngeal structural alterations including nodules, polyps, cysts, papilloma, and cancer
- laryngitis and upper respiratory infections
- vocal abuse and misuse

- Glottal or vocal fry: Popcorn popping or bubbling kind of voice occurring toward the lower end of the pitch range; a slight hoarseness may be heard; not necessarily a disorder of voice as glottal fry is a normal voice characteristic; too frequent production may constitute a clinical problem; the major associated factor is the following: thickness of the vocal folds (ventricular folds in contact with the true folds)

- Tense voice: Voice produced with excessive adduction and medial compression of the folds; voice sounds tense; associated factors include:
  - various organic conditions that promote compensation resulting in hyperadduction
  - faulty learning (functional)

- Spastic voice: Spasticity in voice production; intermittent stoppage of voice because of an extreme degree of tensed vocal fold approximation; a symptom of spasmodic dysphonia; associated factors include:
  - neurologic problems
  - faulty learning (functional)

Voice Disorders of Resonance. Voice characterized by inappropriate resonance; these disorders also may be described as voice quality disorders; include the following:

- Hypernasality: Excessive nasal resonance because of the open velopharyngeal port; associated factors include:
  - craniofacial anomalies including clefts of the soft palate
  - structural problems unrelated to clefts including short hard palate, short velum, partial submucous cleft palate, and deep pharynx

- tonsillectomy and adenoidectomy resulting in reduced tissue mass
- neurologic diseases that cause problems in motor control of the velopharyngeal mechanism (as in dysarthrias)
- Hyponasality: Too little nasal resonance because of limited resonance of the nasal cavity; almost all associated factors are organic:
  - pharyngitis and tonsillitis
  - diseases of the nasal cavity
  - allergies
  - nasal polyps and papillomas
  - foreign bodies in the nasal cavity
  - nasal neoplasm (growth in the nasal cavity)
  - deafness
- Cul-de-sac nasality: "Bottom of the sac" or hollow sounding nasality; associated factors include:
  - excessively posterior carriage of the tongue
  - anterior nasal obstruction
  - faulty learning (functional)
- Assimilative nasality: Nasal resonance in the production of oral sounds that are adjacent to nasal sounds; associated factors include:
  - recent tonsillectomy and adenoidectomy
  - premature opening of the velopharyngeal port (nasality prior to nasal sounds)
  - failure to promptly close the velopharyngeal port (nasality after nasal sounds)

Etiology of Voice Disorders

Note that there is a close interaction between laryngeal pathologies and behavioral patterns; some of the behavioral patterns induce laryngeal pathology. All laryngeal pathologies are described in this section, including those that have behavioral origins.

- Laryngeal pathologies associated with voice disorders; the pathologies involve structural changes in the laryngeal mechanism; pathological changes may have physical or behavioral causes; the deviations in voice parameters are directly related to those pathological structural changes.

Voice Disorders

Laryngeal Pathologies	Potential or Demonstrated Causes	Resulting Voice and Related Problems
Cancer: Carcinoma of laryngeal structures; see Laryngectomy	Smoking, excessive drinking, and genetic predisposition	Hoarseness Swallowing and respiratory problems
Contact ulcer: most often on the posterior third of the vocal folds	Excessive slamming of the folds (behavioral) Gastric reflux (medical) Intubation (medical)	Vocal fatigue Hoarseness Throat clearing Pain in the throat
Retarded laryngeal growth	Endocrine disorders (pituitary disorders in women)	Pitch disorders
Increased mass of vocal folds or slight thickening of folds	Hypothyroidism; lowered estrogen and progesterone during menstruation in women	Hoarseness Lower pitch
Granuloma: firm, granulated, sac-like, vascular growth on the vocal process of the arytenoid process (posterior larynx)	Vocal abuse and misuse Surgical intubation Gastric reflux	Vocal fatigue Throat pain Limited pitch range Hoarseness Frequent throat clearing
Hemangiomas: soft, blood-filled sac on the posterior larynx	Vocal hyperfunction Hyperacidity Intubation	Similar to those under granuloma

(continued)

Voice Disorders

(continued)

Laryngeal Pathologies	Potential or Demonstrated Causes	Resulting Voice and Related Problems
Hyperkeratosis: Pinkish rough growth; leaf-shaped keratinized (horny) cell growth on the folds or inner glottal margins; unilateral or bilateral; may be premalignant	Vocal abuse and misuse Excessive drinking and smoking Exposure to smoke filled environment	Voice quality deviations including hoarseness
Infectious laryngitis: Various types of infection, but mostly common cold	Viral (more often) Bacterial	Hoarseness Low pitch in some cases
Leukoplakia: Patchy, white lesions on vocal folds and under the tongue; may be premalignant	Vocal abuse and misuse Excessive drinking and smoking	Voice quality deviations including hoarseness Diplophonia in some cases Reduced volume
Papilloma: Mulberry- or wart-like growth on the folds and related structures, more often in children	Possibly due to viral infection	Hoarseness Shortness of breath Aphonia in some children
Traumatic laryngitis or functional laryngitis; vocal folds swelling	Vocal abuse (behavioral)	Hoarseness Low pitch

(continued)

Voice Disorders

(continued)

Laryngeal Pathologies	Potential or Demonstrated Causes	Resulting Voice and Related Problems
Vocal fold thickening: Thickening of anterior two thirds of the glottal margins (perhaps a precursor to nodules or polyps); more extensive thickening in other cases	Continuous abuse or misuse (behavioral) Predisposition (genetic) Upper respiratory problems (medical) Postsurgical reaction (medical)	Quality deviations including hoarseness, harshness, and possibly breathiness
Vocal nodules: Typically bilateral, benign, callous-like growth on edges of the vocal folds; often at the midpoint of the folds (anterior and middle third portion), but may vary	Vocal abuse and misuse over a period of time	Hoarseness, breathiness, lower pitch, voice tension, and vocal fatigue Jitters and shimmers Reduced maximum phonation during and (possibly) abnormal s/z ratio Frequent throat clearing
Vocal polyps: Typically unilateral, soft fluid-filled growth on the anterior and middle third of vocal fold edges; may be broad-based sessile or pedunculated	Vocal abuse and misuse over time or due to a single episode of abuse	Hoarseness and breathiness Frequent throat clearing
Webbing: Thin and web-like tissue growth across the vocal folds; may be small or large; usually at the anterior commissure	Congenital formation Irritation of folds due to infection or trauma Postsurgical growth	Severe dysphonia in some cases Respiratory distress (possibly)

V

Voice Disorders

- Laryngeal trauma associated with voice disorders: Externally induced injury to laryngeal structures that result in voice problems;

Laryngeal Trauma	Potential or Demonstrated Causes	Resulting Voice and Related Problems
Injury to larynx	Automobile accidents Assault, gunshot Attempted strangulation Penetration of sharp objects	Varied effects; mild to significant dysphonia
Burning of laryngeal area	Smoke and gas inhalation Harmful chemical ingestion	Varied effects; mild to significant dysphonia
Surgical sequelae: Consequences of certain surgical procedures	Tracheostomy Intubation Long-term use of nasogastric tube	Edema, irritated mucosa, granuloma, web formation, paralysis of folds, and fracture of laryngeal cartilages Mild to severe dysphonia; discomfort

- Neurologic pathologies associated with voice disorders; the pathologies may involve the structure or function of the vocal folds; the basic cause is disordered neural control of the laryngeal mechanism, often due to central nervous system involvement.

Voice Disorders

Neurologic Pathologies	Potential or Demonstrated Causes	Resulting Voice and Related Problems
Unilateral and bilateral adductor paralysis of the vocal folds	Damage to the superior or recurrent branch of the vagus (cranial nerve X) due to trauma, neurological diseases, and surgical accidents	Breathiness, hoarseness, monotone; aphonia in case of bilateral paralysis Flaccid dysarthria including hypernasality and audible nasal emission
Bilateral upper motor neuron lesions (direct and indirect motor pathways)	Variety of causes including vascular and degenerative diseases; tumors; and trauma	Spastic dysarthria Strained-strangled voice, pitch breaks, low pitch, harshness, monoloudness, and hypernasality
Cerebellar lesions	Variety of causes including degenerative and vascular diseases and demyelinating diseases	Ataxic dysarthria Harshness, monopitch, monoloudness Irregular speech rate Occasional tremor
Lesions of the basal ganglia	Variety of causes including such degenerative diseases such as Parkinson's disease and vascular disorders	Hypokinetic dysarthria Monopitch, monoloudness, harshness, breathiness, hypernasality, weak phonation, low pitch

(continued)

(continued)

Neurologic Pathologies	Potential or Demonstrated Causes	Resulting Voice and Related Problems
Amyotrophic lateral sclerosis	Upper and lower motor neuron lesions	Mixed dysarthria (spastic-flaccid) Hypernasality, harshness, monopitch, monoloudness, strained-strangled voice, breathiness, and nasal emission
Multiple sclerosis	Demyelination of various brain structures	Dysarthria (flaccid and spastic-ataxic) Loudness control problems, harshness, impaired pitch control, breathiness, hypernasality, and inappropriate pitch
Spasmodic dysphonia: Adductor type (more common) and abductor type (less common and controversial)	Etiology generally controversial or uncertain Presumed neurologic in most cases Possibly other unknown causes	Strained, struggled, effortful voice production; jerky voice onset; intermittent voice breaks; vocal tremor (adductor type); breathy spasms, failure to maintain voice; worsening symptoms with voiceless sounds (abductor type)

518

Voice Disorders

- Behavioral patterns associated with voice disorders: not associated with pathological changes in the structure of the larynx; the disorders often are described as functional.

Behavioral Patterns	Potential or Demonstrated Causes	Resulting Voice and Related Problems
Speaking at the upper pitch range	Failure to shift to a lower voice Embarrassment about pitch changes at puberty Faulty learning	Falsetto: high pitched breathy voice Downward pitch breaks
Vocal reaction to stressful situations	Negative reinforcement (escape from certain speaking situations) Conversion reaction Combination of stress and organic pathology that disappears (e.g., laryngitis)	Functional aphonia (loss of voice; presence of whisper) or functional dysphonia (some voice production but deviant quality, pitch, and loudness)
Persistence of childhood vocal pitch or use of even higher pitch beyond puberty	Inadequate response to pubertal changes in the larynx Concern about pitch breaks and social reactions to them	Puberphonia: persistent high pitched voice
Use of ventricular folds in voice production	Faulty learning Loading of the ventricular folds on the true folds Disease of the true folds that forces the use of ventricular folds	Ventricular dysphonia: low pitched, monotonous, hoarse voice

Voice Disorders

Assessment Objectives/General Guidelines

- To assess all aspects of voice and its effects on communication
- To work closely with the physician of the patient; in most cases, be a member of a multidisciplinary team
- To be a coordinator of different services, if necessary
- To assist the medical professionals when a diagnosis of voice disorders is of medical significance (e.g., the diagnosis of vocal pathology, including cancer or central nervous system lesion)
- To make periodic assessment of voice in patients under medical treatment
- To integrate voice assessment with medical, psychological, educational, and occupational information of relevance to voice disorder and its management
- Note that careful observation of the patient and listening to his or her speech and voice production is indispensable
- Note that it is necessary to combine clinical judgment (perceptual analysis) with instrumental measures; some instrumental measures may not directly correspond to clinical judgments; some insurance companies may require instrumental measures to reimburse for clinical services
- Note that information from family members should supplement observations of voice parameters, especially when some voice problems may not be consistently observed in the clinic (e.g., in some cases, loudness problem may be more often noticed in natural settings than in the clinic)

Case History/Interview Focus

- See **Case History** and **Interview** under Standard/Common Assessment Procedures

Ethnocultural Considerations

- See Ethnocultural Considerations in Assessment

Voice Disorders

- Note that vocal characteristics including vocal intensity and acceptable levels of nasal resonance may be culturally determined

Assessment

- Interview the client and record a speech and language sample for a complete communication analysis (speech, language, fluency, and voice); see <u>Standard/Common Assessment Procedures</u>
- Keep audiotaped samples of speech and voice to assess changes due to treatment or other factors
- Observe general behaviors
  - general bodily tension; tensed postures; tension in the neck, jaw, and chest; tics
  - signs of neurologic involvement including lack of facial emotional expression (mask-like); tremor, rigidity, flaccidity; paresis, and paralysis
  - extent of mouth opening
  - loud or excessive talking
  - soft or inaudible speech
- Observe general phonatory behaviors
  - frequency of throat clearing and coughing
  - sound initiations: soft and gentle or forceful and with hard glottal attacks
  - emotional expression in speech
  - prosodic features
  - signs of allergy or cold (sneezing, sniffing, nose blowing)
  - flow of speech: smooth, effortless, and fluent, or jerky, effortful, and dysfluent
- Assess vocally abusive behaviors
  - note that, unless the laryngeal pathology is physically based (e.g., cancer), many cases of voice disorders, including some that have laryngeal pathology (e.g., vocal nodules or polyps) have a behavioral origin; vocally abusive behaviors are the main causes of these disorders

Voice Disorders

- assess vocally abusive behaviors through a detailed case history and interview; ask questions about the following vocally abusive behaviors:
  - → excessive talking
  - → excessively loud voice
  - → talking in inappropriate pitch
  - → argumentative behavior patterns
  - → habitually hard and abusive laughing
  - → excessive talking during menstruation
  - → excessive talking during allergy and upper respiratory diseases
  - → frequent shouting, screaming, cheering, throat clearing
  - → occupational use of voice (e.g., teaching, preaching, sports coaching, singing, aerobic instruction, pep club activities)
  - → working and talking in noisy conditions (e.g., bar and sports arenas, construction sites)
  - → smoking
  - → working in smoke-filled rooms (e.g., bars and other places with no regulation on smoking), general exposure to second-hand smoke
  - → excessive alcohol intake
  - → persistent, excessive laryngeal tension
  - → inadequate breath support
  - → constant and excessive grunting during exercising and weight lifting
  - → habitual name shouting (calling) from a distance
  - → not drinking enough water
  - → play activity with much vocal activity (e.g., children who make loud mechanical and animal noises as they play)
- ask the client or a family member to document the occurrence of vocally abusive behaviors in natural settings
  - → ask the client or a parent to keep a diary of vocally abusive behaviors for a week
  - → have the person record the frequency of vocally abusive behaviors

→ have the person record the amount of talking on a daily basis

- Assess functional aphonia
  - Obtain first a medical evaluation that clears the patient of organic pathology leading to lack of voice (e.g., bilateral paralysis of the vocal folds due to neurologic diseases)
  - Identify possible stress factors in life through careful and detailed interview
  - During the interview, make some jokes to assess phonation accompanying laughter
  - Take note of phonation during throat clearing; ask the client to demonstrate his or her throat clearing
  - Take note of phonation during coughing; ask the client to demonstrate his or her coughing
- Assess disorders of loudness (intensity)
  - probe the client and the family members about the client's vocal intensity in natural settings
  - observe and make clinical judgments about vocal intensity; note whether loudness of voice is adequate (normal loudness), inadequate (too soft), or inappropriate (too loud)
  - note variations in loudness; note whether a normal loudness level is maintained during conversation; whether variations in loudness are acceptable; and whether loudness varies unpredictably and inappropriately
  - ask the client to vary loudness to assess the range of intensity the patient can exhibit; ask the patient to whisper, speak softly, and to speak as loudly as possible; ask the patient to shout; ask the patient to count from 1 to 20, gradually increasing the intensity as counting is continued
  - use the **Clnical Voice Evaluation Form** described later to make clinical judgments about the client's vocal intensity
  - use the <u>Sound Level Meter</u> to obtain instrumental measures of loudness and evaluate them against normal range of vocal intensity levels in most social situations:
    → typical speech intensity level: 60 dB SPL at about 1 meter

V

Voice Disorders

→ maximum speech intensity level: 100 to 110 dB SPL at about 1 meter

→ minimum speech (not whispered) intensity level: 40 dB SPL

- compare clinical judgments with instrumental measures; make an evaluation
- Assess disorders of pitch (frequency)
  - use voice models to assess the client's pitch levels
    → have recorded models of an adult male and female, and male and female children's voice samples; record the production of prolonged (about 3 sec) vowels; play back an appropriate sample and ask the client to match the pitch

    → tape record a sample of speech; later, play back the tape; at random intervals, match the client's pitch with a piano or a pitch pipe

    → ask the client to vary the pitch, producing the lowest, intermediate, and the highest pitch levels while prolonging vowels

    → ask the client to say "mmmhhumm" in response to a question that is answered *yes* and "hhmm-mmm" in response to a question answered *no*; the pitch of the "mmm" may indicate the client's most desirable (habitual) pitch

    → identify the best pitch (pitch that is produced with little effort and good sound)
  - use one of the <u>Instruments for Voice and Speech Analysis</u> to measure the frequency range, the best pitch, and the habitual pitch of the client (e.g., the Visi-Pitch, Phonatory Function Analyzer, or Fundamental Frequency Indicator)
  - note that normal pitch for an individual is closer to the lowest pitch produced by that person
  - compare the client's habitual pitch with the normative data; see <u>Vocal Fundamental Frequency in Males and Females</u>
- Assess disorders of voice quality
- Listen carefully and take note of:

524

Voice Disorders

- vocal hyperfunction (tensed production of voice with pressed approximation of vocal folds)
- vocal hypofunction (too lax or inadequate approximation of vocal folds)
- breathiness of voice
- vocal spasticity and periodic voice cessation indicating possible neurological involvement
- hoarseness of voice with or without voice breaks and diplophonia
- colds and allergic reactions that may cause temporary hoarseness
- nodules and other laryngeal pathologies that may cause more permanent hoarseness
- jitter and shimmer
- diplophonia
- glottal fry
- Assess disorders of resonance
  - judge hyponasality and hypernasality as you listen to the client's speech; be aware that clinical judgment of nasality may not always be reliable; therefore, in addition to making judgments, tape record the client's production of:
    → prolonged vowels with low pressure oral consonants (e.g., /a/ with *Ollie* or /u/ with *Lulu*)
    → sentences that are devoid of nasal sounds (e.g., *he wore bow tie and cowboy boots; the dishwasher washes the dishes; Bob took Steve to the store*)
    → sentences that are loaded with nasal sounds (e.g., *Nanny makes marshmallows; Jenny and Nancy joined the Navy*)
    → make judgments of nasality by listening to the taped productions
  - have the client produce phrases or sentences devoid of nasal sounds while holding and releasing the nose; reduced nasality while holding the nose suggests hypernasality and velopharyngeal incompetence

V

- have the client produce phrases that are loaded with nasal sounds while holding and releasing the nose; if nose holding and releasing makes no difference, conclude that the problem is denasality
- have the client produce "maybe baby, maybe baby;" the problem is hypernasality if both words sound like *maybe*; hyponasality if both sound like *baby*
- test stimulability for oral sounds; provide models of oral sounds, phrases, and sentences and ask the client to imitate; successful imitation suggests adequate velopharyngeal closure
- use measures of articulation to assess nasal resonance; administer the *Iowa Pressure Articulation Test*; nasal emission during the production of plosives and fricatives suggest velopharyngeal incompetence
- make an oral examination; note a short palate and obvious problems; note that subtle problems of velopharyngeal closure cannot be determined by visual inspection
- use Instruments for Resonance Assessment to evaluate nasal resonance (e.g., the Nasometer from the Kay Elemetrics Corporation)
- make an endoscopic examination or obtain the results of examination from a physician; see Endoscopy
- make a videofluoroscopic examination of the velopharyngeal closure; see Videofluoroscopy
- assess assimilated nasality by having the client produce:
  → words that contain a nasal sound in the initial or final positions (e.g., *nice* and *mice; Ben* and *him)* with enough mouth opening
  → judge assimilated nasality by the presence of nasal resonance on the adjacent oral sounds
- assess cul-de-sac resonance by noting muffled or hollow oral resonance
- Assess maximum phonation duration

Voice Disorders

- to assess general phonatory efficiency and the use of air flow:
  - → ask the client to phonate /s/ and /z/ as long as possible; measure the duration in seconds
  - → obtain measures on at least three trials
  - → compare the durations against norms (about 15 to 20 sec for adults and 10 sec for children); note that the durations may be highly variable and may increase with additional trials
  - → calculate the /s/ and /z/ durations by dividing z durations into /s/ durations
  - → judge the appropriateness of the ratio (about .90 being normal); /z/ durations slightly longer than the /s/ durations; note that laryngeal pathology shortens the /z/ durations resulting in s/z ratios over 1.4
- Make an aerodynamic evaluation
  - measure phonatory air flow rate; use an instrument described under Instruments for Aerodynamic Measures of Phonatory Functions (e.g., a pneumotachometer, Phonatory Function Analyzer, or Aerophone II)
    - → note that normal flow rate is between 100–150 cc per second
    - → flow rate in excess of 300 cc/sec suggests such laryngeal pathology as vocal fold paralysis
    - → markedly reduced flow rates may suggest spasmodic dysphonia
- Measure subglottal air pressure and resistance
  - → place the open end of a small tube in the oral cavity and attach the other end to a pressure transducer
  - → ask the client to produce /pi/ at the rate of 1.5 syllables a second with normal pitch and loudness; evoke at least 10 productions
  - → note that the peak intraoral pressure obtained through this procedure is assumed to equal subglottic pressure (normal average pressures: 5 to 10 cm H_2O)

- Evaluate the voice parameters; use one of the published voice rating scales (Boone & McFarlane, 2000) or the following **Clinical Voice Evaluation Form**

Make an evaluation of each voice parameter; then, if preferred, assign an overall numerical rating to the parameter; use a 5- or 7-point rating scale to assign a number to suggest the severity beyond the categorical, clinical evaluation (e.g., after having evaluated hard glottal attacks as excessive, you also may assign a 5 or a 7 as the highest numerical rating).

Clinical Voice Evaluation Form

Voice Parameter	Clinical Evaluation			Numerical Rating
Hard glottal attacks	❏ none	❏ some	❏ excessive	
Comments:				
Hyperfunctional voice (tensed)	❏ none	❏ occasional	❏ frequent	
Comments:				
Hypofunctional voice (lax, weak)	❏ none	❏ occasional	❏ frequent	
Comments:				
Voice breaks	❏ none	❏ occasional	❏ frequent	
Comments:				
Voice tremors	❏ none	❏ some	❏ frequent	
Comments:				

(continued)

(continued)

Voice Parameter	Clinical Evaluation			Numerical Rating
Breath support	❏ adequate	❏ somewhat inadequate	❏ inadequate	
Comments:				
Loudness	❏ too soft	❏ normal	❏ too loud	
Loudness variations	❏ too few	❏ normal	❏ excessive	
Comments:				
Pitch	❏ too low	❏ normal	❏ too high	
Diplophonia	❏ none	❏ occasional	❏ frequent	
Pitch breaks	❏ none	❏ occasional	❏ frequent	
Pitch inflections	❏ monopitch	❏ normal	❏ uncontrolled	
Comments:				
Quality				
Breathiness Comments:	❏ none	❏ occasional	❏ excessive	
Harshness Comments:	❏ none	❏ occasional	❏ excessive	
Hoarseness Comments:	❏ none	❏ occasional	❏ excessive	
Comments:				

(continued)

Voice Disorders

(continued)

Voice Parameter	Clinical Evaluation			Numerical Rating
Strained/strangled voice	☐ none	☐ occasional	☐ excessive	
Comments:				
Resonance				
Oral	☐ limited	☐ normal		
Nasal	☐ hyponasal	☐ normal	☐ hypernasal	
Comments:				
Muscle tension (face, neck, and shoulders)	☐ lax	☐ normal	☐ excessive	
Comments:				
Body posture during speech:	☐ approriate		☐ inappropriate	
Comments:				

Instrumental Assessment

- Consider supplementing clinical assessment and judgment of voice parameters with instrumental assessment; the following instruments, measures, or procedures are briefly described under their main alphabetical entries:
  - Electroglottography
  - Endoscopy
  - Instruments for Aerodynamic Measures of Phonatory Functions
  - Instruments for Resonance Assessment

Voice Disorders

- Instruments for Voice and Speech Analysis
- Sound Level Meter
- Stroboscopy

Related/Medical Assessment Data
- Obtain medical reports, including those from the patient's otorhinolaryngologist
- Integrate voice assessment with medical assessment data
- Obtain psychological and behavioral assessment data if available and relevant to the case
- Obtain educational information from teachers in the case of children
- Obtain occupational information of relevance from adult clients

Standard/Common Assessment Procedures
- Complete the Standard/Common Assessment Procedures

Analysis of Results
- Integrate information from different sources
- Evaluate your assessment data in light of information from the case history and other professional sources
- Complete a voice profile by summarizing the findings

Diagnostic Criteria/Guidelines
- Clear evidence of deviant voice as indicated by assessment; depending on the client and potential diagnosis, one or more of the following:
  - abnormal loudness
  - abnormal pitch, pitch breaks, pitch deviations
  - deviant voice quality including breathiness, hoarseness, and harshness
  - deviant resonance including hypernasality, hyponasality, assimilated nasality, and cul-de-sac nasality
  - other vocal characteristics including muscle tension, hard glottal attacks, and abnormal aerodynamic measures
  - evidence of vocal abuse or misuse
  - evidence of organic pathology from medical, radiological, and other examinations

Voice Disorders

Differential Diagnosis

- Distinguish various voice disorders (e.g., loudness disorders, pitch disorders, quality disorders, and resonance disorders)
- Distinguish between laryngeal pathologies that accompany or cause voice disorders from the voice disorders per se (note that a vocal nodule or cancer is not a voice disorder but a cause of it)
- Distinguish between voice disorders associated with laryngeal pathologies (e.g., cancer, granuloma, endocrine disorders, hyperkeratosis, papilloma, leukoplakia, vocal VA nodules, polyps, contact ulcers) and functional disorders which are devoid of laryngeal pathologies (e.g., functional aphonia, functional dysphonia, puberphonia); note that many traditionally considered functional voice disorders are associated with laryngeal pathologies (e.g., vocal nodules, polyps, contact ulcers, thickening of the folds); base the distinction on positive evidence of laryngeal pathology and the results of careful procedures that rule it out
- Distinguish between the immediate cause of the voice disorder from its more remote cause; for example, the immediate cause of hoarseness (a voice disorder) may be physical—a vocal nodule; this hoarseness is not functional; the cause of the nodule may be functional (vocal abuse)
- Distinguish between voice disorders with neurologic involvement (e.g., those resulting from lesions of the vagus nerve, upper motor neuron lesions, cerebellar lesions, lesions of the basal ganglia, and such neurologic diseases as amyotrophic lateral sclerosis and multiple sclerosis) and those without such involvement (e.g., functional aphonia or voice disorder associated with vocal nodules); base the distinction on positive neurological findings and associated additional symptoms of Dysarthrias
- Distinguish between voice disorders due to external trauma to the larynx and those with other causes; base the

532

distinction on evidence of external trauma (e.g., accidents, assaults)

- Identify velopharyngeal incompetence by endoscopic and radiological findings

Prognosis

- Variable, depending on the voice disorder, the associated medical condition, and client motivation
- Generally good for improvement in voice with treatment

Recommendations

- Voice therapy for most clients
- No voice therapy for patients with inadequate velopharyngeal incompetence when there has not been necessary medical intervention
- Augmentative and alternative communication for patients with degenerative neuromuscular disorders
- Medical referral before initiating voice therapy
- See the cited sources and *PGSLP* for details

Andrews, M. L. (1999). *Manual of voice treatment: Pediatrics through geriatrics* (2nd ed.). San Diego, CA: Singular Publishing Group.

Boone, D. R., & McFarlane, S. C. (2000). *The voice and voice therapy* (6th ed.). Englewood Cliffs, NJ: Prentice-Hall.

Case, J. L. (1996). *Clinical management of voice disorders* (3rd ed.). Austin, TX: Pro-Ed.

Deem. J. F., & Miller, L. (2000). *Manual of voice therapy*. Austin, TX: Pro-Ed.

Stemple, J. C., Glaze, L. E., & Gerdeman, B. K. (2000). *Clinical voice pathology* (3rd ed.). San Diego, CA: Singular Thomson Learning.

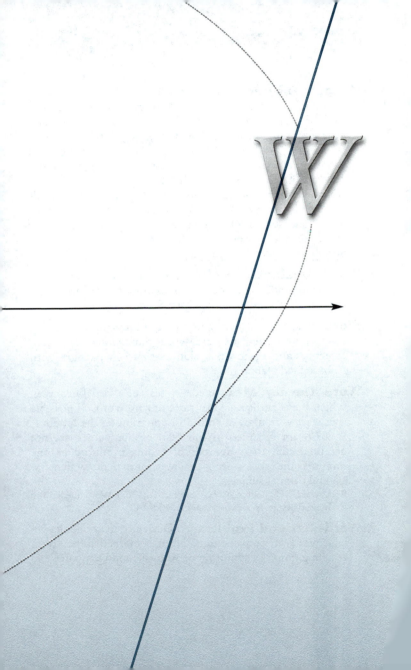

Wilson's Disease.   An inherited, autosomal, progressive neurological disease with a gradual onset; affects metabolism of dietary copper; also known as hepatolenticular degeneration or progressive lenticular degeneration; associated with degeneration of the lenticular nuclei of the basal ganglia; late adolescent or early adult onset; copper deposits in the cornea of the eye; tremor in the outstretched arms; slow movement; rigidity of muscles; drooling; dysphagia; hypokinetic, spastic, and ataxic dysarthrias; ataxia; and subcortical dementia in some cases; for assessment procedures, see mixed dysarthrias under <u>Dysarthria: Specific Types</u> and <u>Dementia</u>.

Word Deafness.   Profound auditory comprehension deficit for spoken words; a less commonly used name for Wernicke's aphasia; see <u>Aphasia: Specific Types</u>.

Word Fluency.   Fluency in rapidly producing words that start with a particular sound, words that belong to a certain category, and so forth; a skill assessed in patients with <u>Aphasia</u> and <u>Dementia</u>.

Word Fluency Measure.   A test of word fluency in which the client is asked to say as many words as possible that start with a given sound in one minute; the letters F, A, or S are specified in the test; proper names are not accepted; the total number of words produced in one minute is the score; norms available for patients with aphasia and normal subjects.

Borkowski, J. G., Benton, A. L. & Spreen, 0. (1967). Word fluency and brain damage. *Neuropsychologia, 5*, 135–140.

Word-Retrieval Problems.   Difficulty in recalling specific words in conversation; often a marked difficulty in recalling nouns; a symptom of <u>Aphasia</u> and <u>Dementia</u>.

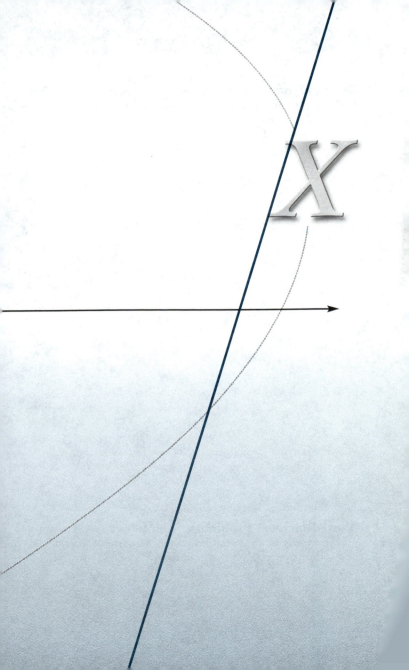

XO Syndrome

XO Syndrome. The same as Turner syndrome (see Syndromes Associated With Communicative Disorders).